MEN'S HEALTH
The Practice Nurse's Handbook

IAN PEATE

BICENTENNIAL
1807
WILEY
2007
BICENTENNIAL

John Wiley & Sons, Ltd

Other Wiley Editorial Offices

John Wiley & Sons Inc., 111 River Street, Hoboken, NJ 07030, USA

Jossey-Bass, 989 Market Street, San Francisco, CA 94103-1741, USA

Wiley-VCH Verlag GmbH, Boschstr. 12, D-69469 Weinheim, Germany

John Wiley & Sons Australia Ltd, 42 McDougall Street, Milton, Queensland 4064, Australia

John Wiley & Sons (Asia) Pte Ltd, 2 Clementi Loop #02-01, Jin Xing Distripark, Singapore 129809

John Wiley & Sons Canada Ltd, 6045 Freemont Blvd, Mississauga, ONT, L5R 4J3, Canada

Wiley also publishes its books in a variety of electronic formats. Some content that appears in print
may not be available in electronic books.

Anniversary Logo Design: Richard J. Pacifico

Library of Congress Cataloging-in-Publication Data

Peate, Ian.
  Men's health : the practice nurse's handbook / Ian Peate.
      p. ; cm.
  Includes bibliographical references and index.
  ISBN 978-0-470-03555-9 (alk. paper)
  1. Men–Health and hygiene.   2. Men–Diseases.   3. Nursing.   I. Title.
  [DNLM: 1. Health. 2. Men. 3. Nursing Care–methods. 4. Genital Diseases, Male–nursing.
  5. Health Promotion.   WY 100 P363m 2007]
  RC48.5.M464 2007
  616.0081–dc22   2007011287

A catalogue record for this book is available from the British Library

ISBN: 978-0-470-03555-9

Typeset in 10/12 pt Times by Thomson Digital.
Printed and bound in Great Britain by TJ International Ltd, Padstow, Great Britain.
This book is printed on acid-free paper responsibly manufactured from sustainable forestry in which at
least two trees are planted for each one used for paper production.

For all the Practice Nurses who are taking forward the role and function of the nurse.

Contents

About the author

Ian Peate, EN(G), RGN, DipN (Lond), RNT, BEd(Hons), MA(Lond), LLM

Address for correspondence:
Associate Head of School
School of Nursing and Midwifery
Faculty of Health and Human Sciences
University of Hertfordshire
Hatfield
Hertfordshire AL10 9AB

Acknowledgements

I would like to acknowledge and thank many fine people for their help and support, and in particular Frances Cohen, Mark Smith and Lyn Cochrane, and Anthony Peate for his help with the illustrations. Without the continued support and encouragement of my partner Jussi Lahtinen my endeavours would never be realised.

I thank the staff at the Royal College of Nursing for their help and the staff at John Wiley & Sons for their expert assistance.

Introduction

Being a man should not seriously damage your health, conclude White and Banks (2004) in their chapter in a men's health text. The maxim is used at the beginning of this text to remind the practice nurse of the fact that being a man in some instances can and does seriously damage their health. Men are much less likely to visit their general practice than women. Those men who are aged under 45 years visit their general practice only half as often as women; it is only when they become older that the gap narrows significantly.

PRACTICE NURSING

The role and function of the practice nurse continues to evolve and change. Most practice nurses are employees of the practice and most practices are run as small businesses with self-employed doctors who contract their services to the NHS; the GP (usually) becomes the practice nurse's boss. Concern regarding the health of men and the provision of services and care to men are just two aspects of the role and function of the practice nurse.

The lack of focus on gender and men by the Department of Health (DH) – for example, in the gender-neutral approach adopted by the *NHS Cancer Plan* (DH, 2000) and some National Service Frameworks – is the antithesis of government attempts to mainstream gender in all aspects of policy (Department of Trade and Industry, Women and Equality Unit, 2003). The important issue of men's health is beginning to receive the attention it deserves; however, men remain visibly absent from most health policy at local and national levels. The practice nurse, at a local level, can intervene and ensure that gender as a determinant of health is raised and included when policy and strategy are being addressed. Men and boys should be actively encouraged to participate in consultations about the development of health services and policy formulation that will meet their needs effectively.

All forms of health service provision must become more accessible to men, and this includes the services provided by the general practice. There are many innovative and creative approaches being made in order to provide men with services that are accessible and 'male-friendly'. Developments may include the provision of services in the workplace, schools, youth clubs, working men's clubs and sports venues – locations where men congregate. The *NHS Improvement Plan* (DH, 2004b) reports that everyone will have fair access to primary care that is near their home or workplace; this may help men, who are notorious for being reluctant users of primary care, particularly if their specific needs are not taken into account.

While this text concerns the health of men, it must be remembered that boys become men. The health of boys also needs to be given serious consideration; for example, they should be encouraged to take a more sensitive approach to risk-taking as well as developing the skills required to ask for and seek help. Boys need at an early age to hear that big boys do cry and that it is acceptable for them to do so.

The vision for the NHS is that it is to move from being a service that does things to its patients to one that is patient led; nurses working in the primary care setting are a part of this vision (DH, 2005). Other factors that are driving evolution and change are, for example, the New General Medical Service Contract (nGMS), the reconfiguration of Primary Care Trusts (PCTs) and Strategic Health Authorities (SHAs) and the advent of Practice Based Commissioning (PBC). PCTs are required to engage with local populations in order to improve health and well-being, commission an equitable range of high-quality services that are responsive and effective, as well as ensuring the direct provision of high-quality responsive and effective services. SHAs are seen as providing strategic leadership, organizational and workforce developments and ensuring that local systems operate effectively and deliver improved performance. SHAs are required to work in partnership with PCTs, as well as having the ability to hold them to account for their performance; the SHA is held to account by the Department of Health.

Ebbett (2007) states that traditionally general practice was seen as the gatekeeper to health services as well as being the patient's advocate; more and more the general practice is taking on a public health role. The advent of the general medical services (GMS) contract (now superseded by the nGMS or GMS2, which is the second version of the GMS contract) has affected all practices; the key aim of the contract is to control workload. There are two areas detailed in the contract: core services and enhanced services.

The role of the practice nurse is changing with nurses taking on more responsibilities and challenges. More practice nurses are taking the opportunity to become nurse practitioners, increasing their prescribing powers, running specialized nurse-led clinics and managing many chronic conditions autonomously. Nurses working in primary care settings have received direction with regard to their work and their career trajectory (DH, 1999, 2002a).

MEN'S HEALTH

Men still experience a poor state of health, with the average male life expectancy at birth being 76 years; male life expectancy is approximately 5–6 years less than women's; this is more profound in men from disadvantaged communities (Baker, 2002), who also suffer a high level of premature deaths from cardiovascular disease, cancer and suicide. Older men are less healthy than older women; they also suffer more strokes, accidents and suicide. Men engage in risk-taking activities that can seriously threaten their well-being and their life – for example, the excessive consumption of alcohol, engaging in high-risk sporting activities – and at the same time are more reluctant than women to seek medical help (Baker, 2004).

Encouraging men to attend the practice is problematic. The older man, for example, may feel that going to see the practice nurse or doctor is an admission of weakness and they may not want to be seen to be giving in to sickness. Often they postpone seeking an appointment until they are very sick. The outcome of these delays in seeking treatment can cause long-term adverse health problems. The practice nurse, if proactive, innovative and creative, has the ability to entice men into the practice or to seek other venues where men would use the services offered. When men do use the services offered by the practice nurse, then it is important that the response made is sensitive and custom-built.

It is well known that the pressure of living in contemporary society brings with it risks to both physical and mental health for both men and women. Women, though, tend to seek help and advice about their problems more readily than men. The rationale for this is unclear; however, the ways in which men view their masculinity may have some bearing on this anomaly. There is an emerging literature that addresses men's health, but this is relatively new. It could be suggested that men's health is in crisis (Gannon et al., 2004). Men have higher rates of morbidity and mortality, and take more risks in nearly all aspects of their lives than women do.

The specific relationship between masculinity and any given health issue is almost always under-recognized and imperfectly understood – and as a result is rarely taken into account in the development of policy and services. Chapter 1 addresses some of the complex issues associated with masculinity and gender and calls for the practice nurse to consider men as a heterogeneous group as well as recognizing that masculinity is not uniform: there may be many types of masculinity. Gannon, Glover and Abel (2004) suggest that the perceived or real crisis faced by men and their health represents long-standing anxieties about the nature of masculinity and the role and function of men in contemporary society.

It is often said that men do not care about their health. This is a myth – one of many that surround men's health. Men do care and do worry about their health. It could be suggested that men often feel they are unable to seek help regarding their health and may not express their fears for a variety of reasons until it is too late. If nurses stereotype men as being unconcerned about their health matters, this can lead to a stifling of the healthcare professional's ability to be creative when working with men (Robertson, 2003). The practice nurse may be able to help promote men's health in many ways, encouraging them to access services and as a result make better use of the services available in the practice setting. Chapter 2 provides insight into gendered health promotion activities. When health promotion activities are carried out in places where men congregate and feel more comfortable – for example, in a pub or a barber shop – tangible benefits are obtained. Often, men hold ingrained attitudes about health, and these attitudes can be difficult to change. The practice nurse is ideally placed to provide positive health education activities that men will relate and adhere to.

Gender inequalities in attempting to access healthcare provision and uptake of services for men and women often occur. The practice nurse must consider gender in order to provide competent healthcare and produce effective policies to support healthcare delivery for the men in the practice population. Chapter 3 encourages the nurse to recognize and take this into account in order to provide effective and gender-sensitive services. A gender duty has now been placed on all public authorities to be proactive in tackling and eliminating discrimination and gender inequality (see the section 'Equality Act 2006 and the gender duty', below). It could be tentatively suggested that if the practice nurse fails to pay attention to the differences between men and women this will reinforce existing gender differences and exacerbate health inequalities; s/he may also be called to account for his/her actions or omissions (NMC, 2004). General practice has a key role to play when attempting to tackle health inequalities; the method adopted will be as complex as the population the practice serves. Understanding the determinants of health as well as the social implications of poor health and the need to motivate and encourage men to present early has the potential to reduce the gulf that exists in relation to male health inequality.

The concept of risk is complex: why people engage in risk and how they may be encouraged to reduce risk challenges all healthcare practitioners. Chapter 4 considers the issue of risk and men as risk takers. People have the ability to make individual choices, and individual choice may be one aspect that persuades men to take part in risk-taking activities; accidents may occur as a result of those risk-taking activities. Similarly it may also be true of the individual's choice to engage in criminal activity as well as be what it is that makes some men victims of criminal activities. Societal factors must also be given due consideration. The pressures society puts on men – for example, how society expects men to behave – can influence significantly risk-taking behaviour. It is not possible, indeed it is erroneous, to attempt to try to understand in isolation why there is an over-representation of men as victims of accidents as well as victims and perpetrators of crime. This must be appreciated in the context of individual choice and societal expectations. Men consume alcohol, smoke cigarettes and use illicit substances more than is good for their health. Use of these substances can contribute to the development of chronic physical conditions such as liver disease, sexual dysfunction as well as self-inflicted injuries and assaults.

Chapter 4 has demonstrated that in many spheres of their lives and for many reasons men are risk takers. Young men and boys are seen as significant risk takers; the risks they engage in at a younger age have the ability to impact on the boy's life as adult. Younger men are often out to impress others, particularly those of the opposite sex, showing strength and bravery by engaging in potentially life-threatening activity, appearing to be emotionally and physically strong, not asking for help and being 'self-contained'. Chapter 5 investigates some risk-taking activities associated with being young and male. Issues are discussed such as eating disorders and the younger male, the impact of underachieving at school with the consequences this brings with it in relation to unemployment at a young age, as well as the sexual, emotional and mental health issues young men may experience and the effects these may have on the person's health and well-being. This chapter also addresses some of the legislative issues pertinent to young men and boys.

The general practice and often the practice nurse are at the centre of contraceptive services; they provide advice, administer treatments and offer follow-up, predominantly to a female audience. Reproductive sexual health, sometimes known as family planning, is constantly changing with new and creative approaches to contraception methods emerging and developing. Chapter 6 addresses contraception from a male perspective. The practice nurse is requested to provide the male patient with a bespoke service, providing the individual with information related to his (and his partner's) individual needs. Legal issues surrounding and concerning children and younger men are discussed. Specific groups of men – for example, those men with learning disabilities who approach the practice nurse for advice concerning contraception – will have particular needs, and these must be taken into account during the consultation; furthermore, there may also be particular aspects of the law that will need to be considered. It is vital that the nurse is aware of sensitivities surrounding the patient's culture, their religious beliefs, special needs and language differences in order to enhance the nurse–patient relationship. As well as providing a high-quality contraceptive service, there is also an opportunity to promote safer sex activities as well as considering offering the patient Sexually transmitted infection (STI) screening opportunities if appropriate.

Chlamydia is the most common STI in the UK. The *Annual Report of the National Chlamydia Screening Programme* (DH, 2006a) describes how only 17 % of those screened opportunistically for chlamydial infection were men, despite chlamydial infection being equally prevalent in both men and women. By 2008 the Department of Health (DH, 2006b) envisages that everybody will be able to access a genitourinary medicine (GUM) clinic within 48 hours. A significant number of patients with STIs first present in primary care. It is therefore very important that the practice nurse is fully familiar with the more common STIs that any patient in the practice may present with. Matthews and Macaulay (2006) note that the role of the practice nurse is becoming increasingly important in detecting and managing STIs in an effort to address and avert the unwelcome costs (physically and economically) of infection. Men remain pivotal in the transmission of STIs; however, the prevalence and incidence of STIs are dependent on sexual behaviour in both males and females. Sexual health is high on the Government's agenda, and Chapter 7 discusses the issue of STIs and the male patient.

Osteoporosis is a disease that is preventable and treatable and is the focus of Chapter 8. The non-pharmacological and pharmacological interventions associated with the disease are outlined. Interventions related to issues associated with nutrition, exercise and lifestyle are discussed. Osteoporosis is not a disease that only affects women; in men osteoporosis is not rare, and nor are the consequences that ensue as a result of the disease. Generally, the osteoporosis spotlight has been on women as it is more likely to occur in the female than the male. The principal focus on females, it could be suggested, has been to the detriment of men, in so far as this may have delayed an understanding of the condition in relation to the male. It is erroneous to apply what is known about osteoporosis in females, without caution, to the male as the female skeleton differs from that of the male. A similar error was made many years ago in relation to heart disease and the belief that what was learnt about male heart disease could be applied to females. While there are similarities in osteoporosis for both men and women there are also differences. The final aspect of Chapter 8 states that our understanding of osteoporosis in men is advancing, but a great deal more using a gender-specific approach is needed in order to further our understanding.

Just as osteoporosis is often understood from the female point of view, the same could be said of obesity in men. Obesity is widely seen as a uniquely female concern. This is highlighted when consideration is given to weight management programmes in primary care. The Men's Health Forum (2005) notes that, despite the much higher prevalence of overweight in men, men are under-represented in primary care weight management programmes: only 26% of participants in the national primary care 'Counterweight' intervention are men. Chapter 9 discusses issues surrounding obesity and overweight. Men, it is noted, are much less likely to have their weight routinely recorded by their general practitioner. Campbell (2006) suggests that weight management should become an essential feature of the practice nurse's work, not an optional extra. Practice nurses should not wait for the patient to raise queries concerning weight-related issues. If men, with the help of the practice nurse, become more aware of the consequences of being overweight or obese, the more likely they will be to seek advice.

It is well known that men are, in general, particularly restrained in seeking help for their health problems; this is particularly the case when it concerns sexual dysfunction – for example, erectile dysfunction. Erectile dysfunction is an important forecaster of early cardiovascular disease and diabetes mellitus. For these facts alone the practice nurse must incorporate the assessment of erectile dysfunction into the everyday management of cardiovascular disease. A number of patients may find it difficult to discuss erectile dysfunction with their partners, let alone with the practice nurse, and because of this the practice nurse should be proactive and not wait for the patient to present with the condition already established. Chapter 10 acknowledges that there are (currently) no endorsed UK guidelines for the assessment and management of erectile dysfunction in the primary care setting. Erectile dysfunction is a common condition and can be easily treated; treatment options are discussed in Chapter 10. Practice nurses can make a difference to the overall well-being of the patient. As they have often developed a role that incorporates health promotion into consultations, they may have longer consultation sessions with patients as well as being multi-skilled and competent practitioners, and they are also often the first point of contact for the patient.

Despite the fact that 28% of men smoke compared to 24% of women, only 46 000 men as opposed to 61 000 women set themselves a quit date to stop smoking when they attended NHS smoking cessation services during a six-month period in 2002. The principal avoidable cause of premature deaths in the UK (DH, 2004a) is smoking. Smoking also has the ability to make men infertile and impact on their reproductive abilities in a variety of ways. Some men may defer consultation as they can perceive infertility to be a threat to their masculinity. With every marker of social disadvantage, smoking rates increase. For example, those from the poorer social classes are more likely to die early due to a variety of factors with the dominant factor in men being smoking. There are other inequalities also evident in relation to smoking. For example, some men with mental health problems and men in prison smoke more than the general population. Chapter 11 focuses on smoking and the impact this has on the male reproductive tract.

Chapter 12 considers the needs of four specific groups of men:

- men who are homeless
- men who are a part of the prison population
- gay men (men who have sex with men)
- asylum-seekers.

It is acknowledged that the practice nurse works with a variety of patients, when working with men s/he will also work with those who are from, or belong to, specific groups, sometimes known as hard-to-reach groups and in certain instances may also be referred to as vulnerable groups. The National Health Service belongs to all of us and this will include those groups who may be classified as hard to reach. Inequality of access to care is problematic for men in general, and it becomes even more of a problem for those men discussed in this chapter. New and innovative ways of providing services that address the needs of these men must be developed if the central premise of primary care is to be respected – fairness, accessibility, responsiveness and efficiency.

Three times more men than women die from suicide (DH, 2002b); the mental health of men and the consequences this may have for him, his partner and family are poorly understood and as a result are often undervalued. In Chapter 13 three issues in relation to the psychological health of men are discussed:

- suicide
- rape
- domestic violence.

Men are prone to specific psychological risk which may require intervention by the practice nurse in order to help men and ease their suffering. The issues men face with regards to their mental health may be managed in the practice setting or the practice nurse may need to refer the patient to the most appropriate healthcare professional. Men are most at risk of depression between the ages of 45 and 64 years, with a second peck when the man is over 85 years. Depression can be triggered by life events, such as becoming unemployed or leaving work when retired and being at home all day. Diagnosing depression in men is problematic, as they can often fail to acknowledge (and recognize) the feelings and emotions they are experiencing. It could be that they have been brought up to deny emotional problems, as this is not how men should feel. Health promotion activities devised and implemented by the practice nurse that attempt to tackle mental ill health must take into account the needs of men and boys, considering the complex issue of masculinity. Caution must be used when attempting to implement approaches that have been used with women in respect to mental health well-being, as these may not be as effective with the male patient; for example, encouraging a man to 'open up' during consultations or to recognize and admit their vulnerability may fail to encourage him to seek and take up any help that may be available.

Men are twice as likely as women to develop, and die from, the ten most common cancers that affect both sexes (Men's Health Forum, 2004). Gender seems to play an important role in some adolescent male cancers, with a particular impact on testicular cancer. This may be due to the reality that early acknowledgement is hindered by some young men's lack of knowledge and their probable reluctance to seek help. The occurrence of bone and brain tumours and leukaemias is twice as high in male adolescents than in females; the reason for this is unknown (Health Development Agency, 2001). Much cancer treatment takes place in the acute care sector; nevertheless, general practice has a key role to play, which may be in the form of detection, referral and also any follow-up review of a patient. Cancer is an important cause of poor health and illness globally. There are many geographical differences noted in incidence, mortality and survival rates. In the UK there are inequalities linked with who gets cancer. Those who live in less affluent and more deprived areas are more likely to get specific types of cancer and, in general, are more likely to die from cancer after being diagnosed with it. The patient may seek support (physical and psychological) from the general practice once a diagnosis has been made. An important role of the practice nurse is to help men to come to terms with the diagnosis and prognosis, acting as advisor and supporter. There will be some men who may require palliative care, and this will involve the management of symptoms – symptom control – and caring for the dying patient and his family. Chapter 14 addresses issues associated with two male-specific cancers: testicular and prostate cancer.

The final chapter, Chapter 15, considers exercise and sports injury. Exercise irrefutably enhances health and well-being and reduces the risks of developing some diseases; most people would concur that exercise provides the person with therapeutic health benefits; despite this many people in the UK choose not to exercise and remain inactive. Men do not engage in sufficient exercise, despite knowing the harmful effects that inactivity can have on their overall health. Choosing not to exercise can lead to difficulties for all organs of the body and all bodily systems as well as causing psychosocial problems. This chapter encourages the practice nurse to spend time with the patient and produce an exercise prescription. As with all forms of prescribing, the nurse must first undertake a detailed assessment of the patient, his needs and aspirations. It could be suggested that those men whose health would benefit most from physical activity appear to be the most resistant to starting or maintaining a programme of exercise. In some instances there may be limitations to the amount and extent of exercise the nurse prescribes based on the patient's medical condition. Excessive exercise has the ability to exacerbate physical complications and can cause injury, just as there are side effects and contraindications related to certain types of medication. This is also the case with exercise: there may be risks associated with exercise for some patients, and these issues are discussed in this chapter. The chapter concludes with a brief discussion on sports injuries.

EQUALITY ACT 2006 AND THE GENDER DUTY

The Government has made a commitment to introduce a statutory duty on all public bodies to prohibit sex discrimination in the exercise of public functions through the introduction of the Equality Act 2006. The Equality Act applies to all public bodies, including public bodies such as general practices. Public bodies and authorities must be proactive in challenging and eradicating discrimination as opposed to waiting for individuals to draw their attention to discrimination: the onus is on the public authorities. The following questions (taken from the Equal Opportunities Commission's draft *Code of Practice*) (Equal Opportunities Commission, 2006) in relation to the legislation must be addressed constantly by public bodies when policy is being considered:

- Is there any evidence that women and men have different needs, experiences, concerns or priorities in relation to the issues addressed by the policy?
- Of those affected by the policy, what proportion are men and what women?
- If more women (or men) are likely to be affected by the policy, is that appropriate and consistent with the objective of the policy?
- Could the policy unintentionally disadvantage people of one sex or the other? Is it essential to consider not just the intended consequences but also any unintended consequences and barriers that might prevent the policy being effective for one sex or the other?

Sage (2006) considers what the Equality Act 2006 might mean for general practice. He states that it should mean that women and men get the services that meet their needs and that practices will actively have to address the issue of low male attendance by considering changes to services that make them more accessible to men.

With the introduction of the gender duty (Equality Act 2006) in 2007, this Act imposes a duty – the gender duty – on all public bodies to ensure that the promotion of the integration of gender concerns into policy, strategy generation and monitoring of policies and programmes of healthcare delivery takes place. Failure to adhere to these requirements may lead to public bodies being called to account for their actions or omissions. Gender duty is to ensure that the provisions in the Equality Act 2006 are carried out and enacted.

Understanding that gender is a central determinant of health as well as recognizing gender as an important factor will alert the nurse to the need for the provision of gender-sensitive and -specific services. A gender-sensitive approach can help to alleviate the many inequalities men face when trying to access and when accessing healthcare provision. This approach will also profit the health of women and girls, as there are several important healthcare female-specific issues that are worthy of further attention.

REFERENCES

Baker, P. (2002) *Getting It Sorted: A New Policy for Men's Health*. Men's Health Forum, London.

Baker, P. (2004) Men's health policy. *Journal of the Royal Society for the Promotion of Health*, **124** (5), 205–206.

Campbell, I.W. (2006) Obesity. In (eds S. Chambers, G. Kassianos and J. Morrell) *Improving Practice in Primary Care: Practical Advice from Practising Doctors*. CSF Medical Communications, Long Hanborough, pp. 263–273, Ch 24.

Department of Health (1999) *Making a Difference: Strengthening the Nursing, Midwifery and Health Visiting Contribution to Health and Health Care*. DH, London.

Department of Health (2000) *NHS Cancer Plan: A Plan for Investment, A Plan for Reform*. DH, London.

Department of Health (2002a) *Liberating the Talents: Helping Primary Care Trusts and Nurses to Deliver the NHS Plan*. DH, London.

Department of Health (2002b) *National Suicide Prevention Strategy*. DH, London.

Department of Health (2004a) *Choosing Health: Making Healthier Choices Easier*. DH, London.

Department of Health (2004b) *NHS Improvement Plan: Putting People at the Heart of Public Services*. DH, London.

Department of Health (2005) *Creating a Patient Led NHS: Delivering the NHS Improvement Plan*. DH, London.

Department of Health (2006a) *Annual Report of the National Chlamydia Screening Programme in England 2004/5*. DH, London.

Department of Health (2006b) *Our Health, Our Care, Our Say: A New Direction for Community Services*. TSO, Norwich.

Department of Trade and Industry, Women and Equality Unit (2003) *Delivering on Gender Equality*. DTI, London.

Ebbett, S. (2007) General practice: The NHS – the practice nurse. In (ed. J. Lucas) *New Practice Nurse*. Churchill Livingstone, Edinburgh. pp. 211–215, Ch 35.

Equal Opportunities Commission (2006) *Gender Equality Duty Draft Code of Practice: Great Britain*. EOC, London.

Gannon, K., Glover, L. and Abel, P. (2004) Masculinity, infertility, stigma and media reports. *Social Science and Medicine*, **59** (6), 1169–1175.

Health Development Agency (2001) *Boy's and Young Men's Health: Literature Review. An Interim Report*. HDA, London.

Matthews, P. and Macaulay, H. (2006) Sexually transmissible infections: a primary care perspective. In (eds T. Belfield, Y. Carter, P. Matthews, C. Moss and A. Weyman) *The Handbook of Sexual Health in Primary Care*. Family Planning Association, London. pp. 155–185, Ch 6.

Men's Health Forum (2004) *National Men's Health Week 2004. Briefing Paper: Man and Cancer*. Men's Health Forum, London.

Men's Health Forum (2005) *Hazardous Waist? Tackling the Epidemic of Excess Weight in Men.* Men's Health Forum, London.

Nursing and Midwifery Council (2004) *Code of Professional Conduct: Standards for Conduct, Performance and Ethics.* NMC, London.

Robertson, S. (2003) Men managing health. *Men's Health Journal,* **2** (4), 111–113.

Sage, R. (2006) Men and health: a gender for change? *Nursing in Practice,* July/August, 67–68.

White, A.R. and Banks, I. (2004) Help seeking in men and the problems of late diagnosis. In (eds R.S. Kirby, C.C. Carson, M.G. Kirby and R.N. Farah) *Men's Health,* 2nd edn, Taylor & Francis, London, pp. 1–9, Ch 1.

1 Masculinities and gender

INTRODUCTION

It has been demonstrated that men have higher mortality rates than women and their longevity is reduced in comparison to that of their female counterparts; they are also at greater risk of illness and injury. Over ten years ago it was recognized that a major factor contributing to the poor state of men's health could be risk behaviour, which was associated with traditional 'male lifestyle' (DH, 1993). Baker (2002) points out that across the developed world the health of men is in critical need of attention. Men frequently fail to seek help when their health begins to deteriorate. Men have higher rates of death than women and, it could be argued, have higher rates of serious illness (Hodgetts and Chamberlain, 2002). There are a number of explanations why this may be the case; one reason in particular is that men, it could be suggested, are reluctant to seek help and advice and adopt a stoical stance towards their health and illness (Watson, 2000).

Woolf, Jonas and Lawrence (1996) suggest that health behaviours help to explain gender differences in health and that they are some of the most important factors that influence health. If the nurse is aware of these health behaviours and is able to help men modify them, he/she can provide effective methods of preventing disease. Doyal, Payne and Cameron (2003) point out that longevity and health status are associated with economic status, ethnicity as well as access to healthcare provision. Courtenay (2000) suggests that health behaviours also impinge on longevity and modification of these behaviours is the most effective way to prevent disease.

Understanding masculinity and gender may help the nurse to begin to understand the male population and, as a result, plan appropriate care and care interventions. Masculinity and gender are dynamic entities in which we all play a part, changing over time with experience and reflection. It must be noted that there are intricate and multifaceted links between biological sex, gender and health. According to Galdas, Cheater and Marshall (2005), the role of masculine beliefs and the similarities and differences amongst men of differing background requires further investigation.

NATURE VERSUS NURTURE

White and Johnson (2000) suggest that the debate as to whether masculinity is a social construct, that is nature versus nurture, is secondary to the many complex mechanisms in place that ensure that the archetypal male continues.

Generally there are three primary explanations of human behaviour:

- biological determinism
- social determinism
- free will.

The first two will be discussed and the relationship between them, gender and masculinity, and male behaviour are also outlined.

BIOLOGICAL DETERMINISM

Biological differences allow the classification of men and women; these are predominantly related to reproductive function. Biological determinism is based on the belief that all differences (or characteristics) of men and women are a result of biology. This approach is also known as genetic determinism.

This approach asserts that certain behaviours are acceptable because 'boys will be boys' – this is 'natural' and is often genetically determined. Gross (2005) asserts that this principle has the ability to remove guilt and responsibility, for example, 'it is in my genes'.

Biological factors, in both sexes, have an influential impact on health; it has to be remembered, however, that this is not confined to reproductive characteristics alone. Doyal (2001) points out that there are a wide range of genetic, hormonal and metabolic influences that play a significant part in shaping distinctive male patterns of morbidity and mortality, for example, cancer of the prostate.

Little consideration is given to the wider variety of behaviours associated with masculinity or femininity or how masculinity or femininity relate to each other when in different settings. Biological determinism is powerful, and has the potential to undermine how men and women behave. Taken to its logical conclusion biological determinism dissociates the environmental and social factors associated with human nature.

SOCIAL DETERMINISM

The opposite of biological determinism is social determinism. This approach suggests that it is social interaction and social construction that determine individual behaviour. As with behavioural determinism, if taken to its logical conclusion social determinism would establish that the human being acts in accordance with his/her social conditioning, as opposed to any genetic predisposition. Socially constructed gender difference is also responsible for determining if an individual can realize their potential for a long and healthy life (Annandale and Hunt, 2000).

Examination of both doctrines would reveal that they are too general in scale to be reliable explanations of, and for, human behaviour. The nurture/nature dichotomy is problematic: what characterizes human behaviour and development is that they are an array of many interacting as well as intersecting causes. Both approaches are inadequate when attempting to understand or explain the diversity of masculinities.

Neither theory is able to provide a satisfactory explanation of, or for, the broad range of behaviours among men and women, parochially or globally. The nurse must be aware of the mix of both biological and social pressures in order to improve understanding and care for men and boys as there is unlikely to be one single explanation for issues that face men with respect to their health and well-being.

GENDER AND SEX

Kraemer (2000) notes that males are more vulnerable than females, even from conception, prior to any social effects coming into play. Within much healthcare literature the terms sex and gender are used interchangeably; both are important in understanding health and illness. With rare exceptions the human species comes in two sexes – male and female. This is the biological sex, anatomy as destiny. This male/female dichotomy is challenged, however, when an individual is born with a multiplicity or variation of sex and is forced into either the male or female domain.

Sex is not only determined by the appearance of the external genitalia. Advances in technology have allowed for the determination of sex by analysis of chromosomes: most often most men have external genitalia and one Y and one X chromosome; females usually have external female genitalia with X chromosomes. Not everyone, however, has discernible external genitalia and some have combinations of chromosomes that do not follow the accepted description of man or woman – their sex may be described as atypical. Blackless et al. (2000) suggest that in approximately 1% of live births some element of sexual ambiguity may exist.

GENDER

It has already been stated that there are many sociocultural factors that have the ability to influence health-related behaviour, and gender is one of the most influential of these factors. There are many gender inequalities associated with the provision of healthcare for men and these are discussed in further detail in Chapter 3 of this text. Adult men, for example, make far fewer healthcare visits than their female counterparts. Chapple and Zieband (2002), in a study they have undertaken, have determined that men are hesitant about seeking medical help. The men they interviewed in their study felt that it was not 'macho' to seek advice about health problems. Little is known about why men engage in less healthy lifestyles and why some men adopt fewer health promotion beliefs and behaviours than women (Courtenay, 2000). In 2001 11% of men and 16% of women reported consulting a GP. In the age group 16–44 years this percentage was 8% and 15% respectively (National Statistics, 2001). The increase in consultations for women of this age group may be associated with visits concerning birth control, child-related issues and pregnancy. This highlights how women use primary care services as a point of referral more than their male counterparts.

Most children during developmental phases of their lives acquire a firm sense of themselves as male or female. They acquire what many developmental psychologists term gender identity (Smith *et al.*, 2003). Explanations associated with theories of gender socialization are being criticized and doubt is being cast on the implication that gender represents two fixed, static and reciprocally absolute role containers (Connell, 1995; Courtenay, 2000). The formation of gender identity is a complex process and is much more than the examination of the external genitalia to determine sex. According to West and Zimmerman (1987), gender is something that a person does and does recurrently in interaction with others. Gender does not live within the person; it is the result of social interactions and transactions (Gray *et al.*, 2002). In this way gender can be viewed as a dynamic, gendered, social structure (Crawford, 1995). The actions and interactions are, according to Gerson and Peiss (1985), produced and reproduced through people's actions.

Gender stereotypes are used by society when it attempts to construct gender. Gender is a living system of social interactions. The stereotypes constructed are stereotypes that represent the characteristics that are often believed to be typical of men or women. Society has strong and entrenched beliefs of what men and women should and should not do, what is masculine or feminine. There are several activities that are used in the construction of male gender stereotypes:

- language
- work
- sports
- crime.

The ways men and women engage in the above activities contribute to the definition of an individual's gendered self, as well as conformation of society's expectations.

Courtenay (2000) notes that research (for example, Martin, 1994) has indicated that men and boys are under comparatively greater social pressures than women and girls to endorse society's gendered prescriptions; for example, men are stronger, tougher and self-reliant. These prescribed behaviours are often acted out by men. Wall and Kristjanson (2005) address the issues of men and their experiences of prostate cancer from a masculine perspective. They discuss the findings of several pieces of empirical research that have dealt with the same issues. Gray *et al.* (2000) have noted that, following a diagnosis and treatment of prostate cancer, the men in their study demonstrated a tacit personal and societal expectation that men are expected to cope, adjust, move on and accept the impact the diagnosis and treatment may have on their lives and relationships.

The analysis provided by Gray *et al.* (2000) and Chapple and Zieband (2002) demonstrates how men appear to sign up to cultural expectations; their experiences of prostate cancer become mute and non-emotional; and they have to demonstrate a stoic attitude and appear independent.

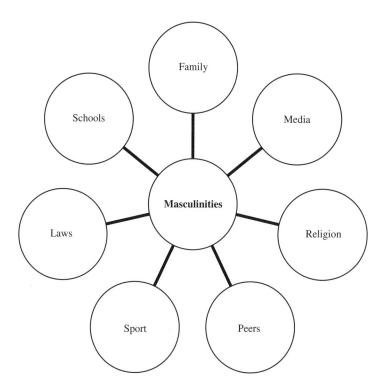

Figure 1.1. Some of the many influences which contribute to gender construction

Gender is taken to mean what it is to be masculine or feminine. This classification is analogous with the male and female classificatory systems used in the biological sexes. Gender roles are a set of norms associated with what it is, or appears to be, male or female. Society in many ways – for example, through the media, family, schooling, linguistics and peer pressure – determines what it is to be male or female, the social construction of gender. These essentialist views are continually reinforced, but are beginning to be challenged more and more (see Figure 1.1).

Consider what messages are being transmitted by the media in advertising, for example; note what it is to be feminine and masculine and in what way families provide role modelling. See Table 1.1 for some common socially constructed features (generalizations) of masculinity and femininity.

The dichotomies noted in Table 1.1 are the result of society's widely shared beliefs of what it is to be feminine or masculine. Society conforms to these stereotypical beliefs and adopts the norms associated with them. Conforming and playing out the stereotypical beliefs result in and reinforce a self-fulfilling prophecy of how we are expected to behave.

Table 1.1. Some common socially constructed
descriptions of masculinity and femininity

Masculinity	Femininity
• Strong	• Soft, gentle
• Powerful	• Weak
• Rational	• Emotional
• Self-reliant	• Dependent
• Breadwinner	• Child-raiser

(Source: Adapted from Laws, 2006)

De Visser and Smith (in press) state that masculinity is characterized by both physical and emotional toughness, risk-taking, predatory heterosexuality and being a breadwinner; competence is displayed in specific social domains, for example in:

• sport
• alcohol and drug use
• sexual activity.

McQueen and Henwood (2002) suggest that masculinity is often set up in binary opposition (see Table 1.1) to their alternatives; the result of this is that anything that is not seen as masculine becomes non-masculine. Hence, it might be suggested that it is non-masculine to be weak or gentle.

Courtenay (1999) points out that men and boys are not passive victims of this socially agreed role; they are neither conditioned nor socialized by their cultures and are actively engaged in exerting power and producing effects in their lives in the construction and reconstruction of dominant norms of masculinity.

MASCULINITIES AND HEALTHCARE PROVISION

Traditionally the terms masculinity and femininity have represented a stable and essential set of gender attributes that distinguish men from women (Sabo and Gordon, 1995). There is no dispute regarding the stability of sex differences as descriptors of physical characteristics; for example, morphology and physiology (Wall and Kristjanson, 2005). Martin (1994), however, challenges the idea that gender is also a fixed and a stable entity. Gender is a dynamic construct and can be produced by individuals who negotiate and transact with their social, cultural and bodily contexts (Courtenay, 2000). As a result of the possibility of these transactions, gender is capable of change over time and according to place; hence temporal and spatial elements emerge as the variables described which alter or have the potential to alter.

The plural masculinities are used to emphasize the case that there is no one pattern of masculinity: just as there is no one fixed pattern of gender, masculinities are not simple settled, homogeneous constructions. Connell (1987) argues for multiple masculinities and, he states, multiple femininities. Frosh, Phoenix and Pattman (2002) and Speer (2001) reveal that there are several different ways of being masculine, although most men appear to aspire to a hegemonic masculinity.

Men have specific roles to play in society and their position within that society is predominantly based on a mythical archetype that is built around ideal body form and body function. Men in society have several, specific roles to play (White and Johnson, 2000).

Being a male patient is one role that men have to learn (Seymour-Smith, Wetherell and Phoenix, 2002), and the practice nurse who has insight into the many roles men have to perform can aim to provide care that is sensitive and appropriate to the male patient. Healthcare beliefs and behaviours can be understood as means of demonstrating gender; the healthcare behaviours and the beliefs men hold have the potential to construct and represent gender, health actions (Courtenay, 2000), and if this premise is accepted, they also become social actions. Health behaviours and beliefs can, unlike social behaviours, such as wearing a dress or wearing a tie, as has already been stated, have a bearing on an individual's health.

Some researchers (Lee and Owens, 2002, for example) suggest that the differences noted between genders are accounted for not by gender but by the behaviours and attitudes related to particular career and lifestyle choices. The shift in perspective means that, in order to understand (or appreciate) fully the way men go about seeking help in relation to their health, the nurse will have to focus their investigations on not only men and their gender differences but also the differences between genders (Galdas, Cheater and Marshall, 2005).

Men are not a homogeneous group of individuals: they are not all the same, but are a heterogeneous entity. Within this heterogeneity there is group variability: not all individual men behave the same. Addis and Mahalik (2003) encourage healthcare providers to take this difference into account when planning and delivering effective healthcare.

The way men seek healthcare advice – health-seeking behaviour – is multifaceted. Sharpe and Arnold (1998) have identified that men consistently ignore health symptoms as well as avoiding seeking help from health services. Sanden, Larsson and Eriksson (2000) note similar findings in their research that was related to men who had discovered a testicular lump. Significant delays in discovering the lump and treatment were found; they attributed this to men's 'wait and see' attitude. Physical problems experienced by the men in their study (Sanden, Larsson and Eriksson, 2000) were seen as things, initially, that would cure themselves such as symptoms associated with a cold, and seeking help was often viewed by these men as strange. Richardson and Rabiee (2001) report similar findings in their investigations; they also note that seeking help from a GP was regarded as unpopular, confiding in the GP was uncomfortable and problems associated with communication, unfamiliarity and feeling vulnerable were cited as reasons for discomfort.

Gascoigne and Whitear (1999) suggest that men in their study who experienced issues associated with testicular cancer associated their reluctance to seek help with feeling embarrassed, appearing foolish and an attempt to normalize their symptoms.

White and Cash (2004) state that normalizing pain (chest pain, for example) or symptoms results in delay in seeking help. These responses are an indication of dominant internalized gender notions of masculinity and masculine identity (Gascoigne and Whitear, 1999). Chapple, Zieband and McPherson (2002) demonstrate that men delay seeking help, and thus treatment, because they did not know the symptoms associated with testicular cancer; they did not want to appear weak, hypochondriacal or lacking in masculinity.

There is evidence to suggest that occupational and socioeconomic status are as important as other variables such as gender when considering the help-seeking behaviours of men (Galdas, Cheater and Marshall, 2005). Socioeconomics are also variables that the nurse has to take into account when considering the help-seeking behaviours of the male patient. Richards, Reid and Murray-Watt (2002), in their study concerning men with chest pain in deprived and affluent areas of Glasgow, determined that men in the deprived area in contrast to those men from the more affluent area tended to normalize their chest pain, which led to a significant delay in seeking help. Social and cultural factors as well as gender have the ability to influence perceptions of symptoms and health behaviours (Richards, Reid and Murray-Watt, 2002; Galdas, Cheater and Marshall, 2005).

HEGEMONIC MASCULINITY

'Heterosexual masculinity', according to Connell (1995), is the most dominant form of masculinity. Hegemonic masculinity is the most culturally dominant of masculinities (Connell, 1987). Subordinate to heterosexual masculinity is homosexual masculinity (Connell, 1995). Courtenay (1999) suggests that hegemonic masculinity has the potential to shape relationships between men and men and men and women, as well as the relationship the male has with his health and his healthcare requirements.

Table 1.2 outlines some characteristics that are associated with hegemonic masculinity. Wall and Kristjanson (2005) describe these characteristics as signifiers of hegemonic behaviour.

Table 1.2. Characteristics or signifiers associated with hegemonic masculinity

- Restricted experience and expression of emotion
- No emotional sensitivity
- Toughness and violence
- Powerful and successful
- Self-sufficient – has no needs and needs no support
- Stoicism
- Being a stud – endorsing heterosexuality
- Misogyny

(Source: Adapted from Wall and Kristjanson, 2005; Frank, 1991; Kiss and Meryn, 2001)

Gray *et al.* (2002) note that hegemonic masculinity is associated with, and incorporates, as a result of its relationship with subordinate masculinities, power and domination, acted out through, for example, aggression, competition, heterosexism and homophobia.

The notion of masculinities as opposed to masculinity moves away from the dated concept of the 'male sex role'. Different circumstances, different cultures and different periods in time construct masculinity differently. They are therefore subject to change; they are fluid and dynamic. The male sex role theory is inadequate when it comes to trying to understand diversity in masculinity (Connell, 1987). Laws (2006) states that for decades researchers and authors have tried to define masculinity. It is difficult, however, to define, as it is a complex concept. However, being able to define masculinity may help healthcare providers to explain and predict male behaviour and as a result of these predictions offer care that is appropriate and meeting individual's needs.

The practice nurse must be constantly aware of this when providing care to men. It should be remembered that there are many different ways that men 'do' masculinity. An increased awareness and insight associated with gender and masculinity can help the nurse understand, for example:

- how men live;
- how and why they encounter high levels of injury;
- why they engage in risk-taking activities;
- patterns of illness and mortality rates;
- drug use and inadequate use of health service provision (Walker, Butland and Connell, 2000; Schofield *et al.*, 2000).

The meaning of masculinity for men who are from a lower social background may differ from the meaning of masculinity for those men from a middle-class background; this may also be the same for those men from very rich economic backgrounds and very poor economic backgrounds. Within the various types of masculinities there can be tensions and contradictions, inconsistencies and disagreements.

In health, there has been much debate around the issue of men's health; contemporary deliberation includes discussion around issues such as identity, sexuality and relationships (Schofield *et al.*, 2000). Doyal (2001) asserts that over the last two decades much activism has taken place by women with regards to the quality of their health and healthcare; she also states that men have also begun to draw attention to the negative effects associated with health and maleness. Links are beginning to emerge between the effects of masculinity on well-being (Schofield *et al.*, 2000). It has been suggested that gender behaviour is socially governed or conditioned – men and women learn as boys and girls what it is to be masculine and feminine; they are actively involved in determining their own gender identities.

Luck, Bamford and Williamson (2000) discuss a 'crisis in masculinity', which is associated with a recognition that there are differences associated with male and female mortality rates. Lyons and Willott (1999) suggest that men are victims of social change and as a result their masculinity is in crisis; they have unequal social relations. Men appear to hold certain abstract ideas with regard to health and these ideas are, according to Watson (2000), enacted in gender-specific ways encouraging and/or constraining the negative and positive effects of health practices. The nurse needs to develop an awareness of how these abstract ideas are enacted in an attempt to provide men with gender-specific healthcare – reacting to their gender-specific needs.

Seymour-Smith, Wetherell and Phoenix (2002) identify that it is not only the way men conceptualize and internalize their health from a gendered perspective but also the way the healthcare professionals approach men's healthcare. These barriers prevent men from addressing their own health; furthermore, they also prevent the healthcare professional from providing appropriate care. Male socialization, and the processes most men go through, has the ability to create difficulties associated with their health. White and Johnson (2000) suggest that as a result of this the maintenance of the male body becomes problematic.

The need for men to ascribe to a socially agreed male role may prevent them from being able to express their needs in association with their illness; they may feel unable to express needs as a result of 'traditional masculinity' (Möller-Leimkühler, 2002).

CONCLUSION

Being male or female influences the understating we have, and the experiences we encounter, of health, as well as the uptake of services and health outcomes; furthermore, gender impinges on the decisions made by those who provide health services. There is much evidence to demonstrate that men die earlier than women and report illness less than women. Much of the theoretical debate describes how men's health behaviours and beliefs are influenced by several factors, such as culture, environment and social class.

Understanding the way men seek help in relation to their health – for example, the way they evaluate symptoms associated with their health and how they arrive at the decision to seek healthcare – can be of value to those who develop strategy, provide policy and offer care. This may encourage men to seek help earlier, and as a result achieve earlier diagnosis and thus treatment.

Men are not a homogeneous group that can be compared with women, and neither should women be compared with men. Nurses are at the vanguard of healthcare provision and must be aware that men can react differently to the way healthcare services are offered as well as health promotion messages as a result of different ages, social and ethnic groups (Galdas, Cheater and Marshall, 2005). Much of the evidence cited in this chapter is based on research associated with homogeneous groups of men, for example, white, middle-class men. More work is needed that takes into account those men from a variety of backgrounds and situations in order to determine if there are any similarities between men.

Masculinity can put male healthcare at a low priority. Men find it difficult as a result of this label to ask for help. The nurse has the skill to encourage men to seek help for their problems, to encourage them to say it's OK to ask for support.

REFERENCES

Addis, M.E. and Mahalik, J.R. (2003) Men, masculinity, and the contexts of help seeking. *American Psychologist*, **58** (1), 5–14.

Annandale, E. and Hunt, K. (2000) *Gender Inequalities in Health*, Open University Press, Buckingham.

Baker, P. (2002) The European Men's Health Forum. *Men's Health Journal*, **1** (2), 43.

Blackless, M., Charuvastra, A., Derryck, A. *et al.* (2000) How sexually dimorphic are we? Review and synthesis. *American Journal of Human Biology*, **12**, 151–160.

Chapple, A. and Zieband, S. (2002) Prostate cancer: embodied experience and perceptions of masculinity. *Sociology of Health and Illness*, **24**, 820–841.

Chapple, A., Zieband, S. and McPherson, A. (2002) Qualitative study of men's perceptions of why treatment delays occur in the UK for those with testicular cancer. *British Journal of General Practice*, **54**, 25–32.

Connell, R.W. (1987) *Gender and Power*, Polity Press, Oxford.

Connell, R.W. (1995) *Masculinities*, Allen & Unwin, Sydney.

Courtenay, W.H. (1999) Stimulating men's health in the negotiation of masculinities. *Society for the Psychological Study of Men and Masculinity Bulletin*, **4**, 10–12.

Courtenay, W.H. (2000) Constructions of masculinity and their influence on man's well-being: a theory of gender and health. *Social Science and Medicine*, **50**, 1385–1401.

Crawford, M. (1995) *Talking Difference: On Gender and Language*, Sage Publications, Thousand Oaks, CA.

Department of Health (1993) *On the State of the Public Health: The Annual Report of the Chief Medical Officer of the Department of Health for the Year 1992*, DH, London.

De Visser, R. and Smith, J.A. Mister In-between: A Case Study of Masculine Identity and Health-Related Behaviour, in press.

Doyal, L. (2001) Sex, gender, and health: the need for a new approach. *British Medical Journal*, **323**, 1061–1063.

Doyal, L., Payne, S. and Cameron, A. (2003) *Promoting gender equality in health school for policy studies*, University of Bristol, Bristol.

Frank, B.W. (1991) Everyday/everynight masculinities: the social construction of masculinity among young men. *Sex Information and Education Council of Canada Journal*, **6**, 27–37.

Frosh, S., Phoenix, A. and Pattman, R. (2002) *Young Masculinities*, Palgrave, Basingstoke.

Galdas, P.M., Cheater, F. and Marshall, P. (2005) Men and health help-seeking behaviour: literature review. *Journal of Advanced Nursing*, **49** (6), 616–623.

Gascoigne, P. and Whitear, B. (1999) Making sense of testicular cancer symptoms: a qualitative study of the way in which men sought help from the health care services. *European Journal of Oncology*, **3** (2), 62–69.

Gerson, J.M. and Peiss, K. (1985) Boundaries, negotiation: consciousness: reconceptualizing gender relations. *Social Problems*, **32** (4), 317–331.

Gray, R.E., Fitch, M.I., Philips, C. *et al.* (2000) Managing the impact of illness: the experiences of men with prostate cancer and their spouses. *Journal of Health Psychology*, **5**, 531–548.

Gray, R.M., Fitch, M.I., Fergus, K.D. *et al.* (2002) Hegemonic masculinity and the experience of prostate cancer: a narrative approach. *Journal of Ageing and Identity*, **7**, 43–62.

Gross, R. (2005) *Psychology: The Science of Mind and Behaviour*, 5th edn, Hodder Arnold, London.

Hodgetts, D. and Chamberlain, K. (2002) The problem with men: working class men making sense of men's health on television. *Journal of Health Psychology*, **7** (3), 269–283.

Kiss, A. and Meryn, S. (2001) Effect of sex and gender type on psychosocial aspects of prostate and breast cancer. *British Medical Journal*, **323**, 1055–1058.

Kraemer, S. (2000) Lessons from everywhere. *British Medical Journal*, **321**, 1609–1612.

Laws, T. (2006) *A Handbook of Men's Health*. Elsevier, Edinburgh.

Lee, C. and Owens, R.G. (2002) *Psychology of Men's Health*. Open University Press, Milton Keynes.

Luck, M., Bamford, M. and Williamson P. (2000) *Men's Health: Perspectives, Diversity and Paradox*. Blackwell Scientific, Oxford.

Lyons, A.C. and Willott, S. (1999) From suet pudding to superhero: representations of men's health for women. *Health*, **3** (3), 283–302.

Martin, J.R. (1994) Methodological essentialism: false difference, and other dangerous traps. *Signs: Western Journal of Women in Culture and Society*, **19**, 630–657.

McQueen, C. and Henwood, K. (2002) Young men in 'Crisis': attending to the language of teenage boy's distress. *Social Science and Medicine*, **55**, 1493–1509.

Möller-Leimkühler, A.M. (2002) Barriers to help seeking by men: a review of sociocultural and clinical literature with particular reference to depression. *Journal of Affective Disorders*, **71**, 1–9.

National Statistics (2001) Living in Britain 2001: General Practitioner (GP) Consultations, http://www.statistics.gov.uk/lib2001/Section3533.html (last accessed May 2006).

Richards, H.M., Reid, M.E. and Murray-Watt, G.C. (2002) Socioeconomic variations in response to chest pain: qualitative study. *British Medical Journal*, **324**, 1308–1310.

Richardson, C.A. and Rabiee, F. (2001) A question of access: an exploration of the factors that influence the health of young males aged 15–19 living in Corby and their use of health care services. *Health Education Journal*, **60** (1), 3–16.

Sabo, D. and Gordon, D.R. (1995) Rethink men's health and illness. In (eds D. Sabo and D.R. Gordon) *Men's Health and Illness*. Sage Publications, Thousands Oaks, CA, pp. 1–21, Ch 1.

Sanden, I., Larsson, U.S. and Eriksson, C. (2000) An interview study of men discovering testicular cancer. *Cancer Nursing*, **23** (4), 304–309.

Schofield, T., Connell, R.W., Walker, L. *et al.* (2000) Understanding men's health and illness: a gender relations approach to policy, research and practice. *Journal of American College Health*, **48** (6), 247–256.

Seymour-Smith, S., Wetherell, M. and Phoenix, A. (2002) My wife ordered me to come: a discursive analysis of doctors' and nurses' accounts of men's use of general practitioners. *Journal of Health Psychology*, **7** (3), 253–267.

Sharpe, S. and Arnold, S. (1998) *Men, Lifestyles and Health: A Study of Health Beliefs and Practices*, Economic and Social Research Council, Swindon (unpublished).

Smith, E.E., Nolen-Hoeksema, S., Fredrickson, B. and Loftus, G.R. (2003) *Atkinson and Hilgard's Introduction to Psychology*, 14th edn, Thompson, New York.

Speer, S. (2001) Reconsidering the concept of hegemonic masculinity: discursive psychology, conversation analysis, and participant's orientations. *Feminism and Psychology*, **11** (1), 107–135.

Walker, L., Butland, D.L. and Connell, R.W. (2000) Boys on the road: masculinities, car culture and road safety education. *Journal of Men's Studies*, **8** (2), 153–169.

Wall, D. and Kristjanson, L. (2005) Men, culture and hegemonic masculinity: understanding the experience of prostate cancer. *Nursing Inquiry*, **12** (2), 87–97.

Watson, J. (2000) *Men's Bodies*. Open University Press, Buckingham.

West, C. and Zimmerman, D.H. (1987) Doing gender. *Gender and Society*, **1** (2), 125–151.

White, A.K. and Cash, C. (2004) The state of men's health on Western Europe. *Journal of Men's Health and Gender*, **1** (1), 60–66.

White, A.K. and Johnson, M. (2000) Men making sense of their chest pain – niggles, doubts and denials. *Journal of Clinical Nursing*, **9**, 534–541.

Woolf, S.H., Jonas, S. and Lawrence, R.S. (1996) *Health Promotion and Disease Prevention in Clinical Practice*. Williams and Williams, Baltimore.

2 Promoting health: the male perspective

INTRODUCTION

In the past most work associated with men's health promotion has adopted a medical model approach focusing on screening for heart disease, hypertension and diabetes. The earliest record of men's health promotion embracing an alternative approach to the medical model was in an article by Moffatt (1980), in which he describes a plan for organizing, implementing and evaluating a Well-Man Clinic.

This chapter is closely related to Chapter 3, where health inequalities are discussed. It considers the health promotion needs of the male patient. Women's and men's needs are different and the service the practice nurse provides must reflect this difference; this also includes health promotion activity (Women's National Commission, 2000). One of the primary aims of any general practice must be the maintenance of health, the prevention of disease and ill health. There are many instances available to the practice nurse to carry out preventative care in daily practice. However, to provide effective health promotion for the male patient the practice nurse must be prepared to invest time and effort into this important activity. Fuller, Backett-Milburn and Hopton (2002) suggest that, for health promotion activities in general practice to succeed, consideration must be given to the view of the patient as well as the attitudes of the healthcare provider. The patient must be central to the decision-making process.

'Adding life to years and not just years to life' is associated with quality of life. The phrase was used in the publication *The Health of the Nation* (DH, 1992), and this, according to Kirby (2004), has led to an increase in health promotion and disease prevention. There are many good reasons why the health of the nation needs to be improved, and Kirby (2004) cites economic reasons as one of them. He suggests that approximately 187 million working days are lost to sickness each year. This equates to £12 million tax on business.

Investing in public health as described in the Government's White Paper *Choosing Health* (DH, 2004a) not only leads to benefits for the NHS, but also to improvement in individual health (King's Fund, 2004). A number of other government policies have also been produced that aim to improve health, for example, *Making a Difference* (DH, 1999a), The NHS Plan (DH, 2000a) and *Shifting the Balance of Power* (DH, 2001).

Nurses have always had a role in promoting the health of the people they care for (Poulton *et al.*, 2000), those working in community settings are continuously involved in health promotion activity, health protection, education and prevention (Department of Health, Social Services and Public Safety and Department of Health and Children, 2001).

It is essential that the nurse has insight and understanding of the various approaches associated with health promoting activities. White (2001) cites Professor Siân Griffith, President of the Faculty of Public Health, who states:

> Men's health is not a medical issue; it is societal. Therefore a much broader approach is needed.

The practice nurse must approach the issue of health promotion from various perspectives (theoretical and practical) if his/her interventions are to be effective. Health promotion is a key activity in enabling men to achieve their full health potential. The Nursing and Midwifery Council (NMC; 2004) states that the nurse must recognize and respect the role of patients and clients as partners in their care and the contribution they can make to it. Nurses, midwives and specialist community public health nurses are also expected to protect and support the health of individual patients and clients; furthermore, they have a duty to help individuals and groups to gain access to health and social care, information and support relevant to the needs of the man.

DEFINING KEY TERMS

The starting point is to define the various key terms that are associated with the promotion of health; there is a plethora of terms that the nurse and other healthcare professionals may use when addressing the healthcare needs of the male patient. Providing strategies for improving the health of men requires the nurse to have an understanding of the various definitions, philosophies, values and beliefs central to the concept of health promotion. Adopting a broader view of health, for example, working in partnership, involving communities, challenging social exclusion and inequalities, provides the opportunity to create a healthy society. Definitions of five key terms will be provided:

- men's health
- health
- health promotion
- health education
- public health.

It must be acknowledged that all terms and concepts associated with the terms above are interdependent on each other. Figure 2.1 demonstrates the inter-relatedness of all of the key definitions.

HEALTH

Health has been defined in many ways over the years, and one basic definition that could be used is that health is the 'freedom from disease and abnormality'. A more

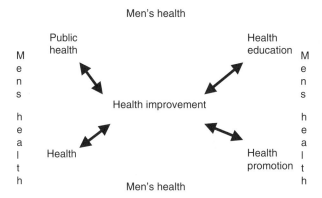

Figure 2.1. Men's health and key definitions

detailed definition became available in 1948 from the World Health Organization (WHO) when health was defined as 'a state of complete mental and physical and social well-being and not merely the absence of disease'; this definition, cited by Lincoln and Nutbeam (2006a), is said to be an absolute definition. Although it is an idealistic definition, it is valuable in so far as it considers health from a variety of perspectives, and health is seen not only as a disease-free state (a quasi medical model approach). Relative definitions of health, according to Lincoln and Nutbeam (2006a), are defined socially and culturally. Different cultures and communities define health differently: the social and cultural contexts are given serious consideration, and because of this it makes the definition of health difficult. Health is now seen as a holistic concept that incorporates the following factors:

- social
- economic
- physical
- sexual
- emotional
- spiritual
- environmental.

The strategies that the nurse employs in order to improve health must also acknowledge and take into account these factors that have the potential to impact on the quality of the man's health.

MEN'S HEALTH

Men's health, according to Banks (2001), is a contradiction in terms because the state of men's health in the UK is poor. One of the factors for this is the lack of knowledge and the limited availability of information regarding men's health in general combined with the low priority it is given in the media in general when compared with the health needs of women. Often the way men view their bodies is different from the way women do.

Frequently men's health is compared to the health of women, and is generally understood in terms of the margins of difference associated with men and women. While there is some value when using this approach it has its limitations and can be misleading. Chapter 1 of this text urged the reader to take account of the diversity that exists between men from different groups and different backgrounds. This is also true of the difference between men and women. It could be suggested that in general men tend to view their bodies as purely functional and expect them to perform whatever role they are asked to perform. They appear to adopt the 'role performance' model of health (Hall, 2003).

There are a number of descriptions of what men's health might be but not many definitions of what it is. There is no agreed definition of what it is that constitutes men's health (Health Development Agency, 2001). Lloyd (1996) suggests that one of the reasons why healthcare professionals have not taken up men's health issues as a concern may be because of this lack of definition. Despite that comment being made by Lloyd (1996) over ten years ago, it could be tentatively suggested that little has changed with regards to providing a definitive definition of this complex concept.

Any definition of men's health must also include the health of young men and boys as good male health starts in youth. The health behaviours of young men and boys must be considered carefully as these behaviours may have an impact on health in later years. Many of the social factors that are responsible for poor male health are first encountered by males in childhood.

A definition of men's health might include one that suggests that it is related to:

> any condition, or determinant that affects the quality of life of men and/or for which different responses are required for older men (or boys) to experience optimal social, emotional or physical health. (New South Wales Health Department, 1999)

At different times in their lives, from childhood to old age, men will have differing health experiences and, as a result of these, differing health needs. The nurse must acknowledge these developmental stages and adapt his/her health promotion activities to reflect the circumstances in which the patient may find himself.

Fletcher (1997) provides a definition that has been adapted from the US Public Health Service's definition of women's health. The Health Development Agency (2001) has adopted Fletcher's (1997) definition in their literature and practice review of boys' and young men's health:

> conditions or diseases that are unique to men, more prevalent in men, more serious among men, for which different interventions are required for men.

Adopting such a definition, suggests the Health Development Agency (2001), allows for a range of conditions, behaviours, underpinning issues and differences in clinical practice, at the same time providing a recognizable framework. They add that the choice of this definition allows for a halfway house approach, between the pure biological definition to men's health and the inclusion of social issues, for example, education, family life and adolescence.

Regardless of the definition chosen, it is no longer acceptable to define men's health merely in the light of male-specific diseases, diseases that uniquely affect the male genital tract, such as testicular cancer and cancer of the prostate. Men's health may include elements of male-specific diseases but it must also take into account the broader context of the term health. Hall (2003) suggests that narrowly defining the health of men in the context of disease is erroneous – the groin, he states, is not where men's health is at. Factors related to a social hierarchy, he continues, such as money, status (i.e. place in the community) and how well a man is loved, are more important than the size of his prostate or his cholesterol levels as predictors in men's health. Harrison and Dignan (1999) note that if healthcare professionals relegate men's health to disease association alone then this would be a retrograde step in an attempt to understand and enhance the concept of health as a whole. O'Dowd and Jewell (1998) also agree that attempting to explain men's health in purely biological concepts of gender is flawed; they ask that men's health be considered in broader contexts, for example, why men take more risks than women, why they may be more reluctant to visit their doctor and how male behaviours are bound up with the notion of masculinity.

HEALTH PROMOTION

A definition of health promotion has been prepared by the WHO (1986) (The Ottawa Charter) as:

> The process of enabling people to increase control over the determinants of health and thereby improve their health.

The key component of this definition is a focus on people and the desire to increase their control over the determinants of health, enabling them to enjoy and improve their health. An alternative definition is provided by Downie, Fyfe and Tannahill (1990):

> Health promotion comprise efforts to enhance positive health and reduce the risk of ill health, through the overlapping spheres of health education, prevention and protection.

Figure 2.2 (below) provides an example of how the three spheres overlap.

THE OTTAWA CHARTER FOR HEALTH

Lincoln and Nutbeam (2006b) demonstrate how health promotion has developed from the nineteenth century up to the 1970s and the 1980s; they state that the WHO

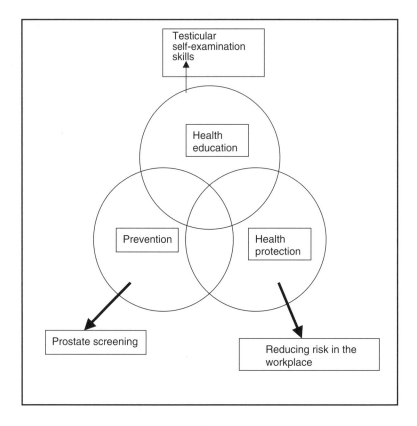

Figure 2.2. The three overlapping spheres (Source: Downie, Fyfe and Tannahill, 1990)

has adopted a key role in association with health promotion activities through the use of various declarations. The Ottawa Charter for Health Promotion (WHO, 1986) was a charter that emerged from a WHO conference on health promotion in 1986. The Ottawa Charter emphasizes the notion of health as more of a resource for living. The following principles of health promotion were defined by the WHO (1986) as:

- involving the population as a whole in the context of their everyday life as opposed to focusing on those at risk of specific diseases;
- directed towards action on the determinants of health, requiring cooperation between sectors and Government;
- combining varied but complementary approaches, including individual communication and education, legislation, financial/monetary measures, and organizational and community development;
- effective community participation;
- involvement of health professionals, particularly in primary healthcare.

Attempting to improve the health status of men will mean that changes will need to be made to the structures and social contexts that are damaging to health. Partnerships will need to be formed and fostered in order to enhance the health of men. This approach (one of partnership) is reinforced by the *Jakarta Declaration on Leading Health Promotion* (WHO, 1997). Five priority areas are cited:

1. Promote social responsibility of health.
2. Increase investments for health development.
3. Consolidate and expand existing partnerships.
4. Increase community capacity and empower the individual.
5. Secure an infrastructure for health promotion.

This declaration has acknowledged that health promotion activities may be outside the direct control of nurses and other healthcare workers. Accepted structures and social contexts must be challenged by the practice nurse in attempting to improve health. Partnership arrangements with other Government sectors that sit outside of healthcare, for example, cross-Government initiatives and inter-sectoral partnerships are required to deliver a truly responsive and enhanced healthcare system.

HEALTH EDUCATION

Downie, Fyfe and Tannahill (1996) provide three basic orientations for health education:

- disease orientation
- risk factor orientation
- health orientation.

The three orientations are described in Table 2.1.

Table 2.1. Three orientations for health education

Orientation	Explanation
Disease orientation education	The aim of this approach is to prevent specific diseases. Emphasis is on the measurement of success in terms of progress towards target rates for both morbidity and mortality.
Risk factor orientation education	Elimination of particular risk factors are addressed in order to prevent associated diseases.
Health orientation education	The key aim is to improve positive health as well as to prevent ill health. This approach acknowledges the need to take into account physical, mental and social aspects of health in both a positive and negative manner.

(Source: Adapted from Downie, Fyfe and Tannahill, 1996)

Edmonds *et al.* (2006) point out that all three orientations have a valid place but it must be acknowledged that a comprehensive and collaborative approach is required to address the complexities associated with most health-related issues.

Tannahill (1985) suggests that health education is:

> communication activity aimed at enhancing well being and preventing or diminishing ill-health in individuals and groups, through favourably influencing knowledge, beliefs, attitudes and behaviour of those with power and of the community at large.

The model used by Tannahill defines the content of health promotion as opposed to the practice; his model delineates the boundaries of health promotion and includes negative and positive aspects of health, as well as taking on a political dimension.

Health education can be seen as a communication activity, primarily aimed at enhancing well-being and preventing ill-health. This is conducted through positively influencing the knowledge, beliefs, attitudes and behaviour of the community. An example of health education might be the promotion of testicular self-examination.

PUBLIC HEALTH

Hayes (2005) states that the term public health is not easy to define as it will mean different things to different people depending on their:

- wealth
- health
- environment
- education
- social, political and cultural context.

A popular definition comes from Acheson (1988), who defines public health as:

> the science and art of preventing disease, prolonging life and promoting physical health through the organised efforts of society.

Public health, according to Hayes (2005), has four essentials associated with it:

- to enhance the health and well-being of the population
- to prevent disease and minimize its consequences
- to extend valued life
- to diminish inequalities in health.

Public health is concerned with a number of themes such as environmental movements, political parties and international agencies, such as the United Nations (Naidoo and Wills, 2000). Public health concerns the improvement of the health of a population, as opposed to treating the diseases of individual patients; it is, therefore, as diverse as the public it addresses. The functions of public health can be seen in Table 2.2 (below).

Table 2.2. The functions of public health

- Health surveillance, monitoring and analysis
- Investigation of disease outbreaks, epidemics and risk to health
- Establishing, designing and managing health promotion and disease prevention programmes
- Enabling and empowering communities to promote health and reducing inequalities
- Creating and sustaining cross-Government and inter-sectoral partnerships to improve health and reduce inequalities
- Ensuring compliance with regulations and laws to protect and promote health
- Developing and maintaining a well-educated and trained, multi-disciplinary public health force
- Ensuring the effective performance of NHS services to meet the goals in improving health, preventing disease and reducing inequalities
- Research, development, evaluation and innovation
- Quality assuring the public health function

(Source: Department of Health, 2004b)

Davies and Macdowall (2006) state that since the nineteenth century public health has improved dramatically. Public health has grown and will continue to grow and the practice nurse has an important role to play in its development.

SOCIAL DETERMINANTS OF HEALTH

Recognition that social and environmental factors decisively impact on people's health, according to the World Health Organization (2005), is ancient. Health and well-being are influenced by many factors, within and outside the individual's control. If the practice nurse is aware of the social determinants, then he/she can plan health promotion activities for the patient with these factors in mind. Social determinants of health are also pertinent in understanding why health inequalities exist.

The different layers of influence on an individual's life are described by Dahlgren and Whitehead (1991); their model, 'the Policy Rainbow', describes factors that are fixed, such as age, sex and genetic make-up; other factors they describe are what they term 'potentially modifiable', and these include individual lifestyle, general socioeconomic status, cultural and physical environments (see also Davies and Macdowall, 2006). The model demonstrates factors that can be changed and modified and some factors that cannot be changed (see Figure 2.3 below).

The model can help to point out the various influences on life and well-being as well as allowing the nurse to identify those factors that are fixed, that is, age and sex, and those that are potentially modifiable, that is, work environment and living conditions. The model clearly identifies the inter-relatedness of all of the components: one layer cannot be discussed in isolation from the others.

In Table 2.3 10 key messages on the social determinants of health are provided. Using these 10 messages may help policy-makers (nurses) to understand and address the health of men in a more appropriate manner.

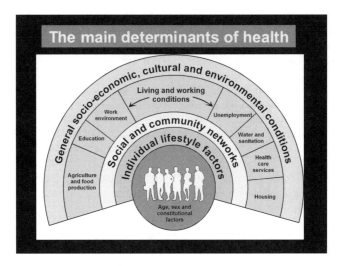

Figure 2.3. The 'Policy Rainbow' (Source: Dahlgren and Whitehead, 1991. The Institute for Further Studies)

HEALTH PROMOTION MODELS

Models provide a plan for investigating and guiding practice, and there are a number of health promotion models available that underpin health promotion activity. Unfortunately the subject of health promotion models is too complex to cover here in depth and the reader is advised to seek other sources to gain insight and understanding.

Table 2.3. Ten key messages on the social determinants of health

1. Health policy and activity must not be confined to the health system; it must run across and include the social and economic determinants of health
2. Stress harms health and should be minimized
3. A good start in life lasts a lifetime; therefore children and parents should be supported
4. Social exclusion and misery cost lives
5. Stress in the workplace creates disease
6. Job security increases health, well-being and satisfaction
7. Friendship, good social relations and strong supportive networks improve health at home, at work and in the community
8. Individuals turn to alcohol, drugs and tobacco and suffer from their use, which is itself influenced by the wider social setting
9. Healthy food is a political issue
10. Healthy transport means reducing driving and encouraging more walking and cycling, backed up by better public transport

(Source: Adapted from Wilkinson and Marmot, 1998)

Nursing models provide the nurse with a mental picture of nursing, according to Newton (1991); they help to direct and organize activity. Models are only conceptualizations of reality. For example, a map of the London underground is only a model of a very complex transport network; the map helps passengers get around the underground system. Sometimes models can oversimplify complex issues such as health promotion. Naidoo and Wills (2001) state that models are abstract representations of real circumstances that assist critical thinking and analysis. Table 2.4 provides a brief insight into five approaches to health promotion.

Table 2.4. Five approaches to health promotion

	Aim	Health promotion activity	Important values
Medical	Freedom from medically defined disease and disability, that is, cirrhosis of the liver	Promotion of medical interventions to prevent ill health	The patient is compliant and passively submits to medical procedures
Behavioural	Individual behaviour conducive to freedom from disease	Attitude and behavioural change to encourage adoption of a healthier lifestyle	Healthy lifestyle as defined by health promoter.
Educational	Individuals with knowledge and understanding enabling well-informed decisions to be made and acted upon, that is, providing the patient with information about testicular self-examination	Information about cause and effects of health-demoting factors. Exploration of values and attitudes. Development of skills required for healthy living	The health promoter respects that the individual has the right of free choice. The health promoter takes on the responsibility of identifying educational content
Client-centred	Working with the client on the client's own terms. The client identifies the need for health promotion activity	Working with health issues, choices and actions with which clients identify. Empowering clients	Clients as equals. The client has the right to set the agenda, that is, educational content. Self-empowerment of the client
Societal	Physical and social environment that enables a choice of healthier lifestyle	Political/social action to change physical/social environment	Right and need to make environment health-enhancing

(Source: Adapted from Naidoo and Wills, 2001)

IMPROVING MEN'S HEALTH

Fareed (1993) suggests that ill health among men is a result of their lifestyle and as health educators nurses can address these issues. Men may need help to recognize that stereotypical gender role behaviour may pose a risk to health and because of this attempts must be made to change these behaviours.

Policy development at local, national and international levels must take into account the specific healthcare needs of men. Policy development activity should engender and reflect an awareness of gender as a significant element of holistic healthcare provision. White and Lockyer (2001) point out how the National Service Framework (NSF) for coronary heart disease (DH, 2000b) fails to mention gender difference despite the fact that it is acknowledged that there has been a recognized difference between the age of greatest vulnerability for men and women. The rate of suicide among men is three to four times higher than in women and this fact is not acknowledged in the NSF *Mental Health* (DH, 1999b). Once gender has been recognized at policy level as a significant issue then the practice nurse may find health promotion activities easier to devise and implement as frameworks for action exist in policy format.

Large numbers of men die as a result of cardiovascular disease; however, cardiovascular disease is not a disease that is male-specific: both men and women suffer with diseases associated with the cardiovascular system, despite the fact that more men than women die of cardiovascular disease. An important point is that the interventions the nurse develops may be different for the male and female, as well as taking into account the age and socioeconomic status of the patient. By doing this the nurse is subscribing to an holistic approach to the health needs of the male.

Preventative activities can reduce disease and disability as well as help men to avoid illness. The practice nurse, it has already been said, has the potential to have an impact on the health of the male patient. The nurse can work with the patient and identify risk factors, develop a plan of action addressing the risk factors, work with the patient to implement the plan and then evaluate outcomes.

PROMOTING HEALTH IN THE PRACTICE
SETTING – OVERCOMING BARRIERS, ENHANCING ACCESS

Health for men, from an early age, has often been seen as a domain that belongs to women. Boys, for example, are more often brought to child health clinics by a female relative. Up until the age of 16 years, attendance at the practice is the same for boys and girls as mothers take them both to see the general practitioner (GP) (White, 2001); after 16 years, men have a greater reluctance to attend. The greater use of health services by females in their early years can be attributed to the provision of some specific aspects of service provision, that is, antenatal care, contraceptive services and screening. The male body does not experience the same physiological changes as the female body does, for example, the monthly menstrual cycle and the prospect of pregnancy.

Frosh, Phoenix and Pattman (2002) point out that some men see health as being concerned with female issues and as being something they should not be concerned with. While it appears that a number of men are content with leaving the issue to the female, it is not right that women should hold responsibility for men's health; men should be encouraged and empowered to become better managers of their own health (White and Banks, 2004). However, if some men are content to leave this to the female partner, then it may be practical to advise and make women aware of the need for men to seek health advice sooner rather than later.

Biddulph and Blake (2001) point out that the average young man is unlikely to access any help or support at all if he experiences a problem; more often he will attempt to manage on his own. Encouraging men to attend early for consultation in order to avoid a late presentation for help is complex. White and Banks (2004) suggest that late presentation of men for diagnosis must be seen as an urgent area for health research and policy development. Delay in accessing healthcare provision, according to White (2001), has repercussions on men's health in relation to the degree of morbidity, as well as having financial implications for caring for men when they become chronically sick. The practice nurse must consider ways to make men more aware of the need to present early for diagnosis and the consequences of late presentation and, therefore, late diagnosis.

Changes may need to be made in the way primary healthcare services are provided to men if the aim is to increase uptake of healthcare provision. The following facts are provided by Wilkins (2005) of the Men's Health Forum, highlighting discrepancies in the uptake of health services.

In a study of patients using smoking cessation services during a six-month period in 2002, out of 107 000 people who set themselves a date to stop smoking only 46 000 were men; this was in comparison with 61 000 women (DH, 2002); 28 % of men smoke as compared with 24 % of women (Office for National Statistics, 2003). A pilot programme for the National Bowel Cancer Screening Programme offered voluntary screening to approximately half a million people; among men the uptake was lower than their female counterpart: men accounted for 52 % and women 61 % (DH, 2003a). It must be noted that the death rate for colorectal cancer in men is 24.7 % per 100 000; in women this is 14.7 % per 100 000 (Cancer Research UK, 2007). The National Chlamydia Screening Programme (DH, 2004c) reveals that during its first full year 13 times as many women were screened and treated as men; this equated to 15 241 women and 1172 men. Chlamydia is a sexually transmitted infection (STI) that is equally prevalent in men and women.

The practice nurse must ask, 'What are the connections between the comparative data shown above?' It could be the fact that men delay seeking help and may also find it difficult to seek help. It can be problematic for a male patient deciding to attend a general practice. They may find the practice male-unfriendly, and often the practice has female receptionists, female healthcare assistants and female nurses.

Their first point of contact, according to Jewell (2001), may be off-putting for men, who may have what they see as an embarrassing problem which may nonetheless be life-threatening. The majority of practice waiting rooms display all the 'propaganda' associated with child and women's health (Banks, 2001), adding to the male perception that practices are not male-friendly. Staff attitudes and the lack of choice of a male practitioner can also be a factor that can decide if a man seeks or delays seeking help.

White (2001) identifies the following reasons why men are reluctant to go to their GP:

- a lack of understanding of the processes of making appointments and negotiating with female receptionists;
- inappropriate opening times, which tend to coincide with work commitments;
- an unwillingness to wait for appointments;
- a feeling that the service is primarily for women and children, making sitting in the waiting room uncomfortable for them;
- even the name 'health centre' has been identified as problematic;
- the negative response many men feel they get when presenting with difficulties that are not quickly dealt with;
- a lack of trust in the system, mainly around the issue of confidentiality, especially within the gay community and disclosure of HIV status;
- great fears relating to shame if their concerns are judged to be of little consequence, or having to admit to another person that they may have a problem, and one that they cannot solve;
- lacking the vocabulary they feel they need to discuss issues of a sensitive nature.

Health promotion activities aim to increase the knowledge and understanding of health, illness and health-related procedures or services. The health promotion activities offered by the practice nurse have the potential to correct any misunderstandings that a person may have about their health as well as increasing the uptake of health services and screening. Table 2.5 outlines some of the strategies that may be used to encourage men to access services.

In a consultation exercise undertaken by the Men's Health Forum (Wilkins, 2005) in response to the Department of Health's consultation to 'Your Health, Your Care, Your Say', individuals and organizations were asked to submit their views about the content of the White Paper *Your Health, Your Care, Your Say: A New Direction for Community Services* (DH, 2006). This White Paper sets out the Government's agenda for the strategy of community healthcare services. The results of the consultation exercise provided feedback from men regarding community care services.

Three questions were asked during the consultation period:

1. If you could change one thing about your local GP surgery to make it more likely that men would go there, what would you do?

Table 2.5. Some strategies that may be used to encourage men to attend and access services

Getting men to come in
- Become a male-friendly practice using images men can relate to, that is, posters, information leaflets/patient information should be male-specific. Provide female patients with information on men's health with an aim for them to pass this information on to their partners and family members
- Consider offering evening surgeries and appointments that men may find more convenient, that is, after their work has finished, consider shift patterns some people work and manage appointment times around them
- Think about taking the service to where men work, for example, factories and other places of work
- Advertise your services widely, for example, in places where men congregate, that is, sports settings, social venues

Encouraging men to open up and talk during the consultation
- Determine the specific needs the men attending your surgery have, that is, initiate a needs analysis, ask men what it is they expect from you as a healthcare provider
- Establish rapport and build up a relationship to understand the whole person
- Initiate discussion – using your interpersonal skills
- Advertise the confidential nature of the services you offer

Succeeding in encouraging men to return
- Ask the man to book another appointment after the consultation
- Explain the importance of returning for follow-up consultations
- Evaluate the services you are offering, are they what the patient wants? Can you offer anything else the patient may feel you have omitted?
- Refer to appropriate agencies
- Provide the patient with information about how to contact you in the future. This can be done using a variety of media, that is, written, SMS text messaging, e-mail, World Wide Web addresses

Helping men to make changes
- Try to work with the patient to identify any barriers to changing behaviour. The barriers may come from within or be extraneous barriers
- Identify common ground with the patient to reduce anxiety and make suggestions to what changes to make first
- Motivate the patient to make a commitment to change, explaining to him the benefits that may come from the proposed change
- Provide useful network contacts, that is, appropriate local networks/support groups
- Encourage ongoing dialogue (see above – encouraging men to return)
- Monitor changes in health behaviour providing useful feedback

(Source: Adapted from Hall, 2003)

2. If you could change one thing about your local GP surgery to make it more likely that *you* would go there, what would you do?
3. Use your imagination: if you could introduce a new service that would improve the health of men into your local community, what would it be?

Three broad categories emerged:

1 When am I supposed to go?

Access was the most popular response to what would make the difference both for them personally and for men in general. Conflict between working time and surgery times were common responses. More flexible opening hours, particularly in the evening and at weekends, were cited many times by men as one way to make them more likely to attend.

2 Why is it so difficult?

Attitudinal and structural problems when using primary care services were seen as off-putting. The failure of primary care to see itself as a service provider geared to the needs of men was noted. Bureaucracy, queuing and delays as barriers to accessing services and ineffective infrastructure can all have an impact on men's desire to attend. The reception process is perceived to lack confidentiality and/or being unwelcoming and obstructive. Some GPs may be dismissive, condescending or unsympathetic, and the whole process of engaging with primary care seems to be impersonal.

3 What about us blokes?

Nearly 50% of respondents felt that primary care was unwelcoming to men. Some men felt primary care was primarily designed for women and children. It was suggested by a number of men that changes should be made in relation to the primary care experience – for example, staffing and decor – to make it more male-friendly.

Those who responded to the question about the new service they would like to see in their own community called for (among other things) regular, informal health checks delivered in a male-friendly environment, often asking for these services to be moved away from primary care settings.

The findings from this small-scale consultation activity demonstrated that the men consulted were dissatisfied with primary care when looking at service provision from a male perspective. It could be tentatively suggested from the results of the consultation that primary care does not engage with men anywhere near as effectively as it might (Wilkins, 2005).

CONSULTING WITH MEN

Practice nurses are experienced practitioners who adopt a patient-centred approach to care; the same principles should also be implemented when providing care for men. Courtenay (2000) points out that men receive significantly less physician contact time in medical consultations than women. Men, he continues, are provided with fewer and briefer explanations from both a simple and technical perspective. Less advice is given to men regarding changing risk factors despite men's greater involvement in high-risk behaviours (Courtenay, 2000). Look around your own GP practice. This may confirm the fact that men are less likely to use GP services.

Effective communication skills are required by the practice nurse in order to identify the patient's problem more effectively and accurately. Maguire and Pitceathly (2002) suggest that there are key tasks in communication with patients (see Table 2.6 below). The tasks listed could be adopted and adapted by the practice nurse when s/he consults with the patient.

Hall (2003) suggests that at different times in their lives, from childhood to old age, men have differing health experiences, health needs and different degrees of interest in improving their health; he adds that there are age categories that are applicable to men's health:

- young boys
- older boys
- young adults
- older adults
- elderly men.

Table 2.7 (below) provides a checklist that discusses these specific ages. The checklist can be used by the practice nurse as a guide to assess needs and create with the patient a plan of care.

Table 2.6. Key tasks in communication with patients

- Eliciting (a) the patient's main problems; (b) the physical, emotional and social impact of the patient's problems on the patient and his family
- Tailoring information to what the patient wants to know; checking his understanding
- Eliciting the patient's reactions to the information given and his main concerns
- Determining how much the patient wants to participate in decision-making (when it comes to what treatment options are available to him)
- Discussing treatment options so that the patient understands the implications
- Maximising the chance that the patient will follow agreed decisions about treatment and advice about changes in lifestyle

(Source: Adapted from Maguire and Pitceathly, 2002)

Table 2.7. Some issues that the practice nurse may use to guide assessment

Young boys (0–9 years)

Check

- General health and development
- Weight and height
- Development progress (speech, learning, motor skills)
- Immunization record
- Un-descended testes or inguinal hernias

Discuss

- Social development: self-esteem
- Family relationships
- School

Older boys (10–19 years)

Check

- General health and development
- Weight and height
- Blood pressure
- Mental health: self-esteem
- Evidence of depression, stress, substance abuse
- Immunization record

Discuss

- Family relations
- School and social relationships
- Smoking, alcohol and drug use
- Driving safely
- Accidents and risk-taking
- Sexuality, relationships and STIs
- Diet and exercise

Young adult (20–49 years)

Check

- Blood pressure
- Blood cholesterol (according to local policy)
- Urinalysis for diabetes
- Family history in relation to, for example, bowel cancer, prostate cancer, diabetes, hyperlipidaemia
- Are there any other specific investigations required?
- Mental health: any signs of depression, stress?
- Immunization record

Discuss

- Occupational health and safety
- Employment
- Driving safely
- Sexual health
- Social support, relationships (partner breakdown)
- Suicide, depression, substance abuse
- Parenting
- Diet and exercise
- Smoking, alcohol and drug use

Older adults (50–74 years)

Check

- All the above items associated with the younger adult
- Prostate disease, prostate-specific antigen, digital rectal examination, ultra-sound sonography if indicated
- Diabetes, urinalysis, blood glucose
- Are there any other specific investigations required?

Discuss

- Diet and exercise
- Smoking, alcohol and drug use
- Family relationships and social support
- Preparation for retirement
- Sexual health
- Prostate cancer

Table 2.7. (*Continued*)

Elderly men (75+ years)	
Check	Discuss
• Full health assessment (physical and psychological)	• Diet, nutrition and exercise • Relationships – partner/carers • Sexual health • Social relations/isolation/loneliness

(Source: Adapted from Robertson, 2003; Hall, 2003)

PLANNING HEALTH PROMOTION INTERVENTIONS

Planning health promotion activities with men as the focus must be produced and made accessible to them in a format and language they will understand and use. See, for example, the work of Banks (2002); he uses the format of a car repair manual to encourage men to get to know more about themselves and their bodies. The Department of Health (2003b) has produced a toolkit to help healthcare professionals develop and produce effective patient information materials. Table 2.8 (below) provides some idea of what it is that the patient may want to know if diagnosed and what they wish they had been told (Crane and Patel, 2005).

It is inappropriate to provide men with modified health promotion materials that have been specifically devised and used with success for women and merely to change the words to relate the material to men. It is important to note that, as Connell (2000) has demonstrated, men do look at themselves in a different way from how women look at themselves.

Prior to embarking on health promotion activity the nurse needs to consider the circumstances surrounding the proposed intervention. This can be termed as the context. Davies and Kepford (2006) point out that an assessment of need is required, identifying the target group for the proposed intervention, the nature of the problem and an awareness of any assets currently in existence.

During the assessment phase, it is prudent to gauge political climate. By doing this, support for the proposed intervention may be forthcoming from those who may hold key decision-making roles. Approvals may be required from key stakeholders,

Table 2.8. What a patient is likely to want to know

• What is it?
• Why have I got it?
• How will it affect me?
• Can it be cured?
• What happens next?
• Might my family get it?

(Source: Crane and Patel, 2005)

for example, those who manage a budget or those who are in a position to grant ethical approval for your undertaking.

You must be sure of your aims and be able to articulate what you wish to achieve. If the aims are clearly articulated at this stage, then the intervention will have more of a chance of succeeding. It is vital to identify resources – both human and material. The interventions must be planned realistically and within confines.

Determining success may be a challenge. Often, the way to demonstrate success is to apply a numeric score/value to the outcome, for example, 16 % more men from black and ethnic minority groups attended the weekly Well-Man Clinic as a result of targeting this specific group. Achieving pre-set targets can also be another way of indicating success.

The final stage of the intervention is the evaluation phase. Nurses are familiar with the evaluation stage of the nursing process and the concepts associated with that process can be applied to the evaluation of health promotion interventions. There are several methods available to the nurse to ensure that evaluation is carried out in a robust and meaningful manner (see, for example, Morgan, 2006).

Men, according to Chell *et al.* (2000), are a notoriously ambivalent group to engage. The practice will need to use innovative and creative strategies to engage those men who are reluctant to attend; the nurse must bear in mind that men have diverse needs and therefore a pragmatic and flexible approach is required.

The Health Development Agency (2001) provides insight into how health promotion activities may have an impact on the state of boys' and young men's health. One of the objectives of the review was to identify gaps in both the literature and practice, considering in particular those boys and young men from vulnerable groups affected by depravation and poverty. The practice nurse may wish to use this review in order to inform his/her practice and proposed interventions.

CONCLUSION

Health can be interpreted in many ways by many people, for example, patients and nurses, and as result of this it is difficult to define. Furthermore, there may be inconsistencies with the definition, values and beliefs held by various parties: the patient and nurse may not share the same perspective.

Health is not only the absence of disease or infirmity. The adoption of a holistic perspective will recognize that physical, psychological, social, economic, cultural, political and environmental factors impinge on health and well-being. These factors impinge on health outcomes for all members of the population, including men.

The provision of male-specific health promotion activities:

- demonstrates (to the male population) that their health needs are important;
- is evidence of the health profession's commitment to improving the health of the male population;
- should help promote the health needs of those most in need: males from deprived socioeconomic backgrounds.

There are many myths surrounding men's health. One of these myths may be that men do not care about their health; men do care and do worry about their health. Often they feel unable to seek help regarding their health and may express their fears for a variety of reasons until it is too late. Robertson (2003) states that stereotyping men as being unconcerned about their health matters can lead to a stifling of the healthcare professional's ability to be creative when working with men. The practice nurse may be able to help promote men's health in many ways, encouraging them to access services and as a result make better use of the services available in the practice setting.

Commitment and involvement of various agencies, both Government and non-Government, are needed if strategies to improve men's health are to succeed, and partnership working with the man at the centre if it is advocated. It is erroneous and detrimental to exclude other populations, for example, women and children (in particular young boys) when devising health promotion activities for the male.

Each practice and each practice nurse must assess the healthcare needs of men in the local population, seek aims and objectives, determine targets and implement health promotion activity. The activity will need to be tailored to meet the needs of the man in partnership with the nurse, other members of the healthcare team and the wider community. Evaluation is vital if lessons are to be learned and good practice promoted.

If health promotion activities directed towards men are to be effective, then the education of nurses, midwives and specialist community public health nurses at both pre-registration and post-registration levels must include the important issue of gender and its association with health and illness.

REFERENCES

Acheson, D. (1988) *Public Health in England*, DH, London.

Banks, I. (2001) No man's land: men, illness and the NHS. *British Medical Journal*, **323**, 1058–1060.

Banks, I. (2002) National Men's Health Press Release, http://www.menshealthforum.org.uk/userpage1.cfm?item_id=915 (last accessed May 2006).

Biddulph, M. and Blake, S. (2001) *Moving Goal Posts: Setting a Training Agenda for Sexual Health Work with Boys and Young Men*. Family Planning Association, London.

Cancer Research UK (2007) www.cancerresearchuk.org/statistics.

Chell, S., Jones, D., Hughes, N. and Saunders, R. (2000) Men's health: slugs and snails? *Practice Nurse*, **11** (17), 6–9.

Connell, R.W. (2000) *The Men and Boys*, Polity Press, Cambridge.

Courtenay, W.H. (2000) Behavioural factors associated with disease, injury and death amongst men: evidence and implications for prevention. *Journal of Men's Studies*, **9**, 81–142.

Crane, R. and Patel, B. (2005) Producing patient literature. *Student British Medical Journal*, **13**, 200.

Dahlgren, G. and Whitehead, M. (1991) *Policies and Strategies to Promote Social Equity in Health*, Institute for Further Studies, Stockholm.

Davies, M. and Kepford, J. (2006) Planning a health promotion intervention. In (eds M. Davies and Macdowall), *Health Promotion Theory*, Open University Press, Maidenhead, pp. 151–168, (chapter 13).

Davies, M. and Macdowall (2006) *Health Promotion Theory*. Open University Press, Maidenhead.

Department of Health (1992) *The Health of the Nation: A Strategy for Health in England*, Her Majesty's Stationery Office, London.

Department of Health (1999a) *Making A Difference: Strengthening the Nursing, Midwifery and Health Visiting Contribution to Health and Social Care*, DH, London.

Department of Health (1999b) *Model Standards and Service Models: Mental Health*, DH, London.

Department of Health (2000a) *The NHS Plan: A Plan for Investment, A Plan for Reform*, DH, London.

Department of Health (2000b) *Model Standards and Service: Coronary Heart Disease*, DH, London.

Department of Health (2001) *Shifting the Balance of Power*, DH, London.

Department of Health (2002) *Statistics on Smoking Cessation in England: April to September 2002*, DH, London.

Department of Health (2003a) *Evaluation of the UK Colorectal Screening Pilot: Final Report*, DH, London.

Department of Health (2003b) *Toolkit for Producing Patient Information*, DH, London.

Department of Health (2004a) *Choosing Health: Making Healthier Choice Easier*, DH, London.

Department of Health (2004b) *Standards for Better Health*, DH, London.

Department of Health (2004c) *Annual Report of the National Chlamydia Screening Programme in England 2003/4*, DH, London.

Department of Health (2006) *Our Health, Our Care, Our Say: A New Direction for Community Services*, DH, London.

Department of Health, Social Services and Public Safety and Department of Health and Children (2001) *A Nursing Vision of Public Health: All-Ireland Statement on Public Health and Nursing*, Department of Health, Social Services and Public Safety, Belfast; Department of Health and Children, Dublin.

Downie, R.S., Fyfe, C. and Tannahill, A. (1990) *Health Promotion Models and Values*, Oxford Medical Publications, Oxford.

Downie, R.S., Tannahill, C. and Tannahill, A. (1996) *Health Promotion Models and Values*, 2nd edn, Oxford University Press, Oxford.

Edmonds, C.B., McClean, J., McGlone, J. and Wilson, L.M. (2006) Disorders of the respiratory system. In (eds M.F. Alexander, J.N. Fawcett and P.J. Runciman) *Nursing Practice: Hospital and Home. The Adult*, 3rd edn. Churchill Livingstone, Edinburgh, pp. 73–157, Chapter 3.

Fareed, A. (1993) Equal rights for men. *Nursing Times*, **90** (5), 26–29.

Fletcher, R. (1997) *Report on Men's Health Services*. Prepared for NSW Department of Health Men's Health Advisory Group, Family Action Centre, University of Newcastle, NSW 2318, Australia.

Frosh, S., Phoenix, A. and Pattman, M. (2002) *Young Masculinities: Understanding Boys in Contemporary Society*, Palgrave, Basingstoke.

Fuller, T.L., Backett-Milburn, K. and Hopton, J.L. (2002) Healthy eating: the views of general practitioners and patients in Scotland. *American Journal of Clinical Nutrition*, **77** (Supplement), pp. 1043S–1047S.

Hall, H.H. (2003) Promoting men's health. *Australian Family Physician*, **32** (6), 401–407.

Harrison, T. and Dignan, K. (1999) *Men's Health: An Introduction for Nurses and Health Professionals*. Churchill Livingstone, Edinburgh.

Hayes, L. (2005) Public health and nurses… What is your role? *Primary Health Care*, **15** (5), 22–25.

Health Development Agency (2001) *Boys' and Young Men's Health: Literature and Practice Review. An Interim Report*, HDA, London.

Jewell, D. (2001) Primary care. (eds N. Davidson and T. Lloyd), *Promoting Men's Health: A Guide for Practitioners*, Bailliere Tindall, London, pp. 151–163, Chapter 14.

King's Fund (2004) *Prevention Rather than Cure – Making the Case for Choosing Health* King's Fund, London.

Kirby, M.G. (2004) Men's health in primary care. In (eds R.S. Kirby, C.C. Carson, M.G. Kirby and R.N. Farah) *Men's Health*, 2nd edn. Taylor and Francis, London, pp. 15–38, Chapter 3.

Lincoln, P. and Nutbeam, D. (2006a) What is health promotion? (eds M. Davies and W. Macdowall) *Health Promotion Theory*, Open University Press, Maidenhead, pp. 7–15, Chapter 1.

Lincoln, P. and Nutbeam, D. (2006b) WHO and international initiatives. In (eds M. Davies and W. Macdowall) *Health Promotion Theory*, Open University Press, Maidenhead, pp. 16–23, Chapter 2.

Lloyd, T. (1996) *A Review of Men's Health*, Royal College of Nursing, London.

Maguire, P. and Pitceathly, C. (2002) Key communication skills and how to acquire them. *British Medical Journal*, **325**, 697–700.

Moffatt, J. (1980) A Well-Man Clinic – Thought for the Future. *Health Visitor*, **53**, 433–434.

Morgan, A. (2006) Evaluation of health promotion. (eds M. Davies and Macdowall). *Health Promotion Theory*, Open University Press, Maidenhead, pp. 168–187, Chapter 14.

Naidoo, J. and Wills, J. (2000) *Health Promotion: Foundations for Practice*, 2nd edn, Bailliere Tindall, London.

Naidoo, J. and Wills, J. (2001) Health promotion. (eds J. Naidoo and J. Wills) *Health Studies: An Introduction*, Palgrave, Houndmills, 2nd edn, pp. 274–307, Chapter 10.

New South Wales Health Department (1999) *Moving Forward in Men's Health*, NSWHD, Gladesville.

Newton, C. (1991) *The Roper, Logan and Tierney Model in Action*, Macmillan, Houndmills.

Nursing and Midwifery Council (2004) *Code of Professional Conduct: Standards for Conduct, Performance and Ethics*, NMC, London.

O'Dowd, T. and Jewell, D. (1998) *Men's Health*, Oxford University Press, Oxford.

Office for National Statistics (2003) *General Household Survey*, ONS, London.

Poulton, B., Mason, C., McKenna, H. *et al.* (2000) *The Contribution of Nurses, Midwives and Health Visitors to the Public Health Agenda*, Department of Health, Social Services and Public Safety, Belfast.

Robertson, S. (2003) Men managing health. *Men's Health Journal*, **2** (4), 111–113.

Tannahill, A. (1985) What is health promotion? *Health Education Journal*, **44** (4), 167–168.

White, A.R. (2001) *Report on the Scoping Study on Men's Health*, Leeds Metropolitan University, Leeds.

White, A.R. and Banks, I. (2004) Help seeking in men and the problems of late diagnosis. (eds R.S. Kirby, C.C. Carson, M.G. Kirby and R.N. Farah) *Men's Health*, 2nd edn, Taylor and Francis, London, pp. 1–9, Chapter 1.

White, A.R. and Lockyer, L. (2001) Tackling coronary heart disease: a gender sensitive approach is needed. *British Medical Journal*, **323**, 1016–1017.

Wilkins, D. (2005) *Response to the 'Your Health, Your Care, Your Say Consultation'*, Men's Health Forum, London.

Wilkinson, R. and Marmot, M. (1998) *Social Determinant of Health: the Solid Facts*, World Health Organization, Geneva.

Women's National Commission (2000) *Treating Women Well – Women and the NHS*, WNC, London.

World Health Organization (1986) *Ottawa Charter for Health Promotion*, WHO, Geneva.

World Health Organization (1997) *Jakarta Declaration on Leading Health Promotion into the 21st Century*, WHO, Geneva.

World Health Organization (2005) *Action on the Social determinant of Health: Learning from Previous Experiences*, WHO, Geneva.

3 Male health inequalities

INTRODUCTION

Gender is an important indicator of health differences nationally and internationally (O'Brien and White, 2003). In order to provide competent healthcare and produce effective policies to support healthcare delivery the nurse must consider gender. Recognizing and taking this into account can help provide effective and gender-sensitive services (Doyal, Payne and Cameron, 2003). Failure to pay attention to the differences between men and women will reinforce existing gender differences and exacerbate health inequalities.

Inequalities do not only vary between men and women but also occur between men – as men are not a homogeneous group. Analysis reveals inequalities between men from different social classes, ethnic and migrant groups (see Chapter 12). It must be remembered that men from black and minority ethnic groups are not homogeneous for health status, disease patterns or health behaviours. There are significant health inequalities among men from black and minority ethnic groups (see Table 3.1).

Kraemer (2000) points out that even from conception, prior to any social effects coming into play, males are more vulnerable than females. At conception there are more male than female embryos. This pole position is, however, quickly challenged as a result of maternal stress during conception, culminating in a reduction in the male to female ratio, suggesting that the male embryo is more susceptible than its female counterpart (Hansen, Møller and Olsen, 1999).

Gender is not the only factor that can impact on health inequalities. One key health indicator is life expectancy. On average, men in the UK die almost five years earlier than women. Living with illness and impairment makes economic hardship much more difficult to avoid. Those with persisting health difficulties and the associated discrimination that this brings have an increased risk of unemployment. They also depend more on welfare benefits as well as experiencing long-term poverty (Power *et al.*, 2002). Those who experience and enjoy good health may be in a better position to:

- control their lives
- live life to the full
- partake in community activity
- perform effectively in society.

Table 3.1. Key facts

- The prevalence for cerebrovascular accident for black Caribbean men showed rates two-thirds higher than the general population, but they had much lower rates of angina (1.9 % compared to 5.3 % of men in the general population)
- South Asian men were 30 % more likely to have ischaemic heart disease than men in the general population
- Among men who had smoked, 35 % of black Caribbean, 35 % of Indian, 21 % of Pakistani and 19 % of Bangladeshi had stopped smoking compared to 54 % of the general population
- Pakistani and Bangladeshi men were more than five times as likely to have diabetes and Indian men were almost three times as likely as the general population

---

(Source: Adapted from DH, 1999c)

This chapter does not just consider health inequalities in relation to men; it also considers health inequality in the population as a whole. Consideration is also given to those who experience health inequalities with learning disabilities or mental health problems. The practice nurse is encouraged to consider the whole spectrum of society and the whole spectrum of men, when considering health inequalities and ways in which they can be addressed and reduced.

A note of caution: when making comparisons between male and female health, it is erroneous to suggest that women's health is the gold standard by which to measure the health of men. Women have as many unmet health needs as men. Although it may be valuable to make a comparison between the sexes when the findings can be illuminating, it is not advocated that funding and other resources be reallocated from women to men. Focusing on the differences between men and women can conceal the differences between men, that is, social class, race and ethnicity.

HEALTH INEQUALITIES

For over one hundred years health inequalities between different groups of the population of the UK have occurred on a regular basis. Health inequalities mean that some population groups are more likely to be sick or are more likely to die younger than others. Every year in the UK many people die or suffer ill health and disability at an earlier age than they should. This should be a concern for every nurse and patient, regardless of gender. The most appropriate interventions (gender-specific and gender-sensitive interventions/ approaches) can lead to a reduction in the inequalities that lead to early unnecessary death and illness, and promote healthier living for longer, for most of the population.

There are many causes of health inequalities, and as a result of these it may be difficult to provide effective solutions to the problems that inequality brings. Health inequalities are often ubiquitously stubborn, persistent and difficult to change (Health Development Agency, 2004; DH, 2003). It is important for the practice nurse to gain as much information about the people s/he cares for in order to identify what the inequalities may be within that population and within a group such as men. When the causes or potential causes are identified, service provision and resources can be directed in the most effective way. The nurse must take into account the determinants of health (see Chapter 2). Ewles (2005) reminds us that consideration of any topic involves many factors (social determinants):

- age
- sex
- genetic make-up
- socioeconomic status
- cultural and physical environment.

Health inequalities are related to a gap that exists between various population groups, for example, those who are better off in a community and those in a community who are worse off, or those from different ethnic backgrounds. Burstrom, Whitehead and Lindholm (2000) suggest that those who are in higher socioeconomic groups have a better chance of staying in employment in the face of long-term illness and impairment than those in poorer groups. Those who have a learning disability, for example, or a mental health problem and are in a lower socioeconomic group will find it difficult to stay in employment.

Health inequalities, wherever they occur in the population, are unacceptable. They can start early in life and unfortunately persist into old age. Inequalities can also impinge on the health of future generations. In childhood, Kuh *et al.* (2004) note, there are socioeconomic gradients in growth and height, in language and cognition as well as social and emotional adjustment, and childhood socioeconomic circumstances affect a range of adult health outcomes. Montgomery, Bartley and Wilkinson (1997) demonstrate that childhood adversity can physiologically stunt growth. Some boys from poorer families grow up to become adolescents and adults who are more likely to experience mental health problems than those in better-off families (Meltzer and Gatward, 2000).

In the UK where a person is born can influence how long they will live. Health is inextricably related to the way people live their lives and the prospects available to them to make healthy choices (DH, 2004a).

POLICY

The NHS has two roles in improving the delivery of healthcare services – ensuring equity of access and in improving the population's health through prevention; it aims to do this through policy development and implementation. The NHS was founded on a principle of equity where provision of services, and access to those services, is based on medical need as opposed to status or ability to pay. The World Health Organization (2000) suggests that, along with the primary goal of better health, health systems should also have the goals related to fairness, responding to the needs of everyone, equally, without discrimination or difference.

A report published as long ago as 1980 (an independent inquiry into health inequalities) pointed to the problem in 'modern Britain' – The Black Report (Department of Health and Social Security, 1980). The inquiry was initially set up to contribute to the development of the Government's strategy for health and action on inequalities in the longer term. Sir Douglas Black the Chair of the committee that produced the report stated:

> Achieving a high standard of health amongst all its people represents one of the highest of society's aspirations. Present social inequalities in health in a country with substantial resources like Britain are unacceptable ...

The Black Report and its successors have been instrumental in keeping health inequalities at the forefront of the public health agenda. Sir Donald made 40 recommendations in the report which ranged from poverty, income, tax and benefits, education and employment to mothers, children and families and ethnicity.

The report largely contributed to the new health strategy *Saving Lives: Our Healthier Nation* (DH, 1999a) together with *Reducing Health Inequalities: An Action Report* (DH, 1999b). The *Action Report* set out what action was being taken across Government to tackle the underlying causes of ill health including socioeconomic factors and it built upon, among other things, the recommendations in Sir Donald's report.

The NHS Plan (DH, 2000) put prevention and inequalities clearly on the agenda both in terms of NHS service delivery as well as with the NHS working with and through other agencies. The Government provided a commitment in *The NHS Plan* that, for the first time ever, local targets for reducing health inequalities would be reinforced by the creation of national health inequalities targets.

Building on the announcement of the targets, the Government completed a public consultation in autumn 2001 on the actions needed to tackle health inequalities and meet the targets. The consultation ranged across Government and across sectors at national, regional and local levels on how these targets would be delivered.

In 1998 the Acheson Report (Acheson, 1998) was produced. This inquiry again considered inequalities in health and advocated that a wide-ranging approach be taken to what constitutes a healthy life. The Acheson Inquiry concluded that:

> Inequalities by socioeconomic group, ethnic group and gender can be demonstrated across a wide range of measures of health and the determinants of health.

The inquiry was initially set up to contribute to the development of the Government's strategy for health as well as action on inequalities in the long term. Forty recommendations were made in the Acheson Report (Acheson, 1998). They included recommendations concerning some of the following:

- poverty
- income
- tax benefits

- education and employment
- issues concerning mothers, children and families
- concerns regarding ethnicity.

Tackling Health Inequalities: A Programme for Action (DH, 2003) takes forward most of the recommendations made in the Acheson Report, which advocated the use of a cross-Government approach to tackling the underlying causes of ill health and the socioeconomic factors that may contribute to ill health. *The NHS Plan* (DH, 2000) once again placed prevention and inequalities on the health agenda, reiterating the need to include other Government agencies in the effort to reduce inequality; and again commitment was made by Government to set local targets to reduce inequalities.

The *Cross Cutting Review* was produced in 2002 (DH, 2002) and assessed progress and agreed priorities, ensuring that further targets were set for further actions. The setting of one national target to reduce health inequalities was agreed:

> By 2010 to reduce health inequalities in health outcomes by 10% as measured by infant mortality and life expectancy at birth.

Local Government has required to adopt the target, which aims to reduce the health gap in childhood and throughout life between socioeconomic groups and the most deprived areas of the country in national Public Service Agreements (PSAs). Local authorities and the NHS are working together to create partnerships that can begin to address inequalities in health. Public health is becoming a core aspect of the public sector and local Government business. This could be termed co-delivery, joint responsibility resting with local Government and Primary Care Trusts (PCTs) to deliver the health improvement and health inequality agenda (Municipal Journal and DH, 2005). The *Spending Review 2004 Public Service Agreement* (DH, 2004b) produced four objectives in relation to the *Cross Cutting Review*'s one national target (see Table 3.2 below).

The evidence reviewed initially in the *Independent Inquiry into Inequalities in Health* (Acheson, 1998), and subsequently by the *Cross-Cutting Review*, demonstrated that in order to achieve the targets and tackle the underlying determinants of inequalities, action will be required across Government. These conclusions have provided the backbone for the *Programme for Action* (DH, 2003).

The White Paper *Choosing Health* (DH, 2004a) provides the opportunity for local authorities and PCT to approach health inequalities jointly. The aim of this White Paper is to improve health and tackle health inequalities.

HEALTH INEQUALITIES: PUBLIC SERVICE AGREEMENT TARGETS

The *Programme for Action* (DH, 2003) reinforces the Government's aim to reduce health inequalities and is supported by the PSAs with the aim of reducing

Table 3.2. *Spending Review 2004, Public Service Agreements*: the four objectives

Objective	Approach
Objective 1: Improve the health of the population: by 2010, increase life expectancy at birth in England to 78.6 years for men and 82.5 years for women	1. Substantially reduce mortality rates by 2010 2. Reduce health inequalities by 10% by 2010 as measured by infant mortality and life expectancy at birth 3. Tackle the underlying determinants and health inequalities
Objective 2: Improve health outcomes for people with long-term conditions	1. To improve health outcomes for people with long-term conditions by offering a personalized care plan for vulnerable people most at risk; and to reduce emergency bed days by 5% by 2008, through improved care in primary care and community settings for people with long-term conditions
Objective 3: Improve access to services	1. To ensure that by 2008 no one waits more than 18 weeks from GP referral to hospital treatment 2. Increase the participation of problem drug users in drug treatment by 100% by 2008; and increase year-on-year the proportion of users successfully sustaining or completing treatment programmes
Objective 4: Improve the patient and user experience	1. Secure sustained national improvements in NHS patient experience by 2008, measured using independently validated surveys 2. Improve the quality of life and independence of vulnerable older people by supporting them to live in their own homes where possible

(Source: Adapted from DH, 2004b)

inequalities by 10% as measured by a reduction in infant mortality and life expectancy at birth. PSAs define the outcomes and targets to be achieved by Government departments in return for resources from the Treasury (Health Development Agency, 2005). The PSA targets are underpinned by two detailed objectives:

• Starting with children under one year, by 2010 to reduce by at least 10% the gap in mortality between routine and manual groups and the population as a whole.
• Starting with local authorities, by 2010 to reduce by at least 10% the gap between areas with the lowest life expectancy at birth and the population as a whole.

For the first time ever the tackling of health inequalities is considered by the Government as one of its top six priorities for the NHS (DH, 2006). Since 2007 each PCT is required formally to review whether they are tackling inequalities. Assessment of whether the targets set have been met is to be carried out and monitored by the Department of Health and the Health Care Commission. The implementation and delivery of Local Delivery Plans (LDPs) will be used to monitor progress and achievement; the initial focus will be on smoking cessation.

INEQUALITY, LEARNING DISABILITIES AND MENTAL HEALTH

Learning disability and problems with mental health occur regardless of gender. Inequalities are also experienced by those with learning disabilities and mental health problems. Some male health inequalities have already been discussed in Chapter 2; consider those inequalities and how they are confounded even further when the patient has a learning disability or mental health problem. Practice nurses must be cognizant of this when providing care for men who may have a learning disability or mental health problem. These groups of men may be overlooked in terms of opportunities for recognizing inequality and in providing an opening to promote healthy lifestyles.

It has been demonstrated that those who are unemployed can suffer the effects of inequalities in many aspects of life. Fryers, Meltzer and Jenkins (2003) point out that mental health problems are more common among people who are unemployed, have fewer educational qualifications, are on low income or have a low standard of living. The Disability Rights Commission (2004a) states that 21 % of those with a mental health problem of working age are in employment compared with 81 % of those who are non-disabled. Lewis *et al.* (1998) estimate that a low standard of living is the primary cause of neurotic disorders in 10 % of all sufferers of the condition in the United Kingdom. Standard of living, they continue, is a more important measure of socioeconomic status than education or social class. The Government has acknowledged that higher rates of mental health problems are associated with being financially worse off (DH, 1999a).

Life expectancy is often used as a key indicator of health. Harris and Barraclough (1998) note that those people who have severe mental health problems are twice as likely to die early than the general population. They also identify that deaths from natural causes were 1.5 times more expected in those who have bipolar disease.

Rates of physical illness are higher than average in people with mental health problems (Seymour, 2003). Mukherjee *et al.* (1996) report that diabetes mellitus is five times more common in those who have schizophrenia, while Henderson and Ettinger (2003) state that development of atypical antipsychotic drugs can be associated with an exacerbation of diabetes.

There are some psychotropic drugs that result in a higher mortality rate (Disability Rights Commission, 2004b). Goldman (2000) points out that adverse interactions between general medical and psychotropic drugs have been reported. Some psychotropic drugs have the ability to cause cardiotoxicity, with potential damaging effects on electrophysiology and myocardial function (Davidson, 2002). Haematological dyscrasias has also been reported in some patients who use antipsychotic drugs (Oyesanmi *et al.*, 1999).

For some people with learning disabilities, morbidity and mortality are related to their impairment. For example, obesity and heart disease are associated with some genetic causes of learning disabilities (NHS Health Scotland, 2004). Poor access to services may occur for a variety of reasons, and as result of this the person may present late and the effects of the illness may be more damaging. Chapter 2 above outlined the potential difficulties associated with men who present late for treatment.

The attitude of the practice nurse and the overall manner of the practice may hinder access to services. Inappropriate stereotypes, negative attitudes and negative assumptions about a person with learning disabilities and their quality of life may prevent patients from accessing and speaking highly of the general healthcare they receive (Beecroft *et al.*, 2001). Difficulties associated with physical access to the practice may also deter the person with learning disabilities from attending as well as previous poor experiences or, according to Alborz *et al.* (2003), fear of the consequences of attending. Not least, concludes Cohen and Phelan (2001), some people may not be registered with general practitioners. The DH (2001), in its publication *Valuing People: A New Strategy for Learning Disability for the Twenty-First Century*, recognizes the shortfalls in access to, and care by, primary care in the United Kingdom for people with learning disabilities and has set the agenda for improving all aspects of care for those with learning disabilities.

Inequality exists when some patients with mental health problems or learning disabilities are denied healthcare on the basis of their condition. The Royal Brompton Hospital (2001) reports that heart surgery has been denied for some people with Down's syndrome and Byrne (2000) and Masterton (2000) note that issues have arisen concerning organ transplantation for those who have mental health problems.

The National Patient Safety Agency (2004) has recognized that problems exist when communicating with healthcare professionals. Symptoms the patients present with may not be communicated in terms that the healthcare professional understands. Healthcare professionals may also erroneously assume that the patient understands more than they do (Alborz *et al.*, 2003). Using effective communication skills and adopting a more proactive approach to the care of men with learning disabilities or mental health problems will require more time for consultations and the practice nurse must factor this into the consultation process. Investing in this can provide a better understanding of the needs of men with learning disabilities or those with mental health problems; it can also enhance and empower the patient, encouraging him to make decisions and to participate actively in his care. The nurse should give consideration to the type of media used to communicate with the individual. Consider, for example, the patient who has difficulty reading or is unable to read. Appointment letters, information leaflets and consent forms may need to be adapted to ensure that the patient understands (Alborz *et al.*, 2003; NHS Health Scotland, 2004). It is advocated that materials should be specifically produced for use in primary care settings, for example, information cards related to male health, regular health checks and healthy lifestyles (National Health Service Executive, 1998).

Cassidy *et al.* (2002) describe how structured health checks have been undertaken by a team of a consultant psychiatrist in learning disability, a GP and a learning disability nurse and then repeated a year later, finding that 94 % of people with learning disabilities were discovered to have a physical health problem that justified intervention. There have been similar findings throughout the United Kingdom (McConkey, Moore and Marshall, 2002; Martin *et al.*, 2004).

TACKLING HEALTH INEQUALITIES

Tackling health inequalities is a complex activity. The challenge is to ensure that future improvements in health over the next 20 years are shared by all (DH, 2003). Roles and responsibilities demand a joinedup approach to ensure that the determinants of health are considered fully. Table 3.3 (below) provides an outline of organizational roles and responsibilities.

The practice nurse needs to develop a range of specific actions in order to address fully the needs and reduce the inequalities experienced by all of those s/he cares for and, in particular, those who have learning disabilities or mental health problems. Expanding the range of services that are on offer to the practice population is to be encouraged; however, Cooper, Melville and Morrison (2004) state that failure to take into account the specific needs of people with learning disabilities or mental health problems may in fact widen the inequality gulf; this could also apply to men from different social, ethnic and migrant groups. The practice nurse has a central role in ensuring that the needs of the whole practice population are met.

Service provision must be matched to need, and the 'one size fits all' approach has to be abandoned as this is a key factor in widening the gap that exists. Reorientation of current services may be required, moving towards a more male-specific prevention and early detection approach, making services more accessible and more flexible and so meeting the diverse needs of the different men in the practice population. Year on year men have been subjected to poorer access to services, more ill health and death, and this, as discussed in Chapter 2, may be as a direct consequence of delayed help-seeking behaviour. By the time the man presents, their condition may have progressed too far for effective treatment.

O'Brien and White (2003) describe gender mainstreaming as a commitment to ensure that men's (and women's) health concerns and experiences are integral to the work of the organization, incorporating all aspects of its activities, from employment issues, through to organizational governance, delivery and outcomes.

Table 3.3. Organizational roles and responsibilities in tackling health inequalities

Organization	Aim
Department of Health	To transform the health and social care systems so that it produces faster, fairer services that deliver better health and tackles health inequalities
Strategic Health Authorities	To ensure that inequalities are addressed strategically
Primary Care Trusts	Lead locally in driving forward health inequalities work with a range of partners. As planners, commissioners and providers of healthcare, PCTs and NHS Trusts should ensure that service modernization narrows health inequalities and does not inadvertently make them worse
Office of the Deputy Prime Minister	To ensure Government targets on health inequalities are met at local level
Government Offices	To ensure Government targets on health inequalities are met at local level
Regional Development Agencies	To address the underlying determinants of health inequalities
Regional Assemblies	To work together with regional partners to address inequalities in health, ensure health issues are promoted, improve the quality of life of citizens and ensure NHS investment contributes to economic, social and physical regeneration
Local Authorities	To deliver services that have an impact on the wider determinants of health
Local Strategic Partnerships	To set local targets for tackling deprivation, including local health inequality targets
Local Authority Overview and Scrutiny Committees	Remit includes public health and inequality issues; councillors are able to scrutinize how local needs are being addressed, how health services are run and how they can be improved

(Sources: Health Development Agency, 2005)

This description of gender mainstreaming could be adopted as a framework by the practice nurse and the practice for ensuring that the issues that concern men are addressed fully.

Griffiths (2001) states that a fundamental task in closing the inequalities gap that exists between men and women and between men and men is to provide joined-up policies from different sectors of society. The root cause of health inequalities – for example, the determinants of health – need to be addressed. Griffiths also suggests that the root cause of many health inequalities in men's health is the lack of employment and resources to live in a way which would result in better health.

CONCLUSION

Generally, the more affluent people are, the better will be their health; conversely, the poorer people are, the worse will be their health. This is further confounded by gender inequalities and inequalities associated with other members of our society such as those with learning disabilities or mental health problems. The challenge is to address these multifaceted health inequalities. In order to do this the nurse needs to devise innovative and creative approaches to begin to reduce the health inequality gap experienced by men and the population as a whole, as change could benefit both sexes.

The Sex Discrimination Act came into force as long ago as 1975. The public sector, according to the Women and Equality Unit (2005), has a big impact on the lives of men; it also has a key role to play in ensuring that equality of opportunity for all regardless of their sex is achieved. The current Government is aiming to make the public sector more responsive to men and women's different needs, reducing inequalities and improving the quality of life for all. The Equality Bill is currently going through Parliament, explaining specific duties and responsibilities, ensuring gender equality between men and women.

The Government has produced a number of key policies, providing a number of challenges designed to reduce inequalities in health. One part of the *Programme for Action* (DH, 2003) demands that regional public health groups with Government offices develop a cross-cutting health inequalities action plan. The action plans are aimed at addressing the underlying determinants of health and include:

- employment
- skills
- housing
- equality
- environment
- transport
- food
- social inclusion
- mental health issues.

The Government polices that have been produced, it could be suggested, need to address health inequalities through a gendered lens, and a refocusing is required to consider gender specifically. Understanding the gender implications could reduce the persistent and stubborn health inequalities felt by all of the population.

It is generally accepted that the role and responsibility of the state is to protect and improve public health. The inequalities identified in this chapter may cause serious difficulty for healthcare providers in order to meet the responsibilities under the new gender equality legislation that is currently progressing through Parliament. The Men's Health Forum (2005) suggests that the Equal Opportunities Commission has already highlighted men's use of primary care as a particular area of concern.

General practice has a key role in tackling health inequalities. The approach used will be as complex as the population the practice serves. Being aware of the determinants of health, the social implications of poor health and the need to motivate and encourage men to present early may reduce the chasm that exists in relation to male health inequality.

REFERENCES

Acheson, D. (1998) *Independent Inquiry into Inequalities in Health Report*, Her Majesty's Stationery Office, London.

Alborz, A., McNally, R., Swallow, A. and Glendinning, C. (2003) *From the Cradle to the Grave: A Literature Review of Access to Health Care for People with Learning Disabilities Across the Lifespan*, National Co-ordinating Centre for NHS Service Delivery and Organisation, London.

Beecroft, N., Becker, T., Griffiths, G. *et al.* (2001) Physical health care for people with severe mental illness: the role of the general practitioner. *Journal of Mental Health*, **10** (1), 53–61.

Burstrom, B., Whitehead, M. and Lindholm, C. (2000) Inequalities in the social consequences of illness: how do people with long-term illness fare on the labour markets of Britain and Sweden? *International Journal of Health Services*, **30**, 435–451.

Byrne, P. (2000) Organ transplantation and discrimination. *British Medical Journal*, **320**, 1600.

Cassidy, G., Martin, D.M., Martin, G.H. and Roy, A. (2002) Health checks for people with learning disabilities. *Journal of Learning Disabilities*, **6** (2), 123–136.

Cohen, A. and Phelan, M. (2001) The physical health of patients with mental illness: a neglected area. *Mental Health Promotion Update*, **2**, 15–16.

Cooper, S.A., Melville, C. and Morrison, J. (2004) People with intellectual disabilities. *British Medical Journal*, **329**, 414–415.

Davidson, M. (2002) Risk of cardiovascular disease and sudden death in schizophrenia. *Journal of Clinical Psychiatry*, **63** (Supplement vol. 9), 5–11.

Department of Health (1999a) *Saving Lives: Our Healthier Nation*, The Stationery Office, London.

Department of Health (1999b) *Reducing Health Inequalities: An Action Report*, DH, London.

Department of Health (1999c) *Health Survey for England: The Health of Ethnic Minority Groups '99'*, The Stationery Office, London.

Department of Health (2000) *The NHS Plan: A Plan for Investment, A Plan for Reform*, DH, London.

Department of Health (2001) *Valuing People: A New Strategy for Learning Disability for the 21st Century*, The Stationery Office, London.

Department of Health (2002) *Tackling Health Inequalities: 2002 Cross-Cutting Review*, DH, London.

Department of Health (2003) *Tackling Health Inequalities: A Programme for Action*, DH, London.

Department of Health (2004a) *Choosing Health: Making Healthier Choices Easier*, DH, London.

Department of Health (2004b) *Spending Review 2004 Public Service Agreement*, DH, London.

Department of Health (2006) *The NHS in England: The Operating Framework for 2006/7*, DH, London.

Department of Health and Social Security (1980) *Inequalities in Health: Report of a Working Group Chaired by Sir Douglas Black*, DHSS, London.

Disability Rights Commission (2004a) *Disability Briefing: January*, DRC, London.

Disability Rights Commission (2004b) *Equal Treatment: Closing the Gap*, DRC, London.

Doyal, L., Payne, S. and Cameron, A. (2003) *Promoting Gender Inequalities in Health*, Equal Opportunities Commission, London.

Ewles, L. (2005) Editor's preface. *Key Topics in Public Health: Essential Briefings on Prevention and Health Promotion*, Elsevier, Edinburgh, xiii–xvii.

Fryers, T., Meltzer, D. and Jenkins, R. (2003) Social inequalities and the common mental disorders: a systematic review of the evidence. *Social Psychiatry and Psychiatric Epidemiology*, **38** (5), 229–237.

Goldman, L.S. (2000) Comorbid medical illness in psychiatric patients, *Current Psychiatry Reports*, **2**, 256–263.

Griffiths, S. (2001) Inequalities in men's health. In (eds N. Davidson and T. Lloyd) *Promoting Men's Health: A Guide for Practitioners*, Balliere Tindall, London, pp. 35–43, Chapter 2.

Hansen, D., Møller, H. and Olsen, J. (1999) Severe peri-conceptional life events and the sex ratio in offspring: follow up study based on five national registers. *British Medical Journal*, **319**, 548–549.

Harris, S.C. and Barraclough, B. (1998) Excess mortality of mental disorder. *British Journal of Psychiatry*, **173**, 11–53.

Health Development Agency (2004) *Health Inequalities: Concepts, Frameworks and Policy*, HAD, London.

Health Development Agency (2005) *Introduction to Health Inequalities*, HDA, London.

Henderson, D.C. and Ettinger, E.P. (2003) Glucose intolerance and diabetes in Schizophrenia. In (eds J.M. Meyer and H.A. Nasrallah) *Medical Illness and Schizophrenia*, American Psychiatric Publishing, Washington, pp. 99–114.

Kraemer, S. (2000) The fragile male. *British Medical Journal*, **321**, 1609–1612.

Kuh, D., Power, C., Blane, D. and Bartley, M. (2004) Socioeconomic pathways between childhood and adult health. In (eds Kuh, D. and Ben-Shlomo, Y.) *A Life Course Approach to Chronic Disease Epidemiology*, 2nd edn, Oxford University Press, Oxford, pp. 371–395, Chapter 16.

Lewis, G., Bebbington, P., Brugha, T. *et al.* (1998) Socioeconomic status, standard of living, and neurotic disorder. *Lancet*, **352**, 605–609.

Martin, G., Philip, L., Bates, L. and Warwick, J. (2004) Evaluation of a nurse-led annual review of patients with severe intellectual disabilities, needs identified and needs met, in a large group practice. *Journal of Learning Disabilities*, **8** (3), 235–246.

Masterton, G. (2000) Psychosocial factors in selection for liver transplantation. *British Medical Journal*, **320**, 263–264.

McConkey, R., Moore, G. and Marshall, D. (2002) Change in the attitudes of GPs to the health screening of patients with learning disabilities. *Journal of Learning Disabilities*, **6** (4), 371–384.

Meltzer, H. and Gatward, R. (2000) *The Mental Health of Children and Adolescents in Great Britain*, Office for National Statistics, London.

Men's Health Forum (2005) *Response to the 'Your Health, Your Care, Your Say Consultation'*, Men's Health Forum, London.

Montgomery, S.M., Bartley, M.J. and Wilkinson, R.G. (1997) Family conflict and slow growth. *Archives of Disease in Childhood*, **77**, 326–330.

Mukherjee, S., Decina, P., Bocola, V. *et al.* (1996) Diabetes mellitus in schizophrenic patients. *Comprehensive Psychiatry*, **37** (1), 68–73.

Municipal Journal and Department of Health (2005) *Health Inequalities: Rising to the Challenge*, Municipal Journal and Department of Health, London.

National Health Service Executive (1998) *Signposts for Success in Commissioning and Providing Health Services for People with Learning Disabilities*, NHSE, London.

NHS Health Scotland (2004) *People with Learning Disabilities in Scotland: Health Needs Assessment Report*, NHS Scotland, Glasgow.

National Patient Safety Agency (2004) *Safeguarding People with Learning Disabilities within the NHS: An Agenda for the National Patient Safety Agency*, NPSA, London.

O'Brien, O. and White, A. (2003) *Gender and Health: the Case for Gender-sensitive Health Policy and Health Care Delivery*, King's Fund, London.

Oyesanmi, O., Kunkel, E.J., Monti, D.A. and Field, H.L. (1999) Hematological side effects of psychotropics. *Psychosomatics*, **40** (5), 414–421.

Power, C., Stansfield, S.A., Matthews, S. *et al.* (2002) Childhood and adult risk factors for socioeconomic differentials in psychological distress: evidence from the 1958 British Birth Cohort. *Social Science and Medicine*, **55**, 1989–2004.

Royal Brompton Hospital (2001) *The Report of the Independent Investigation into Paediatric Cardiac Services at the Royal Brompton Hospital and Harefield Hospital*, Royal Brompton Hospital, London.

Seymour, L. (2003) *Not All in the Mind: The Physical Health of Mental Health Service Users*, Radical Mentalities – briefing paper 2. Mentality, London.

Women and Equality Unit (2005) *Advancing Equality for Men and Women: Government Proposals to Introduce a Public Sector Duty to Promote Gender Equality,* WEU, London.

World Health Organization (2000) *World Health Report 2000: Health Systems: Improving Performance*, WHO, Geneva.

4 Men as risk takers

INTRODUCTION

Chapter 1 of this text outlined the view that males and females are different, and many reasons have been cited for this, for example, from a biological perspective as well as from a social perspective. They also differ in respect to risk: whether it is bungee jumping, driving too fast or posing on a skateboard, the male engages in risk when carrying out these activities.

Over a decade ago the Chief Medical Officer (Calman, 1993) stated that the primary difference between men's and women's health was 'variations in exposure to risk factors' – and this still holds true today. Calman (1993) centred on an individual's lifestyle view of health, addressing the biological and only acknowledging a societal role (Lloyd, 2001).

This chapter focuses on the risks that men take. Risk is defined and the psychological issues that make some men engage in risk-taking behaviours are outlined. Interest about risk-taking and risk-taking behaviours requires an understanding of why some men engage in risk-taking activity and others do not. When the practice nurse has insight and understanding and appreciates the issues underpinning these activities, s/he may be able to develop and implement interventions that can reduce the number of accidents and injuries as a result of risk-taking behaviours. The implications for the health and well-being of the male are described.

RISK-TAKING – WHAT IS IT?

Risk-taking and risk-taking behaviours, according to Gray (2005), are mainly associated with adolescents and young men. Kiddy (2001) points out that adolescence is a transitional phase of life and is very much associated with developments in risk-taking activities, for example:

- smoking
- drinking alcohol
- drug abuse
- sexual health.

Adolescence, suggests Calman (1993), is characterized by experimentation and rapid change. At this stage in life the male adolescent begins to learn new things and takes on board new experiences, behaviours and ideas. The outcome of this can have significant costs for the individual's future physical and mental health.

Purser, Orford and Johnson (2001) suggest that risk-taking:

> involves a range of behaviours often associated with alcohol consumption, including taking drugs they would not have otherwise; having un-protected sex; being involved in an argument or fight; and driving under the influence of alcohol.

Gullone and Moore (2000) have their definition of risk-taking:

> participation in behaviour which involves potential negative consequences (or loss) balanced in some way by perceived consequences (or gain).

Lloyd and Forrest (2001) do not provide a definition of risk but they indicate that the taking of risks is related to how masculinity is socially constructed. They identify four types of risk, that which:

- is socially sanctioned
- involves thrill seeking
- reflects rebellious activity
- is reckless and antisocial.

The major sex differences in death rates, it should be noted, are not in relation to most common causes of death such as cancers and coronary heart disease but in accidents and violence (Lee and Glynn-Owens, 2002).

Societal expectations and hegemonic masculinity appear to encourage men to take physical and psychological risks; physical risk-taking, according to Lee and Glynn-Owens (2002), provides individuals with the ability to demonstrate their competence and courage. Courtenay (2000) develops this concept further by suggesting that men take health risks also by:

- refusing to take time off when they are sick
- being adamant that they need little sleep in order to function
- bragging that alcohol does not impair their ability to drive.

Courtenay (2000) concludes that taking these health risks is one way to validate men as the stronger sex. Stereotyping provides cultural assumptions of what society wants to expect from boys as they grow up and become men: it is accepted that they will become risk takers. The media, for example, reinforces these expectations, encouraging men to drive faster, smoke more, drink more, work the body harder in order to achieve that idealized body shape, become more violent and take more risks: they are encouraged to live up to the 'lad' culture. White (2001) suggests that accidents and risk-taking are closely related to the younger person feeling invulnerable and their desire to be seen as being strong and able.

High levels of risk-taking are evidenced by men's use of health services. Men are less likely than their female counterparts to turn up for GP appointments and are

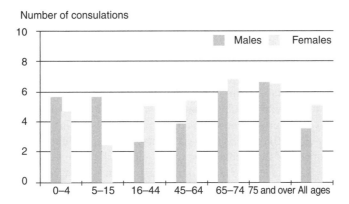

Figure 4.1. The average number of NHS GP consultations per person, per year: by age and sex in the UK (Office for National Statistics, 2006b)

more likely to become more ill by the time they finally get to their practice nurse or GP (Hodge, 2004). Females had more consultations with GPs per year than men (five times compared with three and half for men) and this was most noticeable in the 16–44 year age group (see Figure 4.1).

In 2003/2004, 5 % of people reported consulting a practice nurse during the fortnight before interview. This is less than the average 15 % of people who consulted the GP; nevertheless, the patterns of consultations by age and sex were similar. Females consulted a practice nurse more than men – 7 % compared with 4 % for males. In the age group 16–44 years women were twice as likely as men to have consulted a practice nurse – 5 % for women and 2 % for men. The majority of female consultations in this age group were associated with pregnancy and family planning (Office for National Statistics, 2006b).

The Office for National Statistics (2006b) estimates that 14 % of the population reported visiting an accident and emergency department at least once in the three-month period before interview. Women aged 16–64 years were more likely than men to attend; this resulted in a higher overall attendance rate among females than males – 15 % for females compared with 13 % for males. Attendance at accident and emergency departments in most ethnic minority groups was significantly lower than that of the general population in the 16–34 age group; however, Irish men have similar attendance rates to that of the general population (Erens, Primatesta and Prior, 2000).

The 1999 Health Survey for England (Erens, Primatesta and Prior, 2000) focuses on the health of ethnic minority groups and notes that after age standardization the average annual NHS GP contact rate was found to be higher for black Caribbean men and for Bangladeshi, Pakistani and Indian men when compared with men in the general population. It was noted that Bangladeshi men had more than twice as many contacts per year with the GP than men in the general population.

On a daily basis men are exposed to risk – for example, in the occupations they choose, the modes of transportation used, the games and sporting activities they undertake. Social prescription, according to Lee and Glynn-Owen (2001), in relation to young men in particular suggests that they must 'prove themselves'; they do this very often by taking unnecessary risks. The need to be concerned with caution and safety are often associated with 'femininity' and as Chapter 1 has pointed out this is seen by some males, in particular young males, as inferior. The outcome of relegating 'femininity' to inferior often results in younger men behaving in self-destructive ways. Lantz *et al.* (2001) discuss the issue of macho social conditioning; in this they suggest that aspects of the problem rest in the relationship men have with their bodies. The male body is central to masculinity and men ensure that self-image is in line with what society expects of men.

MALE LIFESTYLES

It has already been noted that men are not a homogeneous group, and the same is said for male lifestyles. Issues related to smoking, use of drugs, alcohol consumption, accidents and criminal activity are discussed here. It has been noted many times that behaviours such as smoking, heavy drinking and drug-taking are harmful behaviours to individuals and other members of society. The White Paper *Choosing Health: Making Healthier Choices* (DH, 2004a) aims to provide actions to reduce the numbers of people who smoke, to encourage and support sensible drinking and to reduce the harm caused by the use of illegal drugs. The support provided and strategies in place include, for example, smoking cessation clinics as well as guidelines for sensible drinking.

Male lifestyle factors that affect men's health must be given consideration when analysing risk and risk-taking, for example, smoking, drinking and the misuse of drugs. The recent trends in smoking, drinking and drug-taking suggest that prevalence remains relatively stable; however, there are differences between gender, age groups and occupational classes (Office for National Statistics, 2006b). Prevalence overall is higher in men than women.

Patel (2000) notes that the factors cited take on different patterns within society: some groups in society appear to be more susceptible than others. It has also been noted that there is an increase in liver disease in South Asian men as a result of an increase in alcohol use; this also brings with it an impact for the overall health of the family.

There are an exceptionally higher numbers of men within the armed forces (predominantly a male occupational group) who smoke. It has been difficult to encourage these men to stop smoking while serving in the forces and even when they leave (Feigelman, 1994).

White (2001) describes another group of men who are higher users of tobacco, alcohol and drugs – gay men. He continues and suggests that this higher use of tobacco, alcohol and drugs increases when these men find themselves marginalized from society. Marginalized group activities, he states, are examples of hidden risk-taking behaviour, particularly when they involve unprotected sex.

SMOKING

Over the last 30 years in Great Britain there has been a substantial decline in the proportion of those over 16 years who smoke. The biggest reduction has been in men. In 1974, 51 % of men aged 16 years and over smoked, compared with 41 % of women. Twenty-six per cent of men and 23 % of women by 2004/2005 were smokers (Office for National Statistics, 2006a). In 2003 male smokers, on average, smoked 15 cigarettes per day, women smoked 13 per day (Office for National Statistics, 2006b). Smoking is strongly associated with socioeconomic classification and is more common among those men in routine and manual occupational groups than those in professional or managerial groups. The Department of Health's *Public Service Agreement 2005–2008* (DH, 2004b) provides a target that aims to reduce adult smoking rates in England to 21 % or less by 2010, this target also specifically aims to reduce prevalence among routine and manual occupational groups to 26 % or less.

ALCOHOL CONSUMPTION

Donaghy and Ussher (2005) state that excessive use of alcohol is an international health concern. In the United Kingdom in 2000 alcohol abuse was responsible for the deaths of 5796 men (Office for National Statistics, 2000); this was a 100 % increase over 20 years (Office for National Statistics, 2004).

The excessive use of alcohol consumption in the population generally should be given serious consideration as excessive amounts can lead to ill health with an increased likelihood of problems such as hypertension, cancer, cirrhosis of the liver, road traffic accidents, antisocial behaviour and stroke (Prime Minister's Strategy Unit, 2004). An understanding of why some men drink excessively and others may not needs to be gained if the nurse is to recognize the implications for effective health education and health promotion initiatives. Young men (those aged between 16 and 24 years) are more likely than young women to drink heavily. In 1995 the Government changed its guidelines on sensible drinking from weekly to daily benchmarks. Regular moderate drinking of between one and two units per day can protect men over the age of 40 years against the risk of death from coronary heart disease and ischaemic stroke (Prime Minister's Strategy Unit, 2004). The Department of Health (1995) currently advises that safe alcohol consumption for men should not exceed between three and four units a day and for the female this is between two and three units daily.[1] The Prime Minister's Strategy Unit (2004) has produced guidelines for reducing the harmful effects of drinking alcohol; similar strategies have also been published in Scotland, Wales and Northern Ireland.

In 2004/2005 two-fifths of men and approximately one-fifth of women in Great Britain exceeded the recommended amount of alcohol on at least one day during the previous week (Table 4.1 below).

[1] Units – A unit of drink contains 8 g of alcohol. This is approximately the amount of alcohol contained in half a pint of beer or cider (ordinary strength), a quarter of a pint of extra strong beer or cider, a small glass (100 ml) of wine, a glass of sherry or port, or a single pub measure (25 ml) of spirits (Royal College of Physicians, 2001).

Table 4.1. Percentages of adults exceeding specified levels of alcohol: by sex and age, 2004/2005 on at least one day in the previous week

	Age				
	16–24	25–44	45–64	65 and over	All aged 16 and over
Males					
More than 4 units and up to 8 units	15	17	19	13	16
More than 8 units	32	31	18	7	22
More than 4 units	47	48	37	20	39
Females					
More than 3 units and up to 6 units	15	16	15	4	13
More than 6 units	24	13	6	1	9
More than 3 units	39	28	20	5	22

(Source: Office for National Statistics, 2006a)

The financial costs in providing nursing, medical and social services for those with alcohol problems run into billions of pounds; the Royal College of Physicians (2001) suggests that this accounts for approximately 12% of the total NHS expenditure in the UK. The personal costs to the individual and his family are incalculable. Figure 4.2 (below) demonstrates death rates from alcohol-related causes.

Alcohol-related deaths in England and Wales have continued to rise since the 1980s, from 5970 in 2001 to 6580 in 2003. The death rate for alcohol-related deaths also increased from 10.7 per 100000 in 2001 to 11.6 per 100000 in 2003. In 2003 males accounted for almost two-thirds of the total number of alcohol-related deaths; these deaths are more common in males than females (Office for National Statistics, 2006a).

Regional variations also exist with higher rates of alcohol-related deaths being reported in the northwest and northeast of England. Lower rates are found in the east, southwest and southeast of England.

BINGE DRINKING

A binge drinker is described as a man who regularly drinks 10 or more units in a single session (Royal College of Physicians, 2001); binge drinking can result in severe impairment of judgement leading to an increase in likelihood of accidents at home, at work, on holiday and on the road (Health Education Authority, 1996; Honkanen, 1993). It can be associated with all ages; however, De Visser and Smith (in press) suggest that it is more likely to occur with younger men, binge drinking during youth is a particular concern as it is a predictor of binge drinking during adulthood (Jefferis, Power and Manor, 2005).

According to De Visser and Smith (in press), the use of alcohol consumption and the behaviour associated with this are influenced by a range of demographic, social

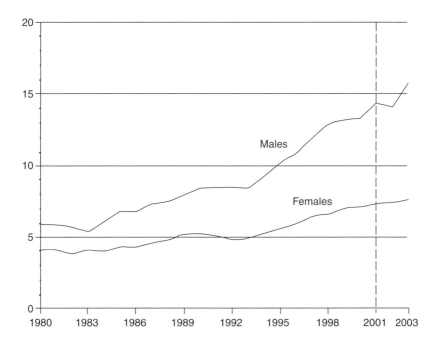

Figure 4.2. Death rates from alcohol related causes by sex per 100000 in England and Wales. Age standardized to the European population. Rates for 2001 are not directly comparable with those for earlier years as a result of a change from ICD 9 to ICD 10. (Source: Office for National Statistics, 2006a)

and attitudinal variables. They continue and suggest that there are other important factors that must also be given consideration that are associated with ethnicity and socioeconomics, for example, the individual, peers, religious and cultural factors. White British teenagers are more likely than their black and Asian peers to have drunk alcohol; Pakistani-British youths are less likely to drink than Indian-British or Chinese-British youths; and Muslim youths are less likely to drink than followers of other religions (Best *et al.*, 2001; Heim *et al.*, 2004; De Visser and Smith, in press). Moore, Smith and Catford (1994) note that binge drinking is associated with men of lower socioeconomic status and Claussen (1999) adds that unemployment is seen as a contributory factor in relation to problem drinking.

Chapter 1 (above) has discussed the issue of masculine identity and how this can impinge on health behaviour. This is also true when alcohol consumption as a male behaviour is concerned. Gender, according to De Visser and Smith (in press) must also be given some consideration at both individual and societal levels. They report that research frequently examines sex differences (i.e. male/female) in drinking behaviour but rarely does it consider gender (i.e. masculine/feminine). As a result of this, some research will not be able to determine if masculinity has an influence on whether some men drink excessively and others do not. Courtenay (2000) and Lee and Glynn-Owens (2002) argue that there is a need for this information as gender is an important influence on health-related behaviours. Men may drink alcohol excessively as a result of a search for their masculine identity; for example, if the definition of maleness (masculinity) is to drink alcohol then this will have an influence on drinking behaviour. Harnett *et al.* (2000) describe excessive drinking as a central component of being a young man, the result of which may mean that this attempt to demonstrate masculinity can lead to sexual violence or economic crime. If alcohol consumption is seen as masculine behaviour, then those men who have insecurities associated with their masculinity may use the consumption of alcohol to demonstrate masculine competence (De Visser and Smith, in press).

Alcohol consumption and the behaviour associated with its consumption, it could be suggested, are socially constructed in an attempt to reinforce masculine identity (Courtenay, 2000). The study undertaken by De Visser and Smith (in press) demonstrates that many men believe alcohol consumption and being able to 'hold your own' are important components of masculinity but they state that not all men express their masculinity by drinking excessively. Abstinence or moderate consumption are also methods of expressing masculinity as there is more than one way to be masculine (Frosh, Phoenix and Pattman, 2002). The links between masculinity and health-related behaviours such as drinking alcohol are not simple; there are a wide range of factors that need to be given consideration (De Visser and Smith, in press).

DRUG USE

Misuse of drugs can also have implications for individual health as well as social consequences. Sixteen per cent of men in England and Wales aged 16–59 years have taken illicit drugs in the previous year. Men outnumber women on all fronts with regards to the use of drugs (see Table 4.2).

Table 4.2. Percentage of the prevalence of drug misuse by those aged 16 to 24 years in England and Wales in the previous year, sex and drug category, 1996 and 2004/2005

	Men		Women	
	1996	2004/2005	1996	2004/2005
Cannabis	30	30	22	18
Ecstasy	9	7	4	3
Cocaine	2	7	—	3
Amphetamines	15	4	9	3
Magic Mushrooms/LSD	9	5	2	2
All Class A drugs[a]	13	11	6	5
Any Drugs	34	33	25	11

(Source: Office for National Statistics, 2006a)
[a]Includes heroin, cocaine, ecstasy, magic mushrooms, LSD and unprescribed methadone

Drugs have been classified under the Misuse of Drugs Act into three categories, A, B and C. These classifications relate to their harmfulness. The most harmful drugs are in Class A followed by Class B and Class C. The classification of certain drugs depends on the method of delivery used. Amphetamines, for example, are a Class B drug if taken orally and if injected become a Class A drug. In January 2004 cannabis was reclassified from Class B to Class C. Table 4.3 provides details of the most-well-known drugs and their classifications.

In 2003 the age-standardized drug-poisoning death rates were higher for males at 6.0 per 100000 than for females – 3.0 per 100000 (Office for National Statistics, 2006b). In 1998 the Government launched a ten-year strategy (this was revised in 2002) to tackle drug misuse (Cabinet Office, 1998). The strategy emphasized the need to reduce the harm caused by drug-taking, suggesting that the most appropriate approach was to attempt to persuade all potential drug users, specifically the young, not to use drugs. The revised strategy also emphasized drug use and those members of society who may be vulnerable.

ACCIDENTS

Men are more likely than women to be affected by a major or minor accident. Risk-taking brings with it the chance of being involved in an accident or death; accidents are the most common cause of death in those men who are aged less than 30 years

Table 4.3. The classification of well-known drugs

Drug	Mode of use	Classification
Speed and other amphetamines	Inject	A
Ecstasy	Oral	A
Cocaine	Sniff or inject	A
Crack	Inject or smoke	A
Heroin	Smoke, sniff or inject	A
LSD	Oral	A
Magic mushrooms	Oral	A
Methadone	Oral	A
Speed and other amphetamines	Sniff or oral	B
Tranquillizers	Oral or inject	B/C (depending on drug)
Anabolic steroids	Oral or injects	C
Cannabis	Smoke or oral	C
Poppers	Sniff	It is an offence to supply these substances if it is likely that the product is intended for abuse
Glue	Sniff	
Gas	Sniff	

(Source: Office for National Statistics, 2006b)

(Kirby, 2004). Throughout the world the leading cause of death and disability are injuries, accidental or non-accidental, and injury that is associated with occupation or social behaviour. White (2001) points out that risk-taking is often, erroneously, seen as a normal part of a young man's life.

The practice nurse should be concerned about accidents and the consequences. As Krug, Sharma and Oranzo (2000) point out, they are a major public health problem, nationally and globally. The problem is a particular issue when it concerns young men, a group that is often neglected in respect to public health issues and initiatives.

Injuries and accidents are discussed and analysed through the lens of language and social debate and are often seen as isolated and unfortunate issues. The causes of accidents and injury are not isolated occurrences; they are often socially constructed and are the result of socially sanctioned patterns of behaviour (Lee and Glynn-Owens, 2002). Road traffic accidents, for example, are usually associated with excessive alcohol use. Deaths related to road traffic accidents are the highest among young men aged between 15 and 34 years of age; they account for one-fifth of deaths in this age group (Office for National Statistics, 2001). Ulleberg (2002) notes that younger drivers are more likely to drive too fast, follow too closely as well as overtake in a more dangerous manner than other drivers would. Young males (i.e. those aged between 20 and 30 years), drivers and riders, are twice as likely to fail a breath test as other road users are, according to the Department for Transport (2005). Mortality as a result of accidents is four times greater in men who are from lower socioeconomic backgrounds than those men from the higher socioeconomic groups, demonstrating that socioeconomic differentials are influential (Griffiths, 2004). According to Begg and Langley (2001), as young men age and approach adulthood their driving improves and they grow out of risk-taking when driving.

Approximately 5000 children die or are seriously injured on Britain's roads each year. Boys have nearly twice as many accidents as girls when they are walking, playing and five times as many when riding bikes. Almost two-thirds of child accident victims are boys. It is also noted that boys are more likely than girls to walk to and from school, to cross roads on their own, to play out in the street and to ride a bike (Automobile Association Motoring Trust, 2003).

The Social Exclusion Unit (2002) notes that a boy from a low-income family is five times more likely than a child from a high-income family to be killed on the road. A boy from an ethnic minority is up to twice as likely to have an accident while walking or playing when compared to the national average (Department of the Environment, Transport and the Regions, 2001).

CRIMINAL ACTIVITY

Crime, just like accidents, also has gendered characteristics. Men, many times over, are more likely to be perpetrators of crime. They are also more likely to be victims of crime and, furthermore, the type of criminal activity is often violent in nature. Lee and Glynn-Owens (2002) suggest that men who engage in violence and criminal activity do so in order to act out hegemonic masculine roles when other strategies for enacting these are not available to them. They also note that when patriarchy and the benefits that this brings with it are unavailable, it is this group of men who are more likely to turn to violence and criminal activity as a way of, or an attempt at, communicating their masculinity. This group is most likely to be single young men. It could be tentatively suggested, therefore, that crime is synonymous with masculinity for some men.

Young men are over-represented in the criminal justice system with 6 % of all 17-year-old boys in England and Wales being found guilty of indictable offences, the highest rate for any age group, and five times the corresponding rate for girls; 80 % of offenders were male, with 11 % under 17 years of age (Office for National Statistics, 2006a). Men in England and Wales in 2004/2005 were almost twice as likely as women to be victims of violent crimes – 5 % as compared to 3 %; younger men aged between 16 and 24 years were at most risk and had experienced a violent crime. Men, and in particular younger men, were more likely to experience violence committed by a stranger. The most common injuries experienced by men were black eyes or bruising. Table 4.4 outlines the types of injury from violent crime by sex.

The most common offences committed by males and females in England and Wales were theft and handling of stolen goods, with men committing over 70 % of

Table 4.4. Types of injury from violent crime by sex 2004/2005

	Domestic	Mugging	Stranger	Acquaintance[a]	All violence
Men					
Minor bruise/ black eye	47	24	30	36	32
Severe bruising	23	14	14	12	14
Scratches	32	15	10	7	11
Cuts	18	15	16	18	17
Broken bones	3	1	3	2	2
Concussion or loss of consciousness	2	2	4	3	3
Other	2	2	10	12	9
Women					
Minor bruise/ black eye	38	11	30	34	31
Severe bruising	27	9	14	19	19
Scratches	17	7	6	16	13
Cuts	14	3	7	19	13
Broken bones	1	1	2	2	2
Concussion or loss of consciousness	1	0	0	3	1
Other	4	3	6	7	5

(Source: Office for National Statistics, 2006a)
[a]Assaults in which the victim knew one or more of the offenders, at least by sight

these offences. Crime is a male preserve (Lloyd, 2001): more men are in prison than women, with white males making up 83 % of the male prison population in England and Wales in 2003, and black males making up the next highest group, followed by Asian and other men. Alcohol is implicated in a number of serious crimes such as homicide, stabbings, beatings, domestic violence and child abuse. The use of illegal drugs is also connected with criminal acts (Griffiths, 2004).

WHY MEN TAKE RISKS – PSYCHOLOGY OF RISK-TAKING BEHAVIOUR

Risk-taking behaviour, suggest Greene *et al.* (2000), has been considered as a personality characteristic, a learned behaviour and developmental phenomenon, and, in relation to adolescence and young men, they suggest that there are three theories why adolescents and young men engage in risk-taking behaviours (see Table 4.5 below). For adolescents (as well as for men in general) risk-taking behaviour is complex and needs to be considered as more than a lack of ability on behalf of the individual to negotiate, apply knowledge and use social skills.

Thom and Francome (2001) describe seven common development predictors that are associated with a number of risk-taking activities:

- disrupted family background
- poor parental supervision and communication
- problems at school
- poor social skills
- physical or sexual abuse in childhood
- having a risk-seeking personality
- having a history of age-inappropriate behaviour.

Understanding the psychological underpinnings as to why adolescents and young men might take risks (or not) could help when providing and devising appropriate healthcare interventions. The nurse must be aware of gender differences associated with males and females; for example, boys appear to be more involved with their own thoughts that lead to a fascination with these thoughts, emphasizing a belief in their own uniqueness and, importantly, their invulnerability (Greene *et al.*, 2000, 1996). It is important, therefore, that the nurse take these gender differences into account when providing separate health promotion messages for boys and girls.

THE ROLE OF THE PRACTICE NURSE

The practice nurse, a public health and primary care worker, is ideally situated to help men and young boys to understand the implications of risk-taking and the

Table 4.5. Three proposed theories associated with risk-taking behaviours

Theory	Characteristics
Sensation-seeking	Sensation-seeking, according to Zukerman (1979, 1994), is generally defined as a trait identified by the seeking of varied, novel, complex and intense experiences as well as the willingness to take risks that will result in those experiences. Behaviours associated with sensation-seeking can be: • Alcohol use (Newcomb and McGee, 1989) • Cocaine use (Ball, 1995) • Risky sexual behaviour (Sheer and Cline, 1994). This theory points to the individual's personality characteristics, attempting to explain that traits of sensation-seeking are present and this type of personality will engage in more risk-taking behaviour than others. Sensation-seeking behaviour reaches a peak during adolescence with the individual wishing to experience novelty, excitement and danger.
Learned behaviour	The key proponent of this theory is that risk-taking is a learned behaviour. The results of this learned behaviour are seen as forms of social deviance, a syndrome of problem behaviour.
Developmental immaturity	Lack of experience is responsible for developmental immaturity; the result of this paucity of experience may lead to errors in judgement. Errors in judgement occur often as a result of the individual's sense of uniqueness or specialness – egocentrism. Egocentrism is defined by Paiget (1929, 1958) as an overall focus on self. Risk, in this context, is seen as normal; it is seen as appropriate behaviour, exploratory behaviour; it is also a negative by product of cognitive development and in particular egocentrism. Risk-taking is deliberate and requires the person to make a decision about how to act, weighing up the pros and cons, the proposed risk against other factors.

(Source: Adapted from Greene *et al.*, 2000; Ulleberg, 2002; Gray, 2005)

consequences for their health. However, before this occurs the nurse must make an exploration of the concepts men and young boys hold in respect to health, risk and their relation to lifestyles.

If the practice nurse is able to begin to understand the views held by men and young boys in relation to risk-taking activity that may result in injury and death, then a concerted effort can be made to provide appropriate health promotion in these areas and in other risk-taking aspects of the person's life such as smoking, alcohol, substance misuse and sexual health.

Providing practical advice to patients is the hallmark of the practice nurse. Practical advice should be provided in such a manner that the patient will wish to take on board the information offered, in a manner the patient understands and is able to use.

The aim should be to provide information and give them the opportunity to improve their knowledge on three levels:

- individual
- educational
- community.

Griffiths (2004) asks that this occurs across the entire age spectrum, commencing in schools.

Alcohol Concern (2001) advocates the use of brief interventions as a way of providing advice and information regarding responsible drinking. A brief intervention, they suggest, may last for 5–10 minutes and can occur once or more than once. The target group are those who drink excessively but are not yet experiencing major problems as a result of their alcohol consumption. The aim is to convince the individual that they are drinking at levels that may be harmful to their health. Often, brief interventions are opportunistic; the person has not already sought help about the alcohol problem and is seeking advice for another problem (Lock *et al.*, 2006). Alcohol Concern (2001) suggests that primary care is an excellent setting in which to deliver a brief intervention. Opportunities to raise issues associated with alcohol can occur:

- during new patient registrations
- Well-Man Clinics
- diabetic clinics
- hypertension clinics
- asthma clinics
- individual consultations.

Lock and Kaner (2000) comment that, despite the potential effectiveness of brief interventions in the primary care setting, practitioners in these areas are not aware of the approach and have failed to incorporate it into routine practice. Table 4.6 (below) provides some strategies that may be used to minimize, for example, the dangers of drinking.

CONCLUSION

Individual choice may be one element that encourages men to engage in risk-taking activities that result in accidents. The same may also be true of the individual's choice to engage in criminal activity and what it is that makes some men victims of crime. Another factor must also be given due consideration, that of the societal influences that are placed on men – how society expects men to behave. The over-representation of men as victims of accidents as well as victims and perpetrators of crime cannot be understood in isolation. This must be appreciated in the context of individual choice.

Table 4.6. Some strategies that may minimize the dangers associated with drinking

---

- Explain the legal limits to the patient
- Encourage the patient to eat and drink something that is easily digested before going out, describe that if the stomach is empty alcohol is absorbed faster
- Drink water in between drinks
- When out with a group, it is wise to nominate a person who has the responsibility to look out for others
- Use a taxi as opposed to walking
- Drink in known venues
- Do not drink and drive

(Source: Adapted from Gray, 2005)

Accidents are a global public health concern and the impact these accidents have on society and the individual has received little attention from an epidemiological perspective. It is suggested that more research is conducted in this important yet neglected area of public health. The high risk of injury and death associated with accidents, particularly in relation to young men, must be given a higher priority by those who work in the sphere of public health.

Excessive alcohol is both a national and international problem. It can result in unnecessary death, ill health, accidents and antisocial behaviour. The reason why some men drink to excess and some men do not is complex. Alcohol consumption is implicated in a number of serious crimes such as homicide, stabbings, beatings, road traffic accidents, domestic violence and child abuse.

Even from a very early age men are exposed to risks and succumb to the effects of these risks more than women do. Data demonstrates this in several aspects of every-day life, for example, road traffic accidents and road accidents. Boys have twice as many accidents as girls while walking or playing and this increases to more than five times as many when riding bikes; furthermore, almost two-thirds of child accident victims are boys.

The practice nurse can provide men with advice and information in an attempt to improve their knowledge related to risk and risk-taking. This should occur across the entire age spectrum, commencing in schools.

REFERENCES

Alcohol Concern (2001) *Fact Sheet 15: Brief Interventions*, Alcohol Concern, London.

Automobile Association Motoring Trust (2003) *The Facts About Road Accidents and Children*, Alcohol Concern, London.

Ball, S.A. (1995) The validity of an alternative five-factor measure of personality in cocaine abusers. *Psychological Assessment*, **2**, 148–154.

Begg, D. and Langley, J. (2001) Changes in risky driving behaviour from age 21 to 26 years. *Journal of Safety Research*, **32** (4), 491–499.

Best, D., Rawaf, S., Rowley, J. *et al.* (2001) Ethnic and gender differences in drinking and smoking among London adolescents. *Ethnicity and Health*, **6**, 51–57.

Cabinet Office (1998) *Tackling Drugs to Build a Better Britain*, The Stationery Office, London.

Calman, K. (1993) *On the State of the Public Health – 1992*, Her Majesty's Stationery Office, London.

Claussen, B. (1999) Alcohol disorders and re-employment in a 5 year follow-up of long-term unemployed. *Addiction*, **94**, 133–138.

Courtenay, W.H. (2000) Constructions of masculinity and their influence on man's well-being: a theory of gender and health. *Social Science and Medicine*, **50**, 1385–1401.

Department of the Environment, Transport and the Regions (2001) Press Release 196, 30th March 2001.

Department of Health (1995) *Sensible Drinking: The Report of an Inter-Departmental Working Group*, DH, London.

Department of Health (2004a) *Choosing Health: Making Healthier Choices Easier*, DH, London.

Department of Health (2004b) *Technical Note for Spending Review 2004: Public Service Agreement 2005–2008*, DH, London.

Department for Transport (2005) *Road Traffic Accidents in Great Britain: 2004: The Casualty Report*, The Stationery Office, London.

De Visser, R.O. and Smith, J.A. Alcohol Consumption and Masculine Identity Among Young Men, in press.

Donaghy, M.E. and Ussher, H. (2005) Exercise interventions in drug and alcohol rehabilitation, (eds G.E.J. Faulkner and A.H. Taylor) *Exercise, Health and Mental Health: Emerging Relationships*, Routledge, London, pp. 48–69, Chapter 4.

Erens, B., Primatesta, P. and Prior, G. (2000) *Health Survey for England: The Health of Minority Ethnic Groups 1999*, The Stationery Office, London.

Feigelman, W. (1994) Cigarette smoking among former military service personnel: a neglected social issue. *Preventative Medicine*, **23**, 235–241.

Frosh, S., Phoenix, A. and Pattman, R. (2002) *Young Masculinities*, Palgrave, Houndmills.

Gray, M. (2005) *Fundamental Aspects of Men's Health*, Quay Books, London.

Greene, K., Krcmar, M., Walters, L.H. *et al.* (2000) Targeting adolescent risk-taking behaviours: the contribution of egocentrism and sensation seeking. *Journal of Adolescence*, **23** (4), 439–461.

Greene, K., Rubin, D.L., Walters, L.H. and Hale, J.L. (1996) The utility of understanding adolescent egocentrism in designating health promotion messages. *Health Communication*, **8**, 131–152.

Griffiths, S. (2004) Men as risk takers. In (eds R.S. Kirby, C.C. Carson, M.G. Kirby and R.N. Farah), *Men's Health*, 2nd edn, Taylor Francis, London, pp. 243–250, Chapter 18.

Gullone, E. and Moore, S. (2000) Adolescent risk-taking and the five-factor model or personality. *Journal of Adolescence*, **23**, 393–407.

Harnett, R., Thom, B., Herring, R. and Kelly, M. (2000) Alcohol in transition: towards a model of young men's drinking styles. *Journal of Youth Studies*, **3**, 61–77.

Health Education Authority (1996) *Think About Drink: There's more to Drink than You Think*, HEA, London.

Heim, D., Hunter, S., Ross, A. *et al.* (2004) Alcohol consumption, perceptions of community responses and attitudes to service provision: results from a survey of Indian, Chinese and Pakistani young people in Greater Glasgow, Scotland, UK. *Alcohol and Alcoholism*, **39**, 220–226.

Hodge, S. (2004) Editorial. *The Journal of the Royal Society for the Promotion of Health*, **124** (5), 194.

Honkanen, R. (1993) Alcohol in home and leisure injuries. *Addiction*, **88**, 939–944.

Jefferis, B., Power, C. and Manor, O. (2005) Adolescent drinking level and adult binge drinking in a national birth cohort. *Addiction*, **100**, 543–549.

Kiddy, M. (2001) Teenage pregnancy: whose problem? *Nursing Times*, **98** (4), 36–37.

Kirby, M.G. (2004) Men's health in primary care. In (eds R.S. Kirby, C.C. Carson, M.G. Kirby and R.N. Farah) *Men's Health*, 2nd edn, Taylor Francis, London, pp. 15–32, Chapter 3.

Krug, E.G., Sharma, G.K. and Oranzo, R. (2000) The global burden of injuries. *American Journal of Public Health*, **90**, 523–526.

Lantz, J.M., Fullerton, J.T., Harshburger, R.J. and Saler, G.R. (2001) Promoting screening and early detection of cancer in men. *Nursing Health Science*, **3**, 189–196.

Lee, C. and Glynn-Owens, R.G. (2002) *The Psychology of Men's Health*, Open University Press, Buckingham.

Lloyd, T. (2001) Men and health: the context for practice. In (eds N. Davidson and T. Lloyd) *Promoting Men's Health: A Guide for Practitioners*, Bailliere Tindall, London, pp. 3–33, Chapter 1.

Lloyd, T. and Forrest, S. (2001) Boys' and Young Men's Health: Literature and Practice Review, Health Development Agency, London.

Lock, C.A. and Kaner, E.F.S. (2000) Use of marketing to disseminate brief alcohol intervention to general practitioners: promoting health care interventions to health promoters. *Journal of Evaluation in Clinical Practice*, **6** (4), 345–357.

Lock, C.A., Kaner, E.F.S., Heather, N. *et al.* (2006) Effectiveness of nurse-led brief alcohol intervention: a cluster randomised control trial. *Journal of Advanced Nursing*, **54** (4), 426–439.

Moore, L., Smith, C. and Catford, J. (1994) Binge drinking: prevalence, patterns and policy. *Health Education Research*, **9**, 497–505.

Newcomb, M.D. and McGee, L. (1989) Adolescent alcohol use and other delinquent behaviors: a one year longitudinal analysis controlling for sensation seeking. *Criminal Justice and Behvior*, **16**, 345–369.

Office for National Statistics (2000) *Mortality Statistics Cause*, Her Majesty's Stationery Office, Norwich.

Office for National Statistics (2001) *Social Focus on Men*, Her Majesty's Stationery Office, Norwich.

Office for National Statistics (2004) *Social Trends 32*, Her Majesty's Stationery Office, Norwich.

Office for National Statistics (2006a) *Social Trends 36*, Her Majesty's Stationery Office, Norwich.

Office for National Statistics (2006b) *Focus on Health*, Her Majesty's Stationery Office, Norwich.

Patel, K. (2000) The missing drug users: minority ethnic drug users and their children. In (eds F. Harbin and M. Murphy) *Substance Misuse and Child Care*, Russell House, Lyme Regis, pp. 39–54, Chapter 2.

Paiget, J. (1929) *The Child's Conception of the World*, Harcourt Brace, New York.

Paiget, J. (1958) *The Growth of Logical Thinking from Childhood to Adolescence*, Basic, New York.

Prime Minister's Strategy Unit (2004) *Alcohol Harm Reduction Strategy for England*, PMSU, London.

Purser, B., Orford, J. and Johnson, M. (2001) *Drinking in Second and Subsequent Generation Black and Asian Communities in the English Midlands*, Alcohol Concern, London.

Royal College of Physicians (2001) *Alcohol: Can the NHS Afford it? Recommendations for a Coherent Alcohol Strategy for Hospitals*, RCP, London.

Social Exclusion Unit (2002) *Making Connections – Transport and Social Inclusion*, SEU, London.

Sheer, V.C. and Cline, R.J. (1994) The development and validation of a model explaining sexual behaviour among college students: implications for AIDS communication campaign. *Communication Research*, **21**, 280–304.

Thom, B. and Francome, C. (2001) *Men at Risk: Risk Taking, Substance Use and Gender*, Middlesex University, London.

Ulleberg, P. (2002) Personality subtypes of young drivers: relationship to risk-taking preferences, accident involvement and responses to a traffic survey campaign. *Transport Research*, **4**, 279–297.

White, A.R. (2001) *Report on the Scoping Study on Men's Health*, Leeds Metropolitan University, Leeds.

Zukerman, M. (1979) *Sensation Seeking: Beyond the Optimal Level of Arousal*, Erlbaum, New Jersey.

Zukerman, M. (1994) *Behavioral Expressions and Biosocial Bases of Sensation Seeking*, Cambridge University Press, New York.

5 Young men and boys

INTRODUCTION

Chapter 4 demonstrated that young men and boys are seen as significant risk takers, and the risks engaged in at a younger age can impact on the boy's adult life. Younger men are often out to impress others, particularly those of the opposite sex, showing strength and bravery by engaging in potentially life-threatening activity, appearing to be emotionally and physically strong, not asking for help and being 'self-contained'.

Risk-taking activities are not the only issues specifically related to being young and male. Other activities, such as eating disorders and the younger male person, the impact of under-achieving at school with the consequential effects of unemployment at an early age, the sexual health of young men and emotional and mental health issues, can also impinge on the person's health and well-being. This chapter describes some of the legislative issues pertinent to young men and boys: mental health issues, issues surrounding male eating disorders and the sexual health needs of young males. Some practical advice is offered regarding the most appropriate and effective uses of resources.

Primary care nursing can be seen as a continuum from individual treatment and care to a population-based approach to improving the health and well-being of the younger man. Those primary care nurses who work in general practice, for example, often focus on the individual aspects of the spectrum, while others such as health visitors and school nurses may spend a lot of their time caring for health needs across a population and leading programmes to tackle them (Department of Health (DH), 2003). The practice nurse also works as a member of a larger multidisciplinary team, potentially making a unique contribution to the care of young men.

The needs of young men in primary care are not always explicitly addressed and there is much that practice nurses can do to meet their additional needs (DH, 2004a). Primary care nurses must ask the question: as professionals do we value young men and boys as members of our society, and if so how can a culture be created in which these people can succeed and achieve their full potential as young men and later as adults? Failure to address their specific needs at this stage of their lives may result in deleterious effects in relation to their future health and well-being. Ensuring that practice nurses are able to meet the needs of young people is critically important. Practice nurses may be the most easily accessible first point of contact a young person has with the health service, and general practice provides valuable opportunities for identifying and acting on behalf of those at risk (Royal College of Nursing (RCN), 2006).

THE YOUNGER MALE

Improving the health of young men and boys is one way of ensuring that in general the health of men improves. It can also begin to address the health inequalities that men throughout their lives may face. The practice nurse needs to formulate health promotion and health education messages that are appropriate and, above all, that will reach the target audience – young men and boys. Nurses must take on board the need to provide services that are tailor-made to meet the requirements of young men, and to encourage them to use those services, expertise must be created that will enable the nurse to work effectively with young men. Activities may need to take place in schools and in places where young men and boys gather and socialize, such as youth groups, taking into account images and the ways in which messages are marketed with the aim to engage these men. Building on what works with young men, and why, may help to attract and encourage men to seek appropriate help early and to talk about what it is that concerns them.

Young men and boys are not an homogeneous group and as such approaches to care must reflect this important consideration. These men come from all spheres of our society. Ethnicity, gender and disability influence individual experiences throughout a person's life. General practice in both rural and urban settings will have patients for whom inequalities in health are both preventable and unfair (DH, 2002). A positive attitude and approach are advocated, offering a provision that seeks to develop emotional and communication skills. The NHS Centre for Reviews and Dissemination (1997) suggests that programmes and interventions that are devised in order to target this group of people must be tailored to the group they are intended to serve. Clustering of risk among young men and boys, which occurs frequently in relation to high-risk activities, may mean that these groups are singled out for specific interventions (British Medical Association (BMA), 2003).

AGE-BASED LEGISLATION

The law recognizes different ages and allows individuals to do different things once they have reached that age. The Children and Young Persons Act 1933, for example, provides that a child aged five years is legally allowed to drink alcohol in private; and, as another example, flying lessons can be taken at any age. At the age of ten a child has full criminal responsibility for their actions and in accordance with the Crime and Disorder Act 1998 can be convicted of a criminal offence. Under the age of four and over the age of 16 years it is legal for a person to enter or live in a brothel (Children and Young Person Act 1933). Table 5.1 (below) provides some legislative issues that are age-related in England.

Table 5.1. Some aspects of age-based legislation in England

Age	Activity	Pertinent legislation
At any age	• Access health records, with exceptions if the content is likely to cause the person or any other person harm	Data Protection Act 1998; Data Protection (Subject Access Modification) (Health) Order 2000
	• Access to education records; however, this can be withdrawn if it is anticipated that this may cause the person or another pupil physical or mental harm	Education (Pupil Information) (England Regulations 2000)
	• Change a name with the consent of every person who has parental responsibility for the young person and if applicable the consent of the person's unmarried father	Children Act 1989
	• Make a complaint if the person feels they have been discriminated against on the basis of race, colour, ethnic or national origin or nationality, sex or marital status	Race Relations Act 1976; Sex Discrimination Act 1984
	• If it is thought that the person is suffering, or at risk of suffering, significant harm and that the person is deemed beyond the control of their parent(s) a care order may be made	Children Act 1989
	• Give evidence in criminal proceedings only if the person understands the questions that are being asked and can give answers to them that will be understood	Youth, Justice and Criminal Evidence Act 1999
	• In some particular circumstances the young person can be made a ward of court until they reach the age of 18 years	Supreme Court Act 1981
10 years	• The person has full criminal responsibility for their actions and could be convicted of a crime	Crime and Disorder Act 1998
	• The young male is deemed capable of committing any sexual offence	Sexual Offences Act 2003

(continued)

Table 5.1. (*Continued*)

Age	Activity	Pertinent legislation
	• Have fingerprints taken with parental consent; have an intimate search carried out without parental consent; have a non-intimate body sample taken if the most senior officer (i.e. superintendent) has reasonable grounds to believe that it will prove or disprove involvement in a recordable offence with parental written consent; have an intimate body sample taken if the superintendent has reasonable grounds to believe that it will prove or disprove involvement in a recordable offence with parental written consent	Police and Criminal Evidence Act 1984; Codes of Practice, 1991
12 years	• If arrested, the person can be kept in police detention and placed in local authority accommodation; this may include secure accommodation if a violent or sexual offence has been committed	Children Act 1960
14 years	• A light-work part-time job may be secured; however, restrictions apply, for example, no more than two hours' work on a school day or Sunday, not allowed to work during school hours, nor can the person work before 0700h or after 1900h. Local authority bylaws may exist	Children and Young Persons Act 1933
	• If convicted of a criminal offence, a maximum fine of £1000 may be imposed	Powers of Criminal Courts (Sentencing) Act 2000
16 years	• The person can enter a bar alone, but can only buy soft drinks	Licensing Act 2003
	• May drink beer, cider or wine with a meal only if accompanied by a person who is aged 18 years or over	Licensing Act 2003
	• Allowed to enter or live in a brothel	Children and Young Persons Act 1933
	• Permitted to hold a licence that allows the person to drive an invalid carriage or a moped, if disabled may also be allowed to hold a licence to drive a car	Road Traffic Act 1988
	• Can work full-time once left school; there are some restrictions, however, on the type of work, for example, unable to work in a casino or betting shop	Education Act 1996

(*continued*)

Table 5.1. (*Continued*)

Age	Activity	Pertinent legislation
	• Can obtain a flight radiotelephony licence for any aircraft	Air Navigation Order 2000
	• Can marry with parental consent; if parental consent is refused, then a court has the power to authorize the marriage	Marriage Act 1949
	• Both males and females may consent to sexual activity involving males and females over 16 years of age	Sexual Offences Act 2003
	• Can buy cigarettes, tobacco and cigarette papers	Children and Young Persons Act 1933
	• Allowed to purchase a knife, knife blade, razor, axe or any other article that has a blade or which is sharply pointed and able to cause injury	Criminal Justice Act 1988
17 years	• Allowed to hold a licence to drive a car, small goods vehicle and an articulated tractor on the road	Road Traffic Act 1988
	• May be subject to police interview or be given a reprimand or warning in the absence of an appropriate adult	Police and Criminal Evidence Act 1984
	• Can purchase any fire arm or ammunition	Fire Arms Act 1968
18 years	• Permitted to buy and drink alcohol in a bar as well as being able to apply for a licence to sell alcohol	Licensing Act 2003
	• Can place a bet and work in a betting office and any other premises where gaming takes place	Gaming Act 1968
	• Will be dealt with in respect to any criminal charges as any adult would be dealt with in the courts	Criminal Justice Act 1991
	• The person has reached the age of majority	Family Reform Act 1969
	• Allowed to vote in both local and general elections	Representation of the People Act 2002
21 years	• Can adopt a child	Adoption and Children Act 2002
	• Can become a Member of Parliament	Parliamentary Elections Act 1695
	• Can become a local counsellor or mayor	Local Government Act 1972

CONSENT, MEDICAL TREATMENT AND EXAMINATION

The issue of consent, medical treatment and the refusal of medical treatment and examination are important aspects of care. This is a complex area of care, and the practice nurse is advised to delve deeper and seek further information and advice if they feel they require clarification on any points of concern. In this section of the chapter a brief overview of key/salient issues is offered.

CONSENT AND MEDICAL TREATMENT

A young person may give consent to surgical, medical or dental treatment; this includes the provision of contraception. The proviso is that the person must be assessed to determine that they have an adequate understanding and intelligence to comprehend fully what is being planned as well as being able to express their own wishes, in this instance the person is said to have capacity to consent. This stipulation emerges from the *Gillick* v. *West Norfolk and Wisbech Area Health Authority* [1985] 2 All ER 402 case. As a result of the Gillick case, the legal position in England and Wales was established. Mrs Victoria Gillick, the mother of a child under 16 years, challenged the decision of the doctor to provide contraception to her child without informing her. The outcome of the case determined that it is legal for those who are less than 16 years of age and fully able to understand what is proposed and its implications are competent to give consent to treatment, regardless of age. The Gillick ruling (known as Fraser competence) means that the consent given cannot be overridden by those with parental responsibility; however, a court has the jurisdiction to overrule this. While the Gillick case was concerned with the provision of contraception, this can be used in other issues regarding consent and competence.

REFUSAL OF TREATMENT

It has already been stated that a young person who is competent can consent to treatment. The young person may also refuse treatment, however; this can be overridden by the person with parental responsibility or a court of law. This is regardless of the young person's ability to demonstrate sufficient understanding. Reversal of the child's decision to refuse treatment is usually done in circumstances where refusal may result in death or permanent disability of the child (see Family Law Reform Act 1969) (Dimond, 2005).

EXAMINATION

Consent to examination follows the same principles associated with Fraser competence (DH, 2001). The proposed examination (medical or psychiatric) of a child can be denied by the parents, who can refuse to let the child be examined. If they refuse, then a court order (directions) may need to be applied for the examination to take place.

Section 54 of the Education Act 1944 contains a general power that allows for children to be examined in school for cleanliness. Medical examinations for any other reason cannot take place without consent.

MENTAL HEALTH ISSUES

Adolescence, according to the Priory Group (2005), is the most tumultuous period of an individual's life. Young men need to learn new social roles. They have to develop new relationships, begin to manage huge physical changes that are occurring to them and start making decisions that will have far-reaching implications for their futures as well as becoming autonomous individuals (RCN, 2004). Adolescence is also seen as an important phase for mental health. Those young men in early adolescence (for example, those aged 11–14 years of age) experience high rates of conduct and emotional disorders. At this stage adult-type depressive disorders begin to make an appearance. The mid- to late-adolescent periods are peak ages for the onset of depressive disorders and schizophrenia as well as other mental disorders (Young Minds, 2002).

The term mental health is problematic as there is no agreed definition. Indeed, Quilgars, Searle and Keung (2005) note that there are several inconsistencies. It is therefore difficult to measure the mental health problems of adolescents. This is further complicated by the fact that the means used to generate data – for example, medical notes – use narrow clinical definitions and only record those people who use the services (BMA, 2003). Practice nurses and other clinical staff often use the term mental disorder and tend to focus on this (Office for National Statistics, 2000). Kurtz (1996) suggests that mental disorders can include:

- emotional disorders such as phobias, anxiety and depression
- conduct disorders
- hyperkinetic disorders such as attention deficit disorder
- developmental disorders
- habit disorders
- eating disorders
- post-traumatic syndromes
- somatic disorders such as chronic fatigue syndrome
- psychotic disorders such as schizophrenia and drug-induced psychosis.

The Royal College of Paediatrics and Child Health (2003) states that young people account for approximately 10–15 % of the UK's total population. They add that this is expected to rise by 8.5 % by the year 2011. The Office for National Statistics (2004) points out that approximately one in ten 5- to 15-year-olds faces handicapping emotional or behavioural problems during the period of time they undertook their survey to gather systematic data on the health of children and young people. Young men who find themselves as children in care, who are homeless and young offenders,

Table 5.2. Those young boys and men who are at high risk of developing mental health problems

- Those who have physical or learning disabilities
- Those who are in care or are care leavers
- Boys who have been excluded from school
- Young men and boys who are in the criminal justice system
- The homeless
- Those who are young carers and, in particular, of a parent with mental illness

(Source: Adapted from Scott, Shaw and Joughlin, 2001)

are especially at high risk of psychiatric disorder (Rutter and Taylor, 2002). It was estimated by Prescott-Clarke and Primatesta (1998) that those boys aged 4–15 years of age were more likely than girls to have conduct and hyperkinetic disorders and peer problems. There are some boys and young men who are known to be at high risk of mental health problems (see Table 5.2).

All primary healthcare providers are encouraged to identify those boys and young men who are at greatest risk and to be attentive of early signs of mental health problems, including emotional problems, which can be less obvious than behavioural difficulties, and to take appropriate action (DH, 2004a). Practice nurses and GPs have a role to play in prevention, early detection and management of mental health problems. It was noted nearly a decade ago that mental health problems often rise as a result of a combination of biological and environmental factors (Acheson, 1998). The practice nurse does not work in isolation and may be required (indeed, is encouraged) to work in partnership with the young man/boy and other agencies, such as social services and education, in order to address fully the needs of the individual (Tamhne, 1997). The nurse is the pivot when issues about the coordination of services are required, ensuring effective working between the various agencies and disciplines, all aiming to address the needs of the patient.

BODY IMAGE AND EATING DISORDERS

The issue of eating disorders often falls under the umbrella term mental health as opposed to nutrition (see, for example, BMA, 2003 and Priory Group, 2005). Much media coverage associated with eating disorders and distorted body image tends to focus on young girls and women. Robinson (2006) points out that most people referred to a specialist eating disorders service are female and make up 90 % of those attending. There is a clear gender bias within the meaning attributed to what are termed eating disorders (Bryant-Jeffries, 2005). It could be suggested that the problem in the male population is overlooked: the lack of recognition that eating disorders in males exist may mean that men may find it difficult to access services. The problem may not be recognized by the practice nurse and as a result the illness may be well established prior to treatment being offered. The first step towards recovery is to acknowledge and recognize that there is a problem.

The recognized gender bias compounds the reporting of an eating disorder, as some men may not possess or be aware of the language required to report and discuss the issues in order to explore it further with the practice nurse (Gillon, 2003). As a result of this very close (yet mistaken) association with eating disorders being solely in the domain of the female, the young man or boy may feel shame and embarrassment and, as a result, reluctance in coming forward for help and advice.

Gillon (2003) suggests that the evidence available regarding anorexia nervosa, bulimia nervosa and compulsive eating points to an increase among males. Practice nurses should be able to recognize the extent to which men and young boys also suffer from eating disorders and provide treatments and services to meet their needs. The Department of Health (2004a) points out that those working in primary care settings should develop the skills in order to recognize inappropriate eating habits, for example, the development of anorexia nervosa and bulimia nervosa, and to make appropriate referrals when specialist input is required.

Most studies related to eating disorders such as anorexia nervosa are based on data that has been obtained from psychiatric care registers or the medical records of patients in hospital (Dhakras, 2005); as a result of this the data must be treated with caution. The real or truer picture of the incidence of eating disorders may be underestimated.

Male eating disorders are illnesses that require treatment and services that will encourage the male to overcome or come to terms with these complex disorders. Gender and sexual orientation are significant factors that affect the incidence and prevalence of eating disorders. The causes of eating disorders (when known) in both males and females have much in common; however, little investigation has been made into the specific treatments and appropriate interventions for men.

Eating disorders are not only about food. They are not only concerned with starving or binge eating, which are often underlying symptoms associated with emotional and psychological disorders (Essex County Council, 1999).

It is difficult to estimate the number of males who have an eating disorder as this will depend on the criteria used to make a diagnosis (Copperman, 2000). Andersen (1999) estimates that the ratio of men to women is 1:6 and 1:20, with approximately 10% of all people with eating disorders being male, which equates to a possible 6000 to 9000 (known) men with an eating disorder in the UK. Most people with eating disorders are female heterosexuals, then gay men, followed by gay women and then heterosexual men (Van Hoeken, Seidell and Wijbrand Hoek, 2005).

Laws (2006) suggests that there are two main forms of eating disorder – anorexia nervosa and bulimia nervosa. There are other types of eating disorders, such as vomiting associated with psychological disturbances, and overeating associated with physiological disturbances (Peate, 2001). Body dysmorphia, also known as reverse anorexia nervosa, is a condition that primarily occurs in men and relates to a feeling that their muscles will never be large enough. Fairburn and Harrison (2003) add

Table 5.3. Risk factors associated with men and the development of problematic eating

- Being overweight as a child
- Being involved in professions where size and shape matter
- Participating in sporting activities where there is a need for the person to be lean
- A greater expectation of thin bodies within homosexual communities

(Source: Adapted from Bryant-Jeffries, 2005)

binge eating to Laws' (2006) main forms of eating disorders. Compulsive overeating or binging is found in approximately over 25 % of obese men in their 30s and 40s; impulsive eating occurs when the man goes beyond the point at which he feels full (Bryant-Jeffries, 2005).

It has already been noted in this chapter that there are risk factors associated with the development of mental illness (see, for example, Scott, Shaw and Joughlin, 2001). The risk factors can be compared with those described by Bryant-Jeffries (2005) (see Table 5.3) for men and the development of problematic eating patterns.

ANOREXIA NERVOSA

The Eating Disorders Association (2006) states that the translation of 'anorexia nervosa' is *loss of appetite due to nervousness*. Commonly, eating disorders occur during the boy's school years and this may be as a result of being called names for being overweight.

Self-starvation and compulsive exercising are key features in anorexia nervosa. They are undertaken as a result of a fear of becoming fat. The person may also hold the belief that they are overweight – a feeling known as body image distortion, when in fact they are normal in weight or underweight. Norman and Ryrie (2004) summarize some of the common features of anorexia nervosa:

- low bodyweight, that is, a body mass index (BMI) score of 17.5 $(\text{kg}\,\text{m}^2)$ or less, or 15 % or more lower than expected for age and height;
- self-induced weight loss – avoidance of 'fattening' foods, vomiting, purging, excessive exercise, use of appetite suppressants;
- body image distortion – fear of fatness, overvalued ideas, imposed low weight threshold;
- men often report a gradual loss of libido due to lowering of their testosterone.

BULIMIA NERVOSA

Bryant-Jeffries (2005) suggests that bulimia nervosa is the most common eating disorder; he states that the illness is often driven by a psychological need to numb pain or depression. It should be noted that while data demonstrates that women show higher levels of depression than men, Luck, Bamford and Williamson (2000) state that depression in men may be masked by alcohol and therefore the incidence of anorexia bulimia (as with other eating disorders) may be underestimated.

Barker (2003) suggests that the individual in cases of bulimia nervosa eats large amounts of food over a short period of time. Having eaten the food he then attempts to rid the body of it by purging – using laxatives, vomiting and over exercising. Chelvanayagam (2006) summarizes some of the features associated with bulimia nervosa. For a person to be diagnosed with bulimia nervosa they usually have the following features:

- persistent preoccupation with eating;
- irresistible craving for food;
- episodes of overeating;
- attempts to counter effects of food – self-induced vomiting, abuse of purgatives (laxatives and diuretics), periods of starvation, use of drugs, for example, appetite suppressants;
- morbid fear of fatness with imposed low weight threshold.

All eating disorders can have a detrimental effect on a young man's or a boy's physical, psychological and social functioning; this often extends to family and friends. If left untreated, the outcome can lead to malnutrition and unnecessary deaths.

ADOLESCENT SEXUAL HEALTH

In the adolescent years it is normal for young men and boys to develop relationships; these are the types of relationship where the boy or young man feels he has been 'swept off his feet'. In healthy relationships of this kind it is important that the individuals involved feel safe, respected and cared about. Young people have the right to enjoy a safe and satisfying sexuality (World Health Organizaton, 2005). For most young people evidence suggests that those who have engaged in sexual intercourse have found it enjoyable, have used protection and have had one partner as part of a steady relationship (West and Sweeting, 2003).

Pressure is often exerted on younger men (by peers, the media and other adults) to be sexually active (Burrack, 1999) and younger people are living in a highly sexualized world, but there appears to be little support available to help them deal with the pressures exerted on them. Often boys turn to alcohol to help them cope and sometimes the alcohol makes them more vulnerable (Childline, 2006). Alcohol is a major factor associated with decision-making and teenage sexual activity.

There are other chapters in this text that specifically address issues related to sexual health (for example, Chapter 6 on issues concerning contraception) and

Chapter 7 addresses sexually transmitted infections (STIs) and the male population. The following section of this chapter provides highlights regarding sexual health and the younger male.

Guidance is lacking for young males on how to make sensible decisions concerning important issues and choices such as sex, alcohol and drugs, according to Childline (2006). The Royal College of Nursing (2006) is of the opinion that it is the school nurse who is ideally placed to provide sexual health and contraceptive advice to young people because of their relationship with this group of the population. Practice nurses, it is suggested, are also in a unique position to raise the issue of sexual health and contraception with younger patients as a result of their privileged relationship with the community as a whole. The school nurse and practice nurse, with other members of the multidisciplinary team (i.e. family planning and sexual health nurses) as well as the school, are encouraged to work as a team in order to assess, supply contraception and condoms, encourage follow-up and to provide onward referral to other appropriate agencies (RCN, 2006; Office for Standards in Education (OFSTED), 2002).

Some elements of the law regarding the younger male have been discussed above. The Sexually Offences Act (2003) provides for the practice nurse when working with young people to offer them confidential advice (and where appropriate) treatment. When parental consent has not been gained the nurse must continue to asses the young person's competence on a case-by-case basis, using the framework and guidance provided under the auspices of the Fraser guidance. Separate legislation may apply to Northern Ireland and Scotland (RCN, 2006) regarding this; the Nursing and Midwifery Council's (NMC; 2004) code of professional conduct applies to all nurses, midwives and specialist community public health nurses in all four countries of the UK. The DH (2004b) provides best-practice guidance for nurses regarding the provision of advice and treatment to young people on contraception, sexual and reproductive health.

The National Survey of Sexual Attitudes and Lifestyles (NATSAL) (2000) reports that, in over 11 000 participants aged between 16 and 44 years, those aged between 16 and 19 years reported first intercourse at younger than 16 years, 30 % for male respondents and 26 % for females. STIs are associated with significant sexual ill health and often the young person may be reluctant to seek help and advice because of the nature of acquisition. Initial symptoms maybe asymptomatic. If left untreated, STIs may go on to cause serious sequelae for both sexes (Simms and Stephenson, 2000). Risky sexual behaviour places individuals at an increased risk of acquiring an STI and an unwanted pregnancy. Behaviours such as unprotected sexual intercourse and high rates of sexual partners increase the risk.

Certain population groups are more likely to engage in risk-taking activity. The Department for Education and Skills (DfES) (2004) suggests that those young people from particular backgrounds or those who have experienced certain significant life events are at risk of having a teenage pregnancy/becoming a teenage parent (see Table 5.4 below).

Table 5.4. Risk factors associated with teenage pregnancy

Sociodemographic factors
- Low income and deprivation
- Those who fail to achieve educationally
- Those who have not experienced education
- Being unmarried
- Being in care
- Involvement in crime
- Ethnicity (i.e. high rates of pregnancy among African Caribbean, Bangladeshi and Pakistani populations)
- Young age at first intercourse
- History of sexual abuse
- Mental health problems
- Smoking
- Poor nutrition

Cognitive factors
- Low expectation/fatalism
- Experimental behaviour
- Cognitive immaturity
- Poor skills base
- Poor knowledge/lack of sex education
- Poor self-esteem

Family factors
- Divorced parents
- Poor parent–child communication

Cultural factors
- Cultural openness
- Peer influence
- Religious influences

(Source: Social Exclusion Unit, 1999; NHS Centre for Reviews and Dissemination, 1997; Chambers, Wakely and Chambers, 2001; Seamark and Pereria-Gray, 1997)

ADVICE ABOUT SEXUAL HEALTH FOR YOUNG PEOPLE

Advising young people about sexual health may include offering support and providing information for them in order to make an informed decision. Young men and boys should be provided with clear and consistent support regarding sex and relationships. For the practice nurse to do this effectively, s/he should allocate time for this important activity. Some young people have reported that they feel rushed and they do not have the time to ask questions (French, 2002). The consultation or advice-giving session may address issues related to the emotional and physical

Table 5.5. Issues the nurse may consider when providing or designing information for young people

---

- Oral information should be supplemented by written information
- Small amounts of information should be provided at any one time in order to improve retention; too much information can be overwhelming
- Some young people may benefit or prefer more technical information supported by statistical data

---

(Source: Free, 2005; Kane, Macdowall and Wellings, 2003)

implications of sexual activity and relationships, the risk of pregnancy and STIs. There should be no coercion or abuse and a mutual agreement to undertake the consultation must have been reached.

During the consultation, the nurse should address the benefits of telling his parents and if appropriate the GP. Explanations provided should inform the young person of other services that may be available, that is, counselling services or other support networks. Wellings *et al.* (2001) highlight the fact that none of the above will diminish the importance of parents talking with their own child about sex and sexual health.

Effective communication skills are key attributes that the nurse needs to possess in order to help young men and boys with issues regarding sexual health and STIs. Free *et al.* (2002) advocate that a non-judgemental approach is used in order to encourage younger people to take up any services on offer. Some young people have reported (Kane, Macdowall and Wellings, 2003) that they feel that healthcare professionals often assume (erroneously) that they have or possess knowledge relating to sexual health and they underestimate the need for more information. Kane, Macdowall and Wellings (2003) note that young people would value most information that is presented in materials specifically produced and designed for them. Young people's information needs differ from other members of the population, and the nurse needs to pitch the information provided at the right level with the appropriate quantity (Free, 2005). Table 5.5 outlines some issues to be considered when designing or providing information for young people (see also Table 5.6 below).

USING RESOURCES

Brown (2001) suggests that, regardless of the practice nurse's experience, s/he may find that working with young men will often push you to the limits of both your patience and skills. He states that any tool that may help to enhance and improve communication with young men should be welcomed; developing and implementing appropriate and effective resources can be a time-consuming activity and thought must be given to the availability of both human and material resources.

Table 5.6. Some points to be taken into consideration in order to make the general practice setting teenage-friendly

- Ensure confidentiality
- Make sure that practice advice is directed towards young men and boys
- Organize a practice meeting with the whole team to discuss how you can all make your practice more teenager-friendly
- Provide education for members of the practice in relation to young men and boys
- Audit the 10- to 18-year-old males in your practice
- Let young men and boys know what your practice provides
- Consider running a 'young person's clinic' or 'young men and boys clinic' in your practice or with other practices
- Involve parents
- Make sexual health and contraceptive services in your practice teenage-friendly
- Offer advice to young men and boys as well as young women and girls for teenagers who become pregnant

(Source: Adapted from Royal College of General Practitioners and Royal College of Nursing, 2002)

The choice of appropriate resources is vital and there are many to choose from, for example:

- books
- magazines
- pod casts
- SMS text messages
- videos
- DVDs
- games
- posters.

Remember that the most important resource is you.

The overall aim and purpose of the activity has to be clearly articulated to all parties involved in the developmental stage. This will provide guidance and direction. It is important to consider the audience. For example, if the practice nurse (together with other agencies if appropriate) is preparing a poster to encourage young men to testicular self-examine and the target group are a group of young Asian men, then this must be depicted in the materials being used. Failure to do this will lead to disenfranchisement. The target audience must be clearly identified. The language used must also be given very careful consideration: aim for a balance between the language the audience is familiar with – slang and street talk – on the one hand and the language you would normally use on the other hand. Consider also regional variations (i.e. accents) as well as cultural differences – yours and theirs. Brown (2001) advises that time is taken to allow for adequate preparation of the resource, in order to increase the man's understanding, as well as ensuring the information-giving event takes place where the target audience is likely to congregate, for example, the mosque, synagogue, sports clubs, music venues, young offenders' institutions.

Evaluating the effectiveness of nursing care is required for developing a sound knowledge base to guide nursing practice. There has been an increase in the emphasis on evaluation and evidence-based practice in healthcare (Swage, 2004; Donaldson, 2004). This is also applicable when the nurse has provided resources that have been used to engage young men in health-promoting activities. Evaluation of care provided is the final stage of the nursing process, and this occurs after monitoring and measuring the effects of nursing interventions. The nurse, in conjunction with the patient, modifies the care delivered. A similar approach can be adapted when evaluating interventions that have been provided to engage men in relation to their health and well-being. The Health Development Agency (2002) has produced detailed descriptions of 12 established projects that have worked and the reasons why these interventions have been successful.

PROVIDING A USER-FRIENDLY SERVICE FOR YOUNG MEN AND BOYS

The Royal College of General Practitioners (RCGP) and the RCN outline points to be taken into consideration (RCGP and RCN, 2002; RCGP, 2002; RCN, 2006) in order to make the general practice more teenage-friendly (see Table 5.6 above).

CONCLUSION

The health and well-being of boys and young men must be taken seriously by practice nurses and other healthcare professionals. Improving the health of young men and boys is one way of making certain that the health of men in general improves. Acknowledging that this group of the population at a young age has specific needs can begin to address the inequalities that men face throughout their life. Creating a culture in which young men can succeed and achieve their full potential demonstrates that they are valued as members of our society.

The *Vienna Declaration on the Health of Men and Boys in Europe* (European Men Health Forum, 2005) ratified the first ever men's health declaration. The contents of the declaration are a good starting point for those practice nurses who are aiming to provide high-quality, inclusive services to young men and boys. The declaration seeks to provide a clear reference for all involved in male health improvement:

• Recognize men's health as a distinct and important issue.
• Develop a better understanding of male attitudes towards health.
• Invest in 'male sensitive' approaches to providing healthcare.

- Initiate work on health for boys and young men at schools and community settings.
- Develop coordinated health and social policies that promote men's health.

There is a growing body of evidence that demonstrates that the ways in which some boys and young men behave are as a result of pressures put on them by society and their peers. These pressures can have an undesirable effect, and the socialization process can impact on men's health in many ways. The stereotypical images nurses and other healthcare professionals have, their attitudes and skills, can also have an adverse effect on the individual's health and well-being.

Young men and boys are often involved in risk-taking activities; these are wide-ranging and include issues relating to diet, mental health and sexual health. Gender features as a major factor in all of these areas.

The number of cases of anorexia/bulimia nervosa in young men and boys is significant and the factors associated with eating orders must be given consideration in order to address the needs of those patients. The negative attitudes of healthcare professionals towards those with an eating disorder can be a barrier to those men seeking help and receiving appropriate care and treatment. Risky sexual health behaviour and the reasons why some young men and boys engage in it is complex. It must be noted that only a small number of young men engage in risky sexual behaviour with a high number of female partners. For a number of young men their ability to express their emotions is problematic and they sometimes fail to do this effectively. This has significant implications for the individual's mental health and well-being. The often heard phrase 'boys will be boys' is a gross generalization of a group that is varied and diverse in nature and behaviour. Young men and boys express their physical and emotional needs in many ways.

The practice nurse must seek out new ways of providing services that are responsive to the needs of this often ignored population – young men and boys. The way the practice welcomes younger males and the resources used to engage these people need consideration. Initiatives must include a range of activities that take into account the all-important issue of gender.

REFERENCES

Acheson, D. (1998) *Independent Inquiry into Inequalities in Health Report*, The Stationery Office, London.

Andersen, A.E. (1999) The diagnosis and treatment of eating disorders in primary care medicine. In (eds P.S. Mehler and A.E. Andersen) *A Guide to Medical Care and Complications: Eating Disorders*, John Hopkins University Press, Baltimore, pp. 1–26, Chapter 1.

Barker, P. (2003) *Psychiatric and Mental Health Nursing: The Craft of Caring*, Hodder, London.

British Medical Association (2003) *Adolescent Health*, BMA, London.

Brown, P. (2001) Developing resources. In (eds N. Davidson and T. Lloyd) *Promoting Men's Health: A Guide for Practitioners*, Bailliere Tindall, London, pp. 89–96, Chapter 7.

Bryant-Jeffries, R. (2005) *Counselling for Eating Disorders in Men: Person Centred Dialogues*, Radcliffe, Oxford.

Burrack, R. (1999) Teenage sexual behaviour: attitudes towards and declared sexual activity. *The British Journal of Family Planning*, **24**, 145–148.

Chambers, R., Wakely, G. and Chambers S. (2001) *Tackling Teenage Pregnancy*, Radcliffe Medical Press, Oxford.

Chelvanayagam, S. (2006) (eds I. Peate and S. Chelvanayagam) *Caring for Adults with Mental Health Problems*, John Wiley & Sons Ltd, Chichester, pp. 117–129, Chapter 8.

Childline (2006) *Casenotes: Alcohol and Teenage Sexual Activity*, NSPCC, London.

Copperman, J. (2000) *Eating Disorders in the UK: Review of the Provision of Health Care Services for Men with Eating Disorders*, Eating Disorder Association, Norwich.

Department of Health (2001) *Twelve Key Points on Consent: the Law in England*, DH, London.

Department of Health (2002) *Addressing Inequalities – Reaching the Hard-to-Reach Groups*, DH, London.

Department of Health (2003) *Liberating the Public Health Talents of Community Practitioners and Health Visitors*, DH, London.

Department of Health (2004a) *Primary Care Version, National Service Framework for Children, Young People and Maternity Services*, DH, London.

Department of Health (2004b) *Best Practice Guidance for Doctors and Other Health Professionals on the Provision of Advice and Treatment of Young People Under 16 on Contraception, Sexual and Reproductive Health*, DH, London.

Department for Education and Skills (2004) *Enabling Young People to Access Contraceptive and Sexual Health Information and Advice: Legal and Policy Framework for Social Workers, Residential Social Workers, Foster Carers and Other Social Care Practitioners*, DfES, Nottingham.

Dhakras, S. (2005) Anorexia nervosa (eds M. Cooper, C. Hooper and M. Thompson) *Child and Adolescent Health: Theory and Practice*, Hodder Arnold, London, pp. 156–164, Chapter 5.

Dimond, B. (2005) *Legal Aspects of Nursing*, 4th edn, Pearson Longman, Harlow.

Donaldson, L. (2004) Clinical governance: a quality concept (eds T. van Zwanenberg and J. Harrison) *Clinical Governance in Primary Care*, 2nd edn, Radcliffe Medical Press, Oxford, pp. 3–16, Chapter 1.

Eating Disorder Association (2006) *What is an Eating Disorder?*, EDA, Norwich.

Essex County Council (1999) *North Essex Mental Health Strategy*, Essex County Council, Colchester.

European Men's Health Forum (2005) *Vienna Declaration on the Health of Men and Boys in Europe*, EMHF, Brussels.

Fairburn, C.G. and Harrison, P. J. (2003) Eating disorders. *The Lancet*, **361**, 407–416.

Free, C., Dawe, A., Masey, S. and Mawer, C. (2002) Young women's accounts of the factors influencing their use and non use of emergency contraception: an in-depth interview study. *British Medical Journal*, **325**, 1393–1396.

Free, C. (2005) Advice about sexual health for young people. *British Medical Journal*, **330**, 107–108.

French, R. (2002) The experience of young people with contraceptive consultations and health care workers. *International Journal of Adolescent Medicine and Health*, **14** (2), 131–138.

Gillon, E. (2003) Can men talk about problems with weight? The therapeutic implications of a discourse analytic study. *Counselling and Psychotherapy Research*, **3** (1), 25–32.

Health Development Agency (2002) *Boys and Young Men's Health – What Works*, HAD, London.

Kane, R., Macdowall, W. and Wellings, K. (2003) Providing information for young people in sexual health clinics: getting it right. *Journal of Family Planning and Reproductive Health Care*, **29**, 141–145.

Kurtz, Z. (1996) *Treating Children Well*, Mental Health Foundation, London.

Laws, T. (2006) *A Handbook of Men's Health*, Elsevier, Edinburgh.

Luck, M., Bamford, M. and Williamson, P. (2000) *Men's Health: Perspectives, Diversity and Paradox*, Blackwell, Oxford.

National Survey of Sexual Attitudes and Lifestyles (2000) *National Survey of Sexual Attitudes and Lifestyles I and II: 2000–2001*, University of Essex, Colchester.

NHS Centre for Reviews and Dissemination (1997) Preventing and Reducing the Adverse Effects of Unintended Teenage Pregnancies. *Effective Health Care*, **3**, 1–12.

Norman, I. and Ryrie, I. (2004) *The Art and Science of Mental Health Nursing: A Textbook of Principles and Practice*, Open University Press, Buckingham.

Nursing and Midwifery Council (2004) *The NMC Code of Professional Conduct: Standards for Conduct Performance and Ethics*, NMC, London.

Office for National Statistics (2000) *The Mental Health of Children and Adolescents in Great Britain: A Summary Report*, ONS, London.

Office for National Statistics (2004) *The Health of Children and Young Children: Mental Health*, ONS, London.

Office for Standards in Education (2002) *Sex and Relationships: A Report from the Office of Her Majesty's Chief Inspector of Schools*, OFSTED, London.

Peate, I. (2001) Male Eating Disorders. *Practice Nursing*, **12** (3), 116–118.

Prescott-Clarke, P. and Primatesta, P. (1998) *Health Survey for England: The Health of Young People 95–97*, The Stationery Office, London.

Priory Group (2005) *Adolescent Angst*, Priory Group, Leatherhead.

Quilgars, D., Searle, B. and Keung, A. (2005) Mental health and well-being. In (eds J. Bradshaw and E. Mayhew) *The Well-being of Children in the UK*, 2nd edn, University of York, York, pp. 134–160, Chapter 6.

Robinson, P.H. (2006) *Community Treatment of Eating Disorders*, John Wiley & Sons Ltd, Chichester.

Royal College of General Practitioners and Royal College of Nursing (2002) *Getting it Right for Teenagers in Your Practice*, RCGP and RCN, London.

Royal College of Nursing (2004) *Adolescent Transition Care: Guidance for Nursing Staff*, RCN, London.

Royal College of Nursing (2006) *Getting it Right for Children and Young People: A Self Assessment Tool for Practice Nurses*, RCN, London.

Royal College of Paediatrics and Child Health (2003) *The Intercollegiate Working Party on Adolescent Health, Bridging the Gaps: Health Care for Adolescents*, RCPCH, London.

Rutter, M. and Taylor, E. (2002) *Child and Adolescent Psychiatry*, 4th edn, Blackwell, Oxford.

Scott, A., Shaw, M. and Joughlin, C. (2001) *Finding the Evidence: A Gateway to the Literature in Child and Adolescent Mental Health*, Royal College of Psychiatrists, London.

Seamark, C.J. and Pereria-Gray, D.J. (1997) Like mother, like daughter: a general practice survey of maternal influences on teenage pregnancy. *British Journal of General Practice*, **47** (416), 175–176.

Simms, I. and Stephenson, J.M. (2000) Pelvic Inflammatory Disease Epidemiology: What Do We Know and What Do We Need to Know? *Sexually Transmitted Infections*, **76**, 80–87.

Social Exclusion Unit (1999) *Teenage Pregnancy: A Report from the Social Exclusion Unit*, The Stationery Office, London.

Swage, T. (2004) *Clinical Governance in Health Care Practice*, 2nd edn, Butterworth-Heinemann, Edinburgh.

Tamhne, R.C. (1997) Who Is Responsible for Child Mental Health? *British Medical Journal*, **315**, 310–311.

Van Hoeken, D., Seidell, J. and Wijbrand Hoek, H. (2005) Epidemiology. In (eds J. Treasure, U. Schmidt and E. Van Furth) *The Essential Handbook of Eating Disorders*, John Wiley & Sons Ltd, Chichester, 11–34, Chapter 2.

Wellings, K., Nanchahal, K., Macdowall, W. *et al.* (2001) Sexual behaviour in Britain: early heterosexual experience. *Lancet*, **358** (9296), 1845–1840.

West, P. and Sweeting, H. (2003) *A Review of Young People's Health and Health Behaviours in Scotland*, Medical Research Council Social Public Health Sciences Unit Occupational Paper No. 10, Glasgow.

World Health Organization (2005) *Sexually Transmitted Infections among Adolescents: The Need for Adequate Health Services*, WHO, Geneva.

Young Minds (2002) *Mental Health Services for Adolescents and Young Adults*, Young Minds, London.

6 Contraception

Young men are half the problem and half the solution (Social Exclusion Unit, 1999)

INTRODUCTION

The Family Planning Association (FPA) (2006a) believes that it is a fundamental right of all men and women to have access to a full choice of contraceptives. This also includes providing them with the information they will require to make an informed choice. Currently, men are often forgotten or ignored when the issue of contraception is discussed, with the burden of family planning falling on women. Men must become more involved in family planning and with the family planning services if this inequitable position is to be rectified. The Department of Health (DH; 2001) provides details of service specifications in relation to the national sexual health and HIV strategy. Issues relating to contraception are within these service specifications (see Table 6.1 below). Chapter 7 discusses sexual health and sexually transmitted infections further.

For contraceptive services to work successfully the practice nurse (and all those involved in family planning) should consider providing services that concentrate on both genders, locally, nationally and internationally. Concerns can be addressed through school and other health service systems with reinforcement through public health education campaigns. A gendered approach is vital if men are to be seen as central to the issues surrounding the reproductive health of the nation as opposed to mere accessories to it.

PROVISION OF CONTRACEPTIVE SERVICES

The main providers of NHS contraceptive services in England are primarily GPs and family planning clinics. Services are also provided by other agencies and voluntary organizations as well as the independent sector. The only detailed data regarding services is from NHS family planning clinics and Brook Advisory Centres. Limited data from general practice and an analysis of NHS prescriptions is becoming available (Health and Special Care Information Centre (HSCIC), 2004). The HSCIC (2004) points out that in England in 2003–2004:

- there were approximately 2.7 million attendances at family planning clinics;
- the number of women attending was estimated at 1.2 million;
- male attenders totalled 106 000;

Table 6.1. Service specifications for levels 1, 2 and 3 – the sexual health strategy

---

Level 1

- Sexual history-taking and risk assessment
- STI testing for women
- HIV testing and counselling
- Pregnancy testing and referral
- Contraceptive information and services
- Assessment and referral of men with STI symptoms
- Cervical cytology screening and referral
- Hepatitis B immunization

Level 2

- Intrauterine device insertion
- Testing and treatment for STIs
- Partner notification
- Invasive STI testing for men (until non-invasive tests are available)
- Vasectomy
- Contraceptive implant insertion

Level 3

- Specialized HIV treatment and care
- Highly specialized contraception
- Specialized infection management, including partner notification
- Outreach contraceptive services
- Outreach for STI prevention
- Special responsibility for service need assessment
- Special responsibility for supporting provider quality and meeting clinical governance requirements

---

(Source: DH, 2001)

- the most common form of primary contraception was oral contraception, accounting for 41 % of clinic attendees;
- the male condom was used by 35 % of attendees.

The number of men attending clinics is a very small percentage of the total number of those attending. In 2003–2004 the number of men opting for vasectomy as a method of contraception was estimated to be approximately 9000; this number has fallen from 21 % in 1993–1994 to about 8 % for 2003–2004 (HSCIC, 2004). Men are more likely than women to have been sterilized for contraceptive purposes. The numbers of male vasectomies increase with the age of the man (Office for National Statistics, 2005).

Contraceptive service provision presents the practice nurse with an opportunity to raise many other health-related issues with the patient. A full health assessment will need to be undertaken and during the consultation a discussion related to sexual health can also occur (Chapter 7 outlines sexual health history-taking). It has been estimated that between 5000 and 10000 cases of people need *in vitro* fertilization treatment because they have had chlamydia in the past (Men's Health Forum, 2006). A sensitive and tactful approach is advocated, one that respects diversity, for example, of language differences, religious beliefs, an individual's special needs and cultural differences.

CONTRACEPTION

It is clear that the practice nurse and other members of the primary care team have a central role to play in the provision of contraceptive services. Practice nurses can offer patients good advice as they often know the individual's circumstances and have access to their health records. The practice nurse is also well placed to provide follow-up and continuity of care. Hannaford (2006) provides a model of good practice for contraceptive services in primary care (see Table 6.2).

The suggestions above can be applied for both men and women who come to the practice to seek advice and treatment. The key aims are to provide the man (and partner if appropriate) with information in an unhurried manner that can help him make the best decision. No one choice of contraception is suitable for every man, and no ideal method exists, Wakely and Chambers (2002) note also that all methods fail – some more than others. The decision as to what type of contraception is appropriate for the individual will centre on a variety of issues, for example:

- method of effectiveness
- perceived safety

Table 6.2. Issues that may be considered when providing contraceptive services in the general practice

---

- Easy access to the practice and the services offered with a guarantee of patient confidentiality
- An unhurried consultation with a knowledgeable practice nurse
- The provision of comprehensive information that has been tailored to meet the needs of each individual or couple, in order to ensure that an informed choice can be made
- The provision of a full range of contraceptive methods (this may require liaison with outside agencies)
- Appropriate assessment before and monitoring during the use of the chosen method of contraception (if appropriate) in an attempt to minimize any real or perceived adverse effects
- Provision of supplementary up-to-date written information for future reference regarding the correct use of the chosen method
- Information about who to contact if problems or concerns arise
- Consideration of other aspects of sexual health
- An opportunity to review the chosen methods of contraception, ensuring that it remains the most appropriate
- Full use of the various skills and resources of the whole practice including doctors

---

(Source: Adapted from Hannaford, 2006)

- known contraindications
- acceptability
- ease of use
- availability.

Hughes (2004) notes that decisions that are made with respect to contraception are based on several factors and can include:

- age
- health
- relationships
- career stage
- financial stability
- lifestyle
- religion
- ethnicity
- perceptions
- anxieties
- embarrassment
- decisions about having children.

It is important that the practice nurse is aware of and understands the way in which the chosen method of contraception operates and is able to teach and advise the patient about how to use the method and where to go to for help and advice should the need arise.

There are six contraceptive methods or groupings, see Table 6.3 (below).

Much research is currently being undertaken in attempting to devise new methods of contraception and to improve on current methods. Historically hormonal contraceptive methods have sat within the female domain; there is, however, a growing interest in the use of approaches focusing on the male. Anderson (2004) points out that the male reproductive system has the potential to provide new hormonal contraceptive methods.

SPERMATOGENESIS

Men, unlike their female counterparts, produce millions of mature gametes daily. Production is continuous; the male begins sperm production during puberty and this continues throughout his life. It has been suggested that the two testes produce over 100 million sperm per day (Hubbard and Mechan, 1997). This section of the chapter provides a brief overview of sperm production – spermatogenesis.

The process of spermatogenesis takes approximately 75 days and results in the production of ejaculated spermatozoa with 23 chromosomes. The process is complex and requires careful regulation; for example, sperm production and survival are dependent upon a constant temperature of around 4 to 7 °C less than the core body

Table 6.3. Six methods of contraception

Hormonal methods
- Combined contraceptive pill (COC)
- Progesterone only pill (POP)
- Injectable hormones
- Hormone implants
- Intrauterine systems (IUS)

Mechanical methods
- Intrauterine contraceptive device (IUD)

Barrier methods
- Diaphragm
- Caps with spermacides
- Sponges
- Male and female condoms

Natural methods
- Fertility devices (persona)
- Coitus interruptus
- Calendar method
- Temperature method
- Cervical mucus method
- Sympto-thermal/multiple index method

Permanent methods
- Male and female sterilization

Emergency methods
- Hormonal
- Post-coital IUD

(Source: Adapted from Hannaford, 2006; Hughes, 2004)

temperature, and this is the reason why the testes are situated in the scrotal sac. The skin on the scrotal sac is thin; therefore heat is easily lost into the surrounding environment when needed.

There are three main phases associated with spermatogenesis:

- proliferation – spermatogonia
- meiosis – spermatocytes
- differentiation – spermatids.

PROLIFERATION – SPERMATOGONIA

Spermatogenesis takes place in the seminiferous tubules of the testes. The process is begun in the basement membrane of each tubule; the primitive stem cells are known as spermatogonia. Spermatogonia are diploid with 46 chromosomes. The cells divide rapidly by meiosis, building up the stem cell line. The spermatogonia differentiate into spermatocytes.

MEIOSIS – SPERMATOCYTES

The matured spermatogonia move away from the basement membrane. Cell division occurs again and primary spermatocytes are formed which are haploid with 23 chromosomes. During this process the cells move closer to the lumen of the seminiferous tubule. The spermatocytes become four spermatids.

DIFFERENTIATION – SPERMATIDS

The spermatids are located immediately adjacent to the lumen of seminiferous tubules. Differentiation occurs at this stage and the spermatids become spermatozoa, each of which contains 23 chromosomes.

The development of spermatids into spermatozoa (sperm) is dependent upon the presence of Sertoli cells; these cells are present in the seminiferous tubules. The spermatids attach themselves to the Sertoli cells; Sertoli cells provide nutrients as well as hormonal signals that will eventually produce developed sperm.

The mature sperm migrate from the seminiferous tubules to the epididymis; in the epididymis the sperm grow and develop and become fertile. The sperm do not become fully motile until they are ejaculated and activated by bio-chemicals in semen and the female reproductive tract. Each sperm consists of:

- a head with acrosome at its tip and a haploid set of chromosomes in a compact and inactive state;
- a mid-piece containing mitochondria and a centriole;
- a tail for motility.

The head of the sperm contains the DNA, the genetic material, and is essential to the nucleus of the spermatid. When the sperm comes into close contact with an egg, the membrane of the acrosome (a helmet-like structure) breaks down, releasing enzymes that aid sperm to penetrate the egg. Mitochondria are wrapped tightly around the mid-piece centrioles providing ATP (adenosine triphosphate) that allow the sperm to use whiplike movements in order to move. See Figure 6.1 below.

CONDOMS

Anderson (2004) suggests that at some point in a man's life he will use a condom; condoms are widely used throughout the world. The use of condoms dates back to 1550 BC in Egypt; they are used internationally as a method of contraception more than any other method (Martin *et al.*, 2000). As a method of contraception, condoms are not foolproof; however, with correct use pregnancy rates as low as 3 % have been

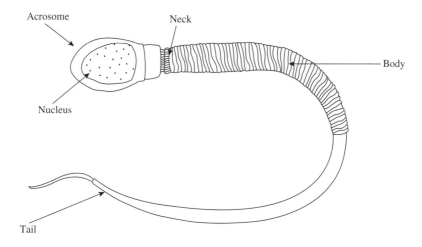

Figure 6.1. The structure of a sperm

reported, with a national trend reflecting approximately 14% in the first year (Fu *et al.*, 1999).

Not all general practices provide condoms; it is, however, important that the practice nurse knows where the patient can obtain condoms free of charge, if they are not available at the practice, for example, family planning clinics and genitourinary medicine clinics. The practice nurse must feel comfortable with discussing condom use and be prepared to suggest ways to the patient as to how he may incorporate their use into lovemaking (Chambers, Wakely and Chambers, 2000).

There has been an increase in the use of condoms nationally and internationally over the last 20 years in an attempt to reduce the incidence of HIV. In making attempts to reduce the incidence of HIV through condom use other potential STIs can also be diminished (Matthews and Ireson, 2006); however, the impact will only be successful if the condom is used correctly. The practice nurse has a vital role to play in enabling the patient to use condoms effectively, the nurse may need to provide the patient with information regarding choice of condom, why condoms may fail and where to go to seek help if this does occur (FPA, 2006b).

The correct choice of condom is vital. Personal choice is an important issue that is given consideration by both males and females. Some types of materials used in condom manufacture have many advantages, for example, enhancing sensation; however, the use of polyurethane in condoms has shown an increased slippage and breakage rate (Frezieres *et al.*, 1998).

Evidence has emerged in a randomized trial demonstrating that synthetic condoms are preferred by two-thirds of males and females (Frezieres and Walsh, 2000). Most male condoms are usually made of latex and are available with a spermicidal preparation as lubricant, which is often nonoxynol-9. Other types of lubricant are used for those who may have skin sensitivities. Figure 6.2 provides details regarding the use of a condom.

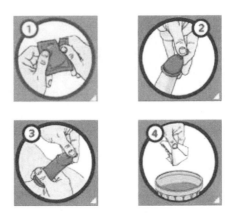

Figure 6.2. How to use a condom (Reproduced by permission of SSL International plc)

PREVENTING CONDOM FAILURE

Condom failure is complex and there are many reasons why condoms fail. Some reasons for condom failure are:

- the type of condom used
- size of condom
- inexperience of user
- anal/vaginal dryness
- excess use of lubrication
- incorrect type of lubrication
- practical difficulties with use, that is, poor manual dexterity and poor eyesight.

The condom should be rolled onto the erect penis prior to the beginning of any genital contact and removed only when all genital contact has ended. When the condom is being removed, it is important to avoid any leakage of ejaculate. The penis should be removed while still erect; leakage of semen can occur if the penis becomes detumescent after ejaculation.

Condoms should only be lubricated with a water-soluble lubricant, for example, Aquagel or KY jelly. The patient should be advised never to use oil-based products as these products will have an adverse effect on the integrity of latex condoms. A list of oil-based products that affect the efficacy of the condom is provided in Table 6.4 (below).

Condoms come in a variety of shapes and sizes and some have a reservoir tip. They can be plain and a number have a ribbed texture that is said to increase sensitivity. They come in a variety of colours and some are flavoured, which should only be used for oral sex. Condom manufacturers produce condoms of differing lengths and widths; most condoms will stretch and fit the length of most penises; the man, therefore, is encouraged to choose the condom that suits him best.

Table 6.4. Some oil-based products that can have an adverse effect on the efficacy of the condom

• Arachis oil	• Low-fat spreads
• Baby oil	• Massage oil
• Bath oil	• Monistat
• Body oil	• Nizoral
• Butter	• Nystain cream
• Cold cream	• Nystavescent
• Cooking oil	• Orthodienoestrol
• Cream	• Orthogynest
• Cyclogest	• Pimafucin cream
• Ecostatin	• Skin softener
• Fungilin	• Sultrin
• Gyno-daktarin	• Sun tan creams
• Hair conditioner	• Vaseline
• Ice cream	• Witepsol-based suppositories
• Lipstick	

(Source: Adapted from Everett, 2004)

In Europe, condoms that carry the European CE (*Conformité Européenne*) mark or the British Standard Kite mark are advocated as this demonstrates that the condoms have been fully tested and have been approved for use. The patient should be advised to check the expiry date on the condom packaging as well as ensuring that it is intact and in good condition. Condoms can deteriorate quickly if they are not stored in ideal conditions; they are adversely affected by heat and light. It is best to avoid storing condoms in a wallet, in the glove compartment of a car or the back pocket. Once the airtight foil package is opened, the condom can deteriorate rapidly.

When the condom is to be opened, it should be opened from the corner of the package, taking care not to rip it with fingernails or the teeth. The condom should be placed over the erect penis and the tip of the condom pinched to expel any air or, if there is no reservoir present, a space for the collection of ejaculate should be made. After ejaculation the used condom should be taken safely from the erect penis, wrapped in tissue or toilet paper and thrown away safely and hygienically; it should not be disposed of in the toilet. Never use a condom more than once. The Family Planning Association (2006a) has provided a checklist that the practice nurse may wish to use when discussing issues about male condom use with the patient (and if appropriate his partner). Check that:

- they know that condoms come in different shapes and sizes;
- previous experience of condom use was positive;
- they have the confidence or language to discuss any problems they may be having with condoms;
- they can read and understand instructions provided by the manufacture and any material you may give them;

- they know how to put a condom on;
- they know where to get condoms from;
- they know they can get a free supply from various NHS services;
- women will be able to influence their partner's use of condoms.

VASECTOMY

The numbers of men opting for vasectomy as a method of contraception during 2003–2004 was estimated to be approximately 9000 (HSCIC, 2004). Men more than women opt to undergo vasectomy for contraceptive purposes and the numbers of male vasectomies increase with the age of the man (Office for National Statistics, 2005). Amundsen and Ramakrishnan (2004) suggest that vasectomy, as a permanent method of contraception, is one of most reliable and cost-effective methods.

Vasectomy is the ligation or the division of the vas deferens, the genital ducts that store and transport sperm to the urethra during ejaculation. The aim is to provide surgical interruption of the vas deferens and the ultimate goal is to arrest the flow of spermatozoa (Peate, 2000). See Figure 6.3.

As with any aspect of contraception the patient (and, if appropriate, his partner) should be given the time to discuss their needs and their individual circumstances. The practice nurse can provide the patient with information and counselling concerning the risks, side effects, failure rates associated with this method of contraception and the possibility of reversal procedures.

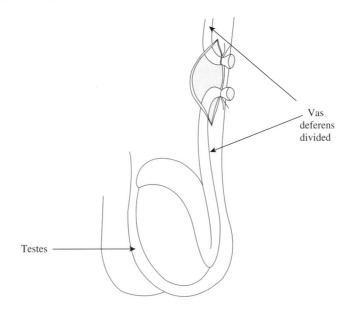

Vas deferens divided

Testes

Figure 6.3. The vas divided

This method of contraception is permanent, and as such it is vital that issues concerning the possibility of relationship breakdown or the loss by death of the partner or one of their children are discussed; also the implications for future pregnancies should be given consideration. A clear explanation must be offered to the man about the nature of the procedure and the processes involved – a simple diagram may enhance this. Some men will need reassurance about the fluid produced on ejaculation after the vasectomy has been performed. It should be explained that the ejaculate will contain fluid that is free from sperm and that the volume of the ejaculate will remain approximately the same and that obstructed sperm are reabsorbed (Laws, 2006). Everett (2004) points out that some men may have fears about their ability to maintain an erection and engage in sexual intercourse following vasectomy. The man should be advised that a vasectomy does not affect libido or the ability to maintain and sustain an erection.

There are issues surrounding the effect a vasectomy may have on the incidence of testicular and prostate cancer. Currently there is no conclusive evidence to demonstrate a link between the two (Everett, 2004; Guillebaud and Hannaford, 2001; Smeltzer and Bare, 2000).

Table 6.5 outlines some information that the patient may require prior to deciding on vasectomy as a method of contraception.

The practice nurse should use his/her professional judgement when providing the information, for example, how much information to give, in what format and to allow the man (and if appropriate his partner) time to make a decision. The man may wish to defer his decision and return at a later date when he has been able to assimilate and fully understand the implications of the vasectomy.

HORMONAL CONTRACEPTION – THE MALE

Creative and innovation approaches to male contraceptive methods are currently undergoing trial, including those that employ hormonal techniques. The use of hormonal contraception and the principles underpinning this practice are not new: over 60 years ago it was established that when men were injected with testosterone preparations they become azoospermic. These early approaches related to male hormonal contraception have developed, and it has been demonstrated that it is possible to provide men with an injection of a high dose of testosterone – an induction dose, and then use a lower dose injection as maintenance.

Anderson (2004) discusses the use of testosterone patch preparations. Trans-dermal testosterone patches have been made available but they require further improvements. The patches can be used on the scrotum and on other parts of the body. Poor concordance may occur and some trans-dermal patches have caused skin irritation (Jordan, 1997; Bennett, 1998).

Testosterone implants have been used in both androgen replacement therapy and also as an aspect of male contraception. Implantation requires a minor surgical procedure in order to insert testosterone pellets. Anderson (2004) suggests that the extrusion rate is below 10%. It has been demonstrated that the use of testosterone

Table 6.5. Some issues that the practice nurse may discuss when providing the patient with information prior to him making his decision to undergo vasectomy

---

Pre-operative counselling is vital for the man to make an informed decision
- The type of anaesthetic that may be used, for example, local or general
- The method of occlusion
  - Ligation and excision of vas deferens
  - Cautery and clipping of vas deferens
  - Cautery and fascial interposition
- The type of dressing that may be applied and the length of time it needs to stay in place
- Expect some swelling and/or bruising around the operation site; this can extend to the umbilicus and thighs
- Pain is expected and is usually relieved by paracetamol, codeine and/or ice packs
- Sutures will dissolve within a week
- Strenuous exercise should be avoided for 2–3 days post vasectomy
- Sexual activity (including masturbation) should not take place before the third day after the procedure as there may be tenderness and soreness
- Current contraceptive use must continue until two successive sperm specimens have proved free of sperm. It may take three months for azoospermia to occur
- Follow-up is required for sperm analysis as sperms may remain viable and motile for some time. It has been suggested that follow-up occurs after six weeks, 12 weeks and six months.
- There is a failure rate associated with vasectomy
- Reversal of the operation is possible, but this is not always 100 % successful
- There are side effects associated with vasectomy
  - Infection
  - Pain
  - Haematoma

(Source: Adapted from Guillebaud and Hannaford, 2001; Weiske, 2001; Laws, 2006; Everett, 2004)

pellets provides a constant delivery of the correct concentration of testosterone, reducing the risk of supra- and sub-physiological testosterone swings seen when using injection preparations (Handelsman *et al.*, 1997). Anderson, Kinniburgh and Baird (2002) are presently investigating the use of implants within a clinically controlled environment; they point out that there are currently some disadvantages using this technique and as a result of this their use outside of a research environment is prohibited.

Just as with females, the use of hormonal approaches to contraception in the male is not without complications and the methods currently under investigation need refinement and fine tuning.

CONCLUSION

The practice nurse is at the centre of contraceptive services, providing advice, administering treatments and offering follow-up. Reproductive sexual health, sometimes known as family planning, is in a constant state of flux with innovative and creative contraceptive methods emerging and developing. The practice nurse must remain ahead of these innovations and developments in order to provide the patient with a high-quality service that reflects contemporary thinking.

In order for the man to make an informed decision, the provision of information is vital. All men need to be provided with tailored information concerning the various methods of contraception available. Providing a bespoke service, with information related to the individual's particular needs, can aid in concordance with contraception. The nurse must cover the benefits, risks and how to deal with the side effects that may occur. A detailed medical history must be taken from the man as part of a routine assessment. Consideration must be given to the law and the legal issue concerning children and younger men. Those men with learning disabilities, for example, who approach the practice nurse for advice concerning contraception may have particular needs that will have to be taken into account. There may also be aspects of the law that need to be considered. To reinforce verbal information provided, and to ensure as much as possible that the man is making an informed decision, this can be reinforced by evidence-based written information, written in such a manner that the man is able to understand and subsequently assimilate the advice.

Being aware of sensitivities surrounding the patient's culture, their religious beliefs, special needs and language differences can enhance the nurse–patient relationship. This can be true in any consultation the practice nurse engages in, including consultations related to contraception. Alongside the provision of a high-quality contraceptive service there is also an opportunity to promote safer sex activities. The practice nurse may also consider offering the patient STI screening opportunities if these are deemed appropriate.

The novel approaches to hormone contraction methods for the male are still in their infancy. However, as science and understanding grows, this may allow men the opportunity to become fully engaged in family planning, encouraging them (if appropriate) to take up their equal share in this important activity. Engaging and serving men with respect to their reproductive needs is also a way of enhancing the reproductive health of women.

Above all, the practice nurse must be deemed competent and demonstrate confidence in the provision of contraceptive services to both men and women, maintaining professional competence (Nursing and Midwifery Council, 2004) and demonstrating an awareness of the advances occurring in this rapidly changing sphere of practice. It is vital that locally agreed protocols are adhered to and provision of care conforms to guidance issued by the Department of Health or other advisory bodies such as the National Institute for Health and Clinical Excellence.

REFERENCES

Amundsen, G. and Ramakrishnan, K. (2004) Vasectomy: a 'seminal' analysis. *Southern Medical Journal*, **97** (1), 54–60.

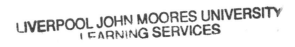

Anderson, P.A. (2004) Male contraception: novel approaches. In (eds R.S. Kirby, C.C. Carson, M.G. Kirby and R.N. Farah) *Men's Health*, 2nd edn, Taylor and Francis, London.

Anderson, P.A., Kinniburgh, D. and Baird, D.T. (2002) Suppression of spermatogenesis by etonogestrel implants with depot testosterone: potential for long-acting male contraception. *Journal of Clinical Endocrinology and Metabolism*, **87**, 3640–3649.

Bennett, N.J. (1998) A burn-like lesion caused by a testosterone trans-dermal system. *Burns*, **24**, 478–480.

Chambers, R., Wakely, G. and Chambers, S. (2000) *Tackling Teenage Pregnancy*, Radcliffe, Oxford.

Department of Health (2001) *The National Strategy for Sexual Health and HIV: Better Prevention, Better Services, Better Sexual Health*, DH, London.

Everett, S. (2004) *Handbook of Contraception and Reproductive and Sexual Health*, 2nd edn, Bailliere Tindall, London.

Family Planning Association (2006a) *Contraception: Family Planning Association Policy Statement*, FPA, London.

Family Planning Association (2006b) *Talking to Clients about Using Condoms*, FPA, London.

Frezieres, R.G. and Walsh, T.L. (2000) Acceptability evaluation of a natural rubber latex, a polyurethane, and new non latex condom. *Contraception*, **61**, 369–377.

Frezieres, R.G., Walsh, T.L., Nelson, A.L. *et al.* (1998) Breakage and acceptability of a polyurethane condom: a randomised controlled study. *Family Planning Perspectives*, **30**, 73–78.

Fu, H., Darroch, J.E., Has, T. and Ranjit, N. (1999) Contraceptive failure rates: new estimates from the 1995 national survey of family growth. *Family Planning Perspectives*, **31**, 56–33.

Guillebaud, J. and Hannaford, P. (2001) Providing high-quality contraceptive services in primary care. In (eds Y. Carter, C. Moss and A. Weyman) *RCGP Handbook of Sexual Health in Primary Care*, Royal College of General Practitioners, London, pp. 83–107, Chapter 6.

Handelsman, D.J., Mackey, M.A., Howe, C. *et al.* (1997) An analysis of testosterone implants for androgen replacement therapy. *Clinical Endocrinology*, **47**, 311–316.

Hannaford, P. (2006) Contraception. In (eds T. Belfield, Y. Carter, P. Mathews, C. Moss and A. Weyman) *The Handbook of Sexual Health in Primary Care*, FPA, London, pp. 57–120, Chapter 3.

Health and Special Care Information Centre (2004) *NHS Contraceptive Services, England: 2003–2004, Bulletin 2005/06 HSCIC*, HSCIC, London.

Hubbard, J. and Mechan, D. (1997) *The Physiology of Health and Illness, with Related Anatomy*, Stanley Thrones, Cheltenham.

Hughes, L. (2004) Women's health. In (eds J. Martin and J. Lucas) *Handbook of Practice Nursing*, 3rd edn, Churchill Livingstone, Ediburgh, pp. 3–27, Chapter 1.

Jordan, W.P. (1997) Allergy and topical irritation associated with trans-dermal testosterone administration: a comparison of scrotal and non scrotal trans-dermal systems. *American Journal of Contact Dermatology*, **8**, 108–113.

Laws, T. (2006) *A Handbook of Men's Health*, Elsevier, Edinburgh.

Martin, C.W., Anderson, R.A., Cheng, L. *et al.* (2004) Potential impact of hormonal male contraception: cross-cultural implications for development of novel preparations. *Human Reproduction*, **15**, 637–945.

Matthews, P. and Ireson, R. (2006) Risk assessment and sexual history: taking in primary care. In (eds T. Belfield, Y. Carter, P. Mathews, C. Moss and A. Weyman) *The Handbook of Sexual Health in Primary Care*, FPA, London, pp. 35–56, Chapter 2.

Men's Health Forum (2006) *Men's Health Forum Report on: Men and Chlamydia: Putting Men to the Test*, MHF, London.

Nursing and Midwifery Council (2004) *Code of Professional Conduct: Standards for Conduct, Performance and Ethics*, NMC, London.

Office for National Statistics (2005) *Contraception and Sexual Health 2004/2005*, ONS, London.

Peate, I. (2000) The testicle. In (ed. P. Downey) *Introduction to Urological Nursing*. Whurr, London, pp. 111–126, Chapter 8.

Smeltzer, S.C. and Bare, B.G. (2000) *Brunner and Suddarth's Textbook of Medical-Surgical Nursing*, 9th edn, Lippincott, Philadelphia.

Social Exclusion Unit (1999) *Teenage Pregnancy*, SEU, London.

Wakely, G. and Chambers, R. (2002) *Sexual Health Matters in Primary Care*, Radcliffe, Oxford.

Weiske, W.H. (2001) Vasectomy. *Andrologia*, **33** (3), 125–124.

7 Sexually transmitted infections

INTRODUCTION

Access to sexual health services needs to be faster and, as part of ensuring this, the Government has provided a comprehensive strategy that aims to improve the sexual health of the nation. Services will be enhanced and as a result it is anticipated that the desired outcome is to improve prevention and access to treatment for sexually transmitted infections (STIs). It is anticipated that by 2008 everybody will be able to access a genitourinary medicine (GUM) clinic within 48 hours (Department of Health (DH), 2006). The cost of STIs is significant (House of Commons Health Committee, 2003) and Matthews and Macaulay (2006) state that the role of the practice nurse is becoming increasingly important in detecting and managing STIs in order to address and prevent the unwanted consequences of infection.

This chapter provides the reader with an outline of key Government policy that has impinged, or has the potential to impinge, on service provision, for example, the *National Strategy for Sexual Health and HIV* (DH, 2001). The provision of high-quality care is dependent upon the practice nurse's ability to undertake a holistic assessment of the patient's needs. In order to undertake an effective assessment of the patient, a detailed sexual health history must be carried out, and this chapter provides the principles underpinning sexual history-taking. An overview of three STIs – gonorrhoea, chlamydia and syphilis – will be described and discussed. Although the issue of HIV will not be covered in depth in this chapter, a short discussion is provided relating to the provision of HIV services in the primary care setting.

THE NATIONAL STRATEGY FOR SEXUAL HEALTH AND HIV

The *National Strategy for Sexual Health and HIV* (DH, 2001) endeavours to apply the values and principles of the *NHS Plan* (DH, 2000) to sexual health and sexual health service provision. Primary care is the key driver for the Government's sexual health strategy. The strategy aims to redesign services around the people who use them as well as:

- improving services
- reducing health inequalities in sexual health
- improving health and sexual well-being.

The practice nurse needs to appreciate the fact that the strategy addresses the needs of the whole nation. If the aims above are to be achieved, then specific approaches will need to be undertaken for men, and a gendered perspective to all aspects of sexual healthcare is vital. There is an opportunity for the nurse to promote holistic, positive sexual health when also addressing the issues of STIs and HIV, focusing on prevention as well as treatment.

The nurse must provide the patient (and his partner(s) if appropriate) with health promotion information that is effective. Provision of competent skilled nursing, as well as a service that is accessible in order to prevent poor sexual health is essential. There is a need to recognize that accessing information can be done in many ways, for example:

- telephone lines
- digital television
- Internet
- SMS messaging
- leaflets
- posters
- one-to-one consultations.

The focus of care must be based on the patient's personal need. To prevent discrimination as discussed in the strategy, information and effective services must be offered in such a way as to avoid discrimination as well as respecting diversity. A gendered approach is therefore required, reflecting a male perspective. The needs of young men, gay men, older men and men from different ethnic groups within the local population must be addressed. If the nurse fails to use an approach that takes into account the needs of men – a targeted approach – then there is a potential that men are likely to miss out on good, effective, preventative sexual healthcare. It should be noted that interventions that do not adopt a local approach may not succeed. Sexual health prevention approaches that are successful with a group of men in Liverpool, for example, may not be effective when used with a group of men from Glasgow.

The practice nurse and all members of the practice should make every effort to engage with men, acknowledging the life experiences of men and using a language that men understand and are familiar with when providing them with, and discussing, information on sexual health issues, and demonstrating gender sensitivity. Men are notorious for not accessing primary care services, and the focus within the strategy is to move services to primary care, which could result in increasing the problems men already have in accessing sexual health services, which are now devolved to primary care. Consideration needs to be given to the reality that some men may not welcome services related to sexual health at a primary care level; they may prefer such services to be provided at a distance from the general practice.

When possible, the practice must invite and involve patients and patient representatives to shape the development of local strategies and plans, ensuring that local gender-sensitive services are available. Such an approach demonstrates a spirit of inclusion in engaging with the local population.

SERVICE PROVISION

A shift in service provision is anticipated: it is no longer practical or economical to deliver services associated with sexual health (and in particular those connected with STI management) in predominantly hospital-based settings. The House of Commons Health Committee (2003) notes that throughout the UK specialist services aimed at providing diagnosis and management of STIs are overwhelmed. Many aspects of sexual healthcare services can, and are, being delivered in a range of settings in an attempt to relieve the pressure on traditional STI service providers. The GP practice is one of those settings where a range of sexual health services can be provided at different levels. The services offered in GP practices by practice nurses can become a reality with the full use of nurse prescribing powers and Patient Group Directions. *Choosing Health* (DH, 2004) recommends the development of locally managed networks for sexual health. The networks aim to provide wide-ranging services that meet the local population's needs.

The new GP contract that came into force in 2004, and subsequent amendments to that contract, provides financial support for some practices wishing to provide enhanced services. The contract provides payment based on the type and quality of services the practice offers (British Medical Association (BMA) and NHS Confederation, 2003). There are three categories of clinical services: essential, additional and enhanced (see Table 7.1 below).

The aims identified in the sexual health strategy propose that a greater role is taken on by the primary care sector. The essential, additional and enhanced services described in Table 7.1 also point to enhancing the roles and functions of those working in primary care in relation to sexual health. The implications, suggests Hughes (2004), are far-reaching. Prior to taking on the additional and enhanced roles and functions, the practice nurse must ensure that s/he is acting within his/her sphere of practice, making known any limitations in their knowledge and skills and taking steps (where appropriate) to put right these discrepancies; this is in line with the Nursing and Midwifery Council's *Code of Professional Conduct* (2004). Section 6.2 states:

> To practise competently, you must possess the knowledge, skills and abilities required for lawful, safe and effective practice without direct supervision. You must acknowledge the limits of your professional competence and only undertake practice and accept responsibilities for those activities in which you are competent.

Failure to take a sexual health history, it could be suggested, is professional misconduct. The nurse is potentially breeching the code of professional conduct in doing the patient possible harm.

HIV

The number of people infected with HIV continues to grow; there is no cure and there is no vaccine available. The introduction of anti-retroviral medications is

Table 7.1. Essential, additional and enhanced services

Essential	Additional	Enhanced
All GP practices must provide essential services covering general day-to-day practice. These essential services include: • The management of patients who are ill or who believe they are ill or with conditions that it is generally believed they will recover from • The general management of chronic disease • The specialist care of patients who are terminally ill	Most practices are able to offer the following service, but have the option to opt out of provision on a temporary or permanent basis if they are experiencing difficulties with, for example, recruitment. • Participation in the NHS Cervical Screening Programme • Contraceptive services • Vaccinations and immunizations • Child health surveillance • Maternity medical services • Minor surgery	These services are optional for GP practices. They are more specialized than those provided through essential or additional services. Essential services may also include services addressing local health needs; these include those services for specific vulnerable groups and the following are some examples: • Specialized sexual health services • Intrauterine contraceptive device fittings • Intrapartum care • Services for drug and alcohol misusers • Minor injuries services

(Source: Adapted BMA and NHS Confederation, 2003)

life-saving in most cases. HIV can be transmitted sexually; it is not (in this text) discussed alongside other STIs. The reader is advised to seek other resources to inform and develop insight and understanding of this complex viral infection.

It is estimated that approximately one-third of those with HIV are yet to be diagnosed and many of these will be using GP services (Madge *et al.*, 2005). HIV that remains undiagnosed, according to Matthews (2006), places the health and life of all in jeopardy. Madge *et al.* (1997) provide evidence to suggest that there are some patients already attending general practice for care who do not know they are HIV-positive.

Many HIV-positive people receive their care and treatment at specific HIV clinics; this care includes general healthcare as well as HIV-specific care. HIV clinics usually provide the HIV-positive person with a range of services that are not HIV-related, for example, flu vaccines, medications for asthma and antidepressants. Barnard (2006) suggests that some clinics are now beginning to limit prescribing to anti-HIV drugs only. This will result in HIV-positive patients having to attend their general practice for treatment not specifically related to anti-HIV medications; not all practice nurses or GPs will have the knowledge and skills to provide care related to HIV, as previously the HIV-positive patient may have used the HIV clinic as a one-stop shop. There are some practices that provide enhanced services; these include addressing the HIV and sexual health specific needs of patients who are HIV-positive.

New roles for the practice nurse will continue to emerge in relation to HIV care; for example, patients will require the continuous monitoring of viral load and CD4 cell count. The practice nurse will need to complement his/her current skills repertoire and consider broader issues that people with HIV may present with. The patient who is HIV-positive may need to be made aware of the advantages of having some HIV services provided by the general practice in conjunction with the HIV clinic. It may be more beneficial for a patient to register with a practice as the practice can more readily assist the patient with referral to district nursing services, and referral to mental health nurses, physiotherapy and chiropody in the community. The practice may be able to offer alternative appointments for the patient (evening appointments). The general practice can provide the patient with prescriptions for non-HIV medicines for longer periods than the HIV clinic can. Unlike an HIV physician, a GP is the only doctor who can make a home visit if the patient is too ill to attend the surgery (National AIDS Manual, 2006). The practice nurse is a very skilled person with much experience, and is able to mobilize services quickly in order to provide ongoing specialist community care nursing to support the patient with a chronic condition at home. In some ways caring for a person with HIV is no different from caring for those with other chronic conditions (Madge *et al.*, 2005). Many of the issues associated with chronic conditions such as HIV, for example depression, are conditions that the practice nurse deals with on a day-to-day basis.

Elford *et al.* (2006) state that nearly one-third of patients, diagnosed with HIV report that they have been discriminated against because of their infection. The survey was undertaken in a northeast London HIV outpatient clinic. Half of those who experienced discrimination reported that this involved a healthcare worker. Out of the sample, gay men were more likely to be discriminated against. It has been unlawful since 2005 under the Disability Discrimination Act 2005 to discriminate against those with HIV; it is also tantamount to professional misconduct (Nursing and Midwifery Council (NMC), 2004). The same standard of service and care that is provided to patients who are HIV-negative must also be provided to those who are HIV-positive.

If the integration of HIV services into primary care is to proceed smoothly and the patient is to receive the best quality care, then effective communication between both primary care and secondary care and vice versa is vital. Education is required in order to equip the practice nurse with the knowledge and skills s/he will require to provide high-quality care that is safe and effective as well as being responsive to the needs of the person with HIV.

SEXUAL HEALTH HISTORY-TAKING

Most practice nurses are adept at assessing and taking a health history in the practice setting; yet, when it comes to sexual health assessment and history-taking this is not always the case. There may be several reasons for this: they may not have been provided with the knowledge and skills required to carry out this important task or it may also be that the nurse feels uneasy about discussing issues related to sex and sexuality (Tomlinson, 2005). Wakely, Cunnion and Chambers (2003) discuss some reasons why uneasiness may be felt when talking to patients about sex:

- fear of offending the patient;
- unfamiliarity with the patient's culture (either their ethnicity or sexual orientation);
- reluctance to become involved in complex and time-consuming issues;
- reticence and embarrassment.

The patient can also be unwilling to talk out about sex because of:

- embarrassment, shame or humiliation;
- unease about their sexuality;
- anxieties about the information being given and confidentiality;
- attending with a partner;
- reservations about being judged inadequate or peculiar.

Johnson *et al.* (2002) suggest that people, including nurses and doctors, regard sexual issues as 'personal', even when these issues are discussed within the confines of the healthcare setting, such as the general practice. Tomlinson (2005) states that patients may feel ashamed, embarrassed or humiliated; the role of the nurse is to be non-judgemental and to put the patient at ease. It has been noted that within primary healthcare settings STI counselling is hardly ever carried out, and when this is done it is often deficient (Haley *et al.*, 1999).

Taking a sexual health history means that the nurse must have the appropriate knowledge, skills and attitudes as well as ensuring that s/he has the time to encourage the patient to be frank and open. Obtaining a sexual health history from the patient can help the nurse diagnose and provide care for him in relation to his sexual problems (Wakely and Chambers, 2002). Failure to take the sexual health history in a confident and competent manner could lead to misunderstanding and ultimately misdiagnosis and therefore inappropriate treatment. Taking the sexual health history competently is therefore crucial to the patient encounter and patient outcome (Matthews, 1998).

The Medical Foundation for Sexual Health (2004) suggests that outcomes of the sexual health history can enable people to receive suitably targeted advice and guidance in relation to the prevention of STIs, HIV or unintended pregnancies. Taking the sexual health history and assessing sexual health is not only about gaining information to determine if the patient has an STI; it is also about the patient's sexual well-being. High-quality care provision means including sexual health in all aspects of patient care; it should be seen as being as important as the physical, spiritual, social and emotional aspects of care (McAndrew, 2000).

Verhoeven *et al.* (2003) and Low *et al.* (2003) suggest that there has been a move towards asymptomatic STIs, for example, chlamydial and gonoccocal infections. A result of this may mean that the practice nurse may encounter more challenges in raising the issue of STIs with patients. Patients may not present with any symptoms, and as such may not have even thought about the issue of an STI, despite the possibility of being infected with one (Matthews and Fletcher, 2001).

Prior to the nurse engaging with the patient there is one obstacle that he may have to face: gaining access to the services that the practice nurse provides. Problems can occur in booking an appointment when wishing to see the nurse. Some surgeries may require the patient to explain to the person taking the booking the reason for the request for consultation (sometimes this is the receptionist). The layout of the surgery and where the reception is based may also be problematic: the patient may fear being overheard by others, and issues concerning confidentiality can arise. It is suggested that the practice display notices and literature that inform the patient that confidentiality will be maintained and that a non-judgemental approach is used by staff; the practice's confidentiality policy should be displayed in the waiting area or made readily available to the patient. Changes should be considered with regards to the layout of the reception area, whereby only one person at a time can stand in front of the receptionist. Such examples can be seen in banks and airports. Issues around confidentiality are cited by young people and gay men as areas of concern (Donovan, Hadley and Jones, 2000; Keogh *et al.*, 2004).

Epstein *et al.* (1997) suggest that it is the history that leads the patient through a succession of questions aimed to build a profile of the patient and their sexual problems. The history-taking episode ends with the nurse having a more in-depth understanding of the patient, and a differential diagnosis may have been arrived at, explaining to the patient about the symptoms he has presented with. The range of questions that are asked when adopting a holistic approach will range from the presenting symptoms to:

- the patient's social history
- educational background
- employment history if appropriate
- psychosocial history
- travel history
- circumstances at home
- family history
- sexual history/activity
- a review of the major organs.

The practice nurse is likely to become more proficient at sexual history-taking by increasing the number of times s/he takes a sexual health history, and the number of times s/he asks patients about their sexual health (Nusbaum and Hamilton, 2002). By incorporating sexual health history-taking into routine history-taking exercises, the nurse can be presented with opportunities to offer preventative care, for example, immunization against hepatitis B and counselling opportunities that are concerned with risk-minimizing sexual behaviours.

The nurse should greet the patient in a relaxed yet confident manner. It is important to demonstrate to the patient that the consultation will be carried out in private and that there will be no disturbances. The way the seating is arranged also needs consideration and if possible place your chair to the side of your desk so that you will be able to observe the patient's body language, but be aware the patient will also be able to observe your body language.

It may be a challenge for the nurse working with the patient to determine what exactly the problem is that the patient is coming to see you about. Often, when discussing issues that provoke embarrassment or shame, the patient will be vague and use nonverbal communication. He may discuss the issue as if it is a 'friend' who is experiencing the problem; he can also be indirect and use euphemisms and innuendo (Peate, 2005a). It is vital that both parties are using the same language when discussing intimate issues, phrases such as 'sore down below' can mean many things to the patient and nurse. Elucidation throughout the consultation is central to effective sexual history-taking. The nurse needs to decide if vernacular terms are to be used during the consultation or if medical terminology is required. The decision is not easy as the nurse may be worried about offending the patient, and professional judgement is called for. Whatever approach is used, the nurse must strive to ensure that both parties are clear and being understood. If misunderstanding occurs, or is likely to occur, ask the patient to explain further, delve deeper and clarify what you think you may have heard. This may be challenging as you may be embarrassed or even shocked about what you are hearing or what you believe you are hearing. Skelton and Matthews (2001) suggest that specialist guidance and specific knowledge may be needed about the range of sexual practices in order to gain an understanding of pertinent issues.

If the nurse conducts sexual history-taking as if asking questions from a questionnaire or a list, to be run through with the patient, this may lose all of its potential value. Asking a lot of questions may mean that the patient will respond with a lot of answers. Problems may be encountered if these approaches are used: the nurse may not have identified the problems the patient is presenting with, s/he did not hear the patient or the patient may not have been given permission to tell his story: effective communication skills are essential. It is often easier for the nurse to avoid asking sensitive questions concerning intimate issues surrounding sex and sexuality and closed questioning can be used by the nurse to limit the patient's responses, avoiding having to get involved as opposed to using open-ended questions inviting the patient to offer more. The use of open-ended questions such as those that do not require a yes/no response are advocated in an attempt to elicit as much information as possible (Carter, Moss and Weyman, 1998). Table 7.2 (below) provides some examples of open, closed and judgemental questions.

Table 7.2. Some examples of open, closed and judgemental questions

---

Closed questions:
'Did you use a condom?'
'Have you had this kind of discharge before?'
'Does is hurt after you have had intercourse?'

Open questions:
'How can I help you?'
'What is the problem?'
'What do you think caused the difficulty?'

Judgemental questions:
'At your age don't you think you should know better?'
'As a healthcare professional don't you think you, of all people, should have known better?'

(Source: Adapted from Tomlinson 1998)

It can help the patient if the nurse makes clear the reason why personal questions need to be asked. For example, 'I am going to ask some questions that are personal. By asking these types of questions I can assess your needs fully and decide on the tests that will be right for you. Therefore I need to ask more about your sex life.'

It is easy to make assumptions about people, and every effort should be taken to avoid this. During the history-taking exercise, avoid using terms that make assumptions about either the patient's sexual behaviour or their sexuality. If asking questions about a patient's sexual orientation, the nurse is advised to use the term 'partner' instead of 'boyfriend' or 'girlfriend', 'husband' or 'wife'. Ask the patient how many partners he has instead of asking him if he is married and/or monogamous. The response he gives you may confirm whether he is married and monogamous or not.

Another area where professional judgement is required is whether to conduct the interview with the patient alone or with his partner present, and this needs much consideration. The patient may not be as forthcoming with important details if his partner is present; on the other hand, joint consultations may provide much valuable information.

A SEXUAL HEALTH HISTORY SUMMARY

Below (Table 7.3) is a checklist (aide-memoire) provided to help you conduct the sexual health history with confidence. It has already been stated that as time goes by and the more sexual health histories you take the more proficient you will become and the more your confidence will grow. The approach you use and the way in which you frame the questions along with the terminology chosen will depend on your assessment of the patient's understanding.

Table 7.3. Checklist of some questions that may help guide and inform the sexual health history

General issues:
- Do you currently engage in sexual activity?
- Are there any concerns you have about your sex life?
- With whom do you have sex, men, women or both?
- Tell me about the sexual activity you have. Do you, for example, engage in oral/anal sex?
- Do you masturbate?
- Are you sexually satisfied?
- Is your sexual activity as frequent as you would like it to be?
- Does your partner prefer more or less sexual activity than you do?
- Do you have orgasms?
- Is there any pain associated with sexual activity – you/your partner?
- Is there anything about your sexual activity that you would want to change?
- Are there any worries you have about your genitals?

STIs:
- Have you ever had an STI?
- Do you think you may be at risk of contracting an STI?
- Tell me how many sexual partners have you had in the last 12 months?
- Do you ever experience a burning sensation when you pass water?
- Have you noticed any discharge from your genitalia?
- Is there a rash or any lumps in the genital area?

Hepatitis:
- Have you ever had a yellowing of the skin or eyes, or have any of your friends told you that you look yellow?
- Have you ever experienced:
  - Upper abdominal pain?
  - Light- coloured stools?
  - Dark urine?
- Has any one ever told you that you have a liver problem or hepatitis?
- Have you been vaccinated for hepatitis?

(Source: Adapted from Wakely, Cunnion and Chambers, 2003; Nusbaum and Hamilton 2002)

When the nurse has completed taking an in-depth sexual health history, the next step, working with the patient, is to come to a decision concerning the most appropriate way forward in order to address and treat the problem. The remaining sections of this chapter discusses the management of three common STIs.

MANAGEMENT OF SEXUALLY TRANSMITTED INFECTIONS

STIs have the potential to cause major public health problems (BMA, 2002):

Table 7.4. First sexual heterosexual experience before 16 years

	Men (%)	Women (%)
General population	27.4	20.4
Black-Caribbean	56.3	22.3
Indian	10.3	1.0

(Source: Wellings *et al.*, 2001)

- Some STIs have potentially serious outcomes for both physical and psychological health.
- Some favour and make possible the transmission of HIV infection.
- Some may cause serious ill health for both mothers and babies.
- Some can cause fertility problems.

The annual number of diagnoses of gonorrhoea has doubled since 1996; with chlamydia there has been an increase of 140% and syphilis has increased by 910%. It is estimated that infection rates will increase further (Terence Higgins Trust, 2004). These increases provide health services with a major challenge and nurses can help to confront this challenge.

Chlamydia, non-specific urethritis (NSU) and wart virus are common STIs. The number of visits made to GUM clinics has increased twofold in the last decade, during which more than a million people visited GUM clinics (DH, 2001). With the implementation of the *National Strategy for Sexual Health and HIV* (DH, 2001) the practice nurse may in the future be caring for an increase in the numbers of patients who attend the surgery with problems that are related to STIs. These increasing trends in STIs may in part be associated with changes in sexual behaviour (Health Development Agency (HDA), 2004). It is estimated that young men experience their first heterosexual sexual encounter at approximately 16 years of age (Wellings *et al.*, 2001). Table 7.4 provides data concerning sexual experiences among the general population and different ethnic groups.

Table 7.5 (below) outlines the number of new diagnoses made at GUM clinics for syphilis, gonorrhoea and chlamydia between 2000 and 2005. The cases reported are underestimations as these fail to capture the number of cases diagnosed in general practice and independent/private centres.

STIs can be classified into four groups (see Table 7.6 below).

ARRIVING AT A DIAGNOSIS

The nurse must examine the patient and carry out a range of diagnostic tests in order to make a diagnosis. A brief outline of the principles underpinning good practice when examining a male patient is now provided.

Local policy and procedure will determine the diagnostic tests that may be required to confirm diagnosis; the nurse must refer to these policies and procedures

Table 7.5. Number of new diagnoses made at GUM clinics for syphilis, gonorrhoea and chlamydia between 2000 and 2005 (UK)

Infection	2000	2001	2002	2003	2004	2005
Syphilis[a]						
Male	398	917	1 482	1 895	2 565	3 100
MSM[b]	181	483	847	1 053	1 371	1 868
Total Male	579	1 400	2 329	2 948	3 936	4 968
Gonorrhoea[c]						
Male	15 234	16 626	17 871	17 398	15 699	14 055
MSM	3 140	3 727	3 618	4 078	3 978	4 352
Total male	18 374	20 353	21 489	21 476	19 677	18 407
Chlamydia[d]						
Male	29 821	33 362	38 675	43 043	48 665	51 980
MSM	1 078	1 516	1 644	2 111	2 222	2 697
Total male	30 899	34 878	40 319	45 154	50 887	54 677

(Source: Health Protection Agency, 2006)
[a]Including primary, secondary and early latent syphilis.
[b]Men who have sex with men.
[c]All cases of uncomplicated gonorrhoea.
[d]All cases of uncomplicated genital chlamydial infection.

used at a local level at all times. The results of the tests carried out can confirm or eliminate possible infections, and because of this it is important that attention is given to policy and procedure. The following should also be considered:

- the timing of the test(s) (if appropriate);
- adequate preparation of the patient for the test(s);
- effective collection and dissemination of the specimens collected.

One aspect of making a diagnosis is to give the patient the results of the test(s) that have been carried out. Providing the patient with his test results must be done with tact and sensitivity, approaching each person as an individual when presenting him with either a positive or negative diagnosis as there may be consequences for the patient with respect to the test results. There may be occasions where referral to another agency, that is, psychosexual counsellor, is needed as the patient may be experiencing issues of a psychosexual nature. The practice nurse must be aware of who s/he can refer the patient to and make that referral for the patient, informing him of the reason why.

Examination of the genitalia is an intimate procedure, and every person has the right to have a chaperone present during the examination (Royal College of Nursing (RCN), 2003); these examinations should be conducted in a sensitive and respectful manner. An explanation of why the examination is needed and what is to be expected should be given; for example, is he required to lie down or stand up for the exami-

Table 7.6. The WHO Classification of STIs with examples of some of the STIs

Viral infections:
- HIV infection
- Acquired Immunodeficiency Syndrome secondary to HIV infection
- Herpes simplex virus infections
- Type 1 Herpes simplex virus infection
- Type 2 Herpes simplex virus infection
- Human papilloma virus infections
- Hepatitis B infection
- Other sexually transmitted viral infections

Bacterial infections:
- Syphilis
- Gonococci infections
- Chlamydiasis
- Trichomonal infection
- Other sexually transmitted bacterial infections

Yeast infections:
- Candidiasis
- Other sexually transmitted yeast infections

Infestations:
- Phthirus pubis crab infestation
- Sarcoptes scabiei infestation
- Other sexually transmitted viral infestations

(Source: WHO, 2000.)

nation? Informed consent must be gained from the patient, and/or the appropriate guardian in the case of those men with learning disability, for example. The patient may wish to ask questions and time must be set aside for him to do this and for the nurse to provide him with answers.

An understanding of the function and anatomy of the male genitalia is required if the nurse is to conduct the examination in a competent and confident manner. Figure 7.1 (below) provides an overview of the male genitourinary tract.

Guidance concerning intimate examinations has been produced by the Royal College of Obstetricians and Gynaecologists (RCOG; 2002). Peate (2005b) provides a discussion of male genital examination in detail. Surprisingly, there are few published guidelines specifically related to examination of the male genitalia (Rogstad, 2003).

Examining the male genitalia may make some patients and nurses feel uneasy, and there may be a concern if, for example, the patient experiences an erection while the examination is in progress. If this does occur, the nurse should explain that this is a normal physiological reaction and the examination should continue and the nurse should proceed in a professional and composed manner (Bickley, 2002).

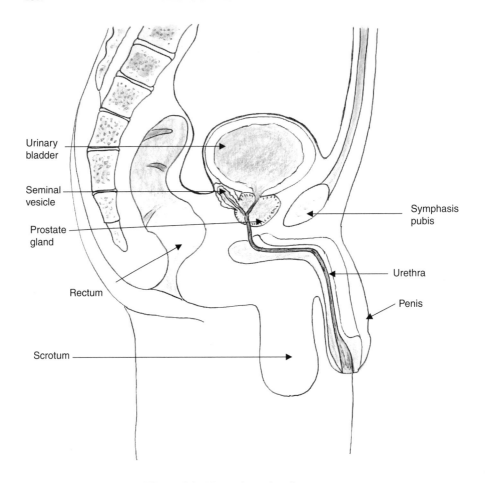

Figure 7.1. The male genitourinary tract

Privacy and dignity must be protected at all times during the examination; the nurse should encourage the patient to relax as much as possible. The nurse's room where the examination is to take place should be warm and it must be free from any disturbances (Collins, 2004). A holistic assessment is required and the nurse should endeavour to respect any cultural customs or traditions (Dean, 2005). A good light source is needed for the nurse to observe the patient adequately (Estes, 2002). All universal precautions apply and gloves should be worn whenever there might be contact with bodily fluids, mucous membranes, or non-intact skin (RCN, 2005; Wilson, 2006); wearing gloves can also highlight the strictly clinical nature of the examination.

Before and during examination, Peate (2005b) suggests that the nurse should:

- explain to the patient why the examination is needed and what technique s/he intends to use, that is, will the patient be expected to stand/sit/lie?

- give the patient an opportunity to ask questions;
- ensure that the patient gives his consent for the examination to take place; local policy may require the nurse to gain written consent prior to the examination/investigation;
- offer information and give explanations in such a manner that the patient understands and has a clear idea of what to expect;
- provide the patient with the opportunity to have a chaperone present during the investigation regardless of organizational constraints; if a chaperone cannot be supplied, then the nurse must consider, with the patient's agreement, delaying the investigation to a later time in the day or a later date; details of this discussion should be recorded; if the patient refuses an examination this should be documented in the notes;
- not assist the patient in removing clothing unless assistance is required;
- ensure that there are no unnecessary interruptions;
- make certain that the patient's privacy and dignity are protected;
- take into account the wishes of the patient.

The appropriate equipment should be available in the room prior to the examination beginning; this will avoid having to stop the examination if any additional equipment is required. The reason for the examination, the site of the infection and the investigation required determine the exact type of equipment that will be required. For the male patient, French (2004) suggests the following equipment:

- a plastic loop for insertion into the urethra for specimen collection and analysis;
- urine collection apparatus for urinalysis, microscopy, sensitivity and culture;
- Dacron-tipped throat swab;
- Proctoscope for rectal examination and a plastic loop for specimen collection and analysis for those men who report anal sex;
- specific equipment for analysis of prostatic fluid that has been expressed via the urethra following direct prostate massage.

As STIs are often found in conjunction with other STIs, the confirmation of one infection should be followed by other tests for other infections. Matthews and Macaulay (2006) suggest that regardless of the diagnosis, even when this is pubic lice for example, other tests for other infections should be carried out.

SYPHILIS

Syphilis is caused by infection from *Treponema palladium*. This is a mucocutaneous STI. Syphilis is divided into:

- primary
- secondary
- tertiary (early and late syphilis).

The primary stage often consists of a painless single ulcer (chancre) at the site of inoculation; this may be accompanied by regional lymphadenopathy. The chancre may go unnoticed by the patient as it is often asymptomatic. Often the chancre is classically located in the anogenital region. The chancre may also be atypical; for example, they may be multiple, painful and purulent.

The secondary stage has many clinical manifestations (multi-system involvement) and they include a generalized polymorphic rash (this is often noted on the soles and palms – usually the rash is non-itchy), mouth ulcers, condylomata lata, mucocutaneous lesions, patchy alopecia, generalized lymphadenopathy, meningitis, splenomegaly and hepatitis.

The third stage is a non-infectious stage. Patients rarely present with tertiary syphilis. Manifestations include gummatous syphilis, neuro syphilis and cardiovascular syphilis. This latent stage can be divided into early and late syphilis.

SITES OF INFECTION

- genitalia
- anal region
- fingers (rare)
- oral cavity
- eye lid
- nipple
- any part of the skin or mucous membrane.

MODES OF TRANSMISSION

Syphilis is primarily transmitted sexually, with an incubation period of up to 9–90 days (see Table 7.7). Vertical transmission from mother to foetus can occur at any stage.

Table 7.7. Classification and stages of syphilitic infection

Time after exposure	Stage of infection
9–90 days	Primary
6 weeks to 6 months	Secondary
2 years	Latent (early)
Over 2 years	Latent (late)
3–20 years	Neuro syphilis
Over 10–40 years	Cardiovascular syphilis
3–12 years	Gummatous syphilis

(Source: Adler and French, 2004)

DIAGNOSIS

A detailed sexual health history should be taken. The patient should be asked about the presence of ulcers and if these are single or multiple, painful or painless, rash, joint pain and malaise. Careful physical examination is required paying attention to lymph node enlargement. The buccal mucosa, palate and tonsils should also be examined for signs of ulceration. Conlon and Snydman (2004) maintain that diagnosis must be confirmed by laboratory tests.

If the general practice does not have the appropriate facilities, it may be advisable to refer the patient to a local GUM clinical where further investigation, treatment and partner notification can be undertaken (Khot and Polmear, 2006). Syphilis serology is always required in line with local policy as most cases of syphilis are detected on serological testing (Clutterbuck, 2004). Swabs can be taken from the ulcer/erosion site; the swab should be obtained using the materials supplied in commercial testing kits, and transported in the medium provided in the kit. Firm but gentle pressure is required to take the swab from the base of the ulcer in order to obtain a satisfactory sample. The specimen is usually taken for herpes simplex identification also.

TREATMENT

Penicillin is the drug of choice for all stages of syphilis. Table 7.8 (below) describes the drugs used in the treatment for some stages of syphilitic infection.

PARTNER NOTIFICATION

The patient should be encouraged to refer sexual partners for assessment and, if appropriate, treatment. Referral to a GUM clinic for partner notification may be required (Khot and Polmear, 2006).

ISSUES TO BE CONSIDERED

Syphilis is strongly associated with an increased risk of HIV transmission; it is not uncommon for a simultaneous diagnosis of syphilis and HIV to be made (Clutterbuck, 2004). The patient should also be asked to undergo tests for other potentially coexisting STIs, for example, gonorrhoea, chlamydial infection, HIV and hepatitis serology if indicated.

Treatment reactions can occur, such as the Jarisch–Herxheimer reaction; this acute reaction may occur approximately eight hours after treatment of early syphilis and resolve within a day. The patient may complain of:

- myalgia
- fever

Table 7.8. Standard treatment for some forms of syphilis

Stage of infection	Standard treatment	Alternatives	Points for consideration
Primary and secondary	Benzathine penicillin 2.4 megaunits intramuscularly as a single dose or aqueous procaine penicillin 600 000 units intramuscularly per day for 10 days	Doxycycline 100 mg orally twice per day for 14 days	• May require daily injection • Injections can be painful • There are treatment reactions • Use of doxycycline does not necessitate injections
Latent early (less than two years)	Benzathine penicillin 2.4 megaunits intramuscularly as a single dose or aqueous procaine penicillin 600 000 units intramuscularly per day for 10 days	Doxycycline 100 mg orally twice per day for 14 days	
Latent late (more than two years)	Aqueous procaine penicillin 900 000 units intramuscularly per day for 17 days or Benzathine penicillin 2.4 megaunits intramuscularly weekly over two weeks (three injections)	Doxycycline 100 mg orally twice per day for 30 days	

(Source: Adapted from Adler and French, 2004)

- chills
- rigors
- worsening of lesions.

The patient may require aspirin in order to relieve the symptoms. In more severe cases serious complications can arise and the patient should be hospitalized.

Procaine psychosis – the result of intravenous procaine injection and a hypersensitive reaction to penicillin – may also occur. If these drugs are given in the general practice the nurse must always ensure that resuscitation equipment and drugs are available prior to treating the patient with parenteral penicillin (Clutterbuck, 2004).

The nurse should advise the patient to avoid unprotected sexual intercourse until they and their partner(s) have completed their treatment. Follow-up is required to determine if the patient has completed treatment; often this is best managed in the GUM clinic. For those patients who have late syphilis they will require ongoing clinical care and assessment and this must be provided by the most appropriate clinician (Peate, 2005a). Repeat serology is also required.

GONORRHOEA

Gonorrhoea is the clinical disease that is a result of infection from *Neisseria gonorrhoeae*, a gram-negative diplococcus. Gonorrhoea is a frequently diagnosed STI. This is a highly infectious bacterial STI and is associated with significant morbidity.

SIGNS AND SYMPTOMS

Clinical manifestations may be systematic, local, uncomplicated or complicated. In men, uncomplicated local infections often occur urethrally. The patient may complain of dysuria, urethral discharge and epididymitis, with an accompanying tachycardia and pyrexia. Often the man will notice staining in his underwear as a result of mucopurulent or purulent discharge. This infection may also be asymptomatic. If the man engages in anal sex, then he can present with anal discharge with an accompanying perianal pain. Those who perform oral sex can present with pharyngeal infections, with many of these infections being asymptomatic.

MODES OF TRANSMISSION

Infection occurs when secretions through inoculation are transmitted from one mucous membrane to another. Often this occurs through sexual contact, for example, vaginal, anal and oral sex. Cross infection from the fingers to the eye may also happen as well as vertical transmission.

MAKING A DIAGNOSIS

A full sexual health history is needed to help the nurse make a definitive diagnosis; however, confirmation is made by confirming the presence of *Neisseria gonorrhoeae*. Specimens can be collected from the:

- urethra
- rectum
- oropharynx.

The practice nurse must adhere to local guidelines and policy with regards to specimen collection and transportation in order to ensure that a correct diagnosis is made.

TREATMENT AND NURSING CARE

The patient will require the nurse to provide him with detailed explanations regarding his condition. Verbal explanations should be supplemented with written information produced in such a way that the patient understands and can assimilate it. There are commercially produced leaflets that are available for the public, for example, those produced by the Family Planning Association. Sexual intercourse should be avoided until both the patient and his partner(s) have been treated and have attended for follow-up.

Treatment for each person is provided following an individual assessment, with the drug of choice being ciprofloxacin 500 mg orally as a single dose or ofloxacin 400 mg as a single dose. The causative organism *Neisseria gonorrhoeae* can complicate the treatment as the organism is able to develop multiple resistance to antimicrobial agents (Health Development Agency, 2004). The prescribing of antimicrobials must take into account local antimicrobial sensitivities if treatment is to be effective.

POTENTIAL COMPLICATIONS

When the infection transluminally spreads from the urethra, it can involve the epididymis and the prostate gland. Skin lesions, as a result of disseminated gonoccocal infection, can occur and may result in athralgia and tenosynovitis (Association for Genitourinary Medicine and the Medical Society for the Study of Venereal Diseases, 2002).

NOTIFICATION OF PARTNERS

The practice nurse should encourage the patient to refer his sexual partner(s) and contacts for assessment and evaluation in order for treatment to be offered if appropriate. The practice nurse may need to contact an experienced sexual health adviser for guidance regarding methods and ways of contacting and notifying partners.

CHLAMYDIA

Chlamydia trachomatis is the organism responsible for the infection chlamydia. This organism is an intracellular pathogen and types D to K are found in genital infections.

SITES OF INFECTION

- urethra
- rectum
- pharynx
- conjunctiva.

MODES OF TRANSMISSION

The primary mode of infection is through vaginal intercourse. The infection can also be transmitted through anal and orogenital sex. Vertical transmission can also occur.

SIGNS AND SYMPTOMS

It is estimated that 50% of men with chlamydia are asymptomatic. There may be urethral discharge with subsequent underwear staining. Some men have severe dysuria while others may not. Anal discharge and anorectal discomfort may occur where there is rectal infection. The patient may inform the nurse that he has a sore throat; however; in many cases of pharyngeal infection these are asymptomatic.

POTENTIAL COMPLICATIONS

There are many potential complications associated with chlamydial infection. The list below is not exhaustive and identifies some of the complications for both male and female patients:

- pelvic inflammatory disease
- Fitz-Hugh–Curtis syndrome
- tubal damage
- long-term pelvic pain
- vertical transmission to neonate
- epididymo-orchitis
- Reiter's syndrome.

Untreated chlamydia may make a person with HIV more infectious. Chlamydia has the ability to cause breaks in the mucous membranes of the affected area and as a result increases the number of HIV-infected cells in those areas (Men's Health Forum, 2006).

NOTIFICATION OF PARTNERS

The patient should be offered the opportunity to refer his partners(s) and contacts for assessment and treatment. Advice may need to be sought from an experienced sexual health adviser.

SPECIFIC ISSUES ASSOCIATED WITH THE MALE PATIENT AND CHLAMYDIA

According to the Men's Health Forum (2006) the most effective way to reduce chlamydia is to prevent infections. It suggests that the most effective way to do this is to improve public awareness and increase the use and availability of barrier contraception.

It has already been noted that chlamydia is the most common STI that is diagnosed at GUM clinics. As a result of this the public health White Paper *Choosing Health: Making Healthier Choices* (DH, 2004) has made sexual health one of its priority areas. Additional funding has been made available as well as a stronger commitment to speed up the rollout of the National Chlamydia Screening Programme. The programme aims to increase the level of screening of the population overall; however, the programme has failed (thus far) to screen men in large enough numbers to stem the number of infections (Men's Health Forum, 2006).

The *National Chlamydia Screening Programme Report* (DH, 2005) demonstrates that only 12.5 % of those tested under the National Chlamydia Screening Programme were men. Improved screening in non-traditional settings is central to increasing the number of men who are screened and treated. Some general practices currently offer screening to their practice population; however, these services do not always consider gender. Providing screening services aimed particularly at men could improve uptake; by making determined efforts to increase the numbers of men screened, the practice can contribute to the overall reduction in the rates of infection. If men remain infected with chlamydia, they will continue to infect women as a result of the symptomatic nature of the infection in men. Women who are screened and treated for chlamydia will only be re-infected by men who are failing to be offered screening.

CONCLUSION

There is evidence to suggest that a significant number of patients with STIs first present in primary care (Clutterbuck and Ross, 1997). It is imperative that the practice nurse is fully conversant with the more common STIs that any patient in the practice may present with. It is unwise to limit recognition of an STI on the basis of discharge only; the symptoms of STIs are varied and subtle, and some are insidious in nature. Delivering the Government's sexual health strategy is exciting, and at the same time a challenging undertaking for all of those who work in the primary care setting, including the practice nurse.

It is widely accepted that assessment and history-taking are central to making a correct diagnosis; this is also true of sexual health assessment and sexual health history-taking. Embarrassment, lack of knowledge and skills are issues that can impede sexual health history-taking. The more often the practice nurse carries out a holistic assessment of the patient including assessment of sexual health, the more proficient s/he will become.

HIV is one of the most important communicable diseases in the UK. HIV causes serious mortality and significant morbidity. HIV is now treatable but it must be remembered that there is no cure and currently no vaccine available. The provision of high-quality STI diagnosis and management (including care for those with HIV) in the primary care setting is possible.

REFERENCES

Adler, M. and French, P. (2004) Syphilis: clinical features, diagnosis, and management. In (eds A. Adler, F. Cowan, P. French, H. Mitchell, and J. Richens) *ABC of Sexually Transmitted Infections*, 5th edn, BMJ Books, London, pp. 49–54, Chapter 12.

Association for Genitourinary Medicine and the Medical Society for the Study of Venereal Diseases (2002) *Clinical Effectiveness Guidelines*, MSSVD, London.

Barnard, E.J. (2006) Better practice. *AIDS Treatment Update*, **158**, 4–7.

Bickley, L.S. (2002) *Bates' Guide to Physical Examination and History Taking*, 8th edn, Lippincott, Philadelphia.

British Medical Association (2002) *Sexually Transmitted Infections*, BMA, London.

British Medical Association and NHS Confederation (2003) *Investing in General Practice: The New General Medical Services Contract*, BMA and NHS Confederation, London.

Carter, Y., Moss, C. and Weyman, A. (1998) *Royal College of General Practitioners Handbook of Sexual Health in Primary Care*, RCGP, London.

Clutterbuck, D. (2004) *Sexually Transmitted Infections and HIV*, Elsevier Mosby, Edinburgh.

Clutterbuck, D. and Ross, D. (1997) Sources of information on genitourinary medicine clinics. *International Journal of STD and AIDS*, **8** (8), 532.

Collins, E.M. (2004) Male genitalia, hernia and rectal examination (ed. Altman, G.B.) *Delmar's Fundamental and Advanced Nursing Skills*, Thompson, New York, pp. 90–98, Chapter 1.

Conlon, C.P. and Snydman, D.R. (2004) *Mosby's Color Atlas and Text of Infectious Diseases*, Mosby, Edinburgh.

Dean, J. (2005) Examination of patients with sexual problems (ed. J. Tomlinson) *ABC of Sexual Health*, 2nd edn, BMJ, London, pp. 17–24, Chapter 5.

Department of Health (2000) *The NHS Plan: A Plan for Investment, A Plan for Reform*, DH, London.

Department of Health (2001) *Better Prevention, Better Services, Better Sexual Health: The National Strategy for Sexual Health and HIV*, DH, London.

Department of Health (2004) *Choosing Health: Making Healthier Choices*, The Stationery Office, London.

Department of Health (2005) *National Chlamydia Screening Programme Report 2004/05: Looking Back, Moving Forward, Annual Report of the NCSP in England, 2005/05*, DH, London.

Department of Health (2006) *Our Health, Our Care, Our Say: A New Direction for Community Services*, DH, London.

Donovan, C., Hadley, A. and Jones, M. (2000) *Confidentiality and Young People: Toolkit for General Practice, Primary Care Groups and Trusts*, Royal College of General Practitioners and the Brook Advisory Centre, London.

Elford, J., Anderson, J., Ibrahim, F. and Bukutu, C. (2006) Discrimination Experienced by People Living with HIV. *HIV Medicine*, **7**(Supplement 1), abstract, 93.

Epstein, O., Perkin, G.D., de Bono, D.P. and Cookson, J. (1997) *Clinical Examination*, 2nd edn, Mosby, London.

Estes, M.E.Z. (2002) *Health Assessment and Physical Examination*, 2nd edn, Thompson, New York.

French, P. (2004) Examination techniques and clinical sampling. In (eds M. Adler, F. Cowan, P. French, H. Mitchell, and J. Richens) *ABC of Sexually Transmitted Infections*, 5th edn, BMJ Books, London, pp. 15–16, Chapter 4.

Haley, N., Maheux, B., Rivard, M. and Gervais, A. (1999) Sexual risk assessment and counselling in primary care: how involved are general practitioners and obstetrician-gynaecologists? *American Journal of Public Health*, **89**, 899–902.

Health Development Agency (2004) *Prevention of Sexually Transmitted Infections (STIs): A Review of Reviews into the Effectiveness of Non-Clinical Interventions: Evidence Briefing*, HAD, London.

Health Protection Agency (2006) *All New Diagnosis Made at GUM Clinics: 1996–2005. United Kingdom and Country Specific Tables*, HPA, London.

House of Commons Health Committee (2003) *Sexual Health: Third Report of Session 2002–2003*, The Stationery Office, London.

Hughes, L. (2004) Women's health (eds J. Martin and J. Lucas) *Handbook of Practice Nursing*, 3rd edn, Churchill Livingstone, pp. 3–27, Chapter 1.

Johnson, A.M., Mercer, C.H., Erens, B. *et al.* (2002) Sexual behaviour in Britain: partnerships, practices and HIV risk behaviours, *Lancet*, **358**, 1835–1842.

Keogh, P., Weatherburn, P., Henderson, L. *et al.* (2004) *Doctoring Gay Men: Exploring the Contribution of General Practice*, Sigma, London.

Khot, A. and Polmear, A. (2006) *Practical General Practice: Guidelines for Effective Management*, 5th edn, Butterworth-Heinemann, London.

Low, N., Connell, P., McKevitt, C. *et al.* (2003) 'You Can't Tell by Looking': pilot study of a community-based intervention to detect asymptomatic sexually transmitted infections. *International Journal of STD and AIDS*, **14**, 830–834.

Madge, S., Olaitan, A., Mocroft, A. *et al.* (1997) Access to medical care one year prior to diagnosis in 100 HIV: positive women. *Family Practice*, **14** (3), 255–257.

Madge, S., Matthews, P., Singh, S. and Theobald, N. (2005) *HIV in Primary Care*, Medical Foundation for AIDS and Sexual Health, London.

Matthews, P. (1998) Sexual history taking primary care (eds Y. Carter, C. Moss and A. Weyman) *Royal College of General Practitioners Handbook of Sexual Health in Primary Care*, Royal College of General Practitioners and Family Planning Association, London, pp. 17–50, Chapter 2.

Matthews, P. (2006) The Diagnosis of HIV in a Primary Care Setting (eds T. Belfield, Y. Carter, P. Matthews, C. Moss and A. Weyman) *The Handbook of Sexual Health in Primary Care*. Family Planning Association, London, pp. 187–208, Chapter 7.

Matthews, P. and Fletcher, J. (2001) Sexually transmitted infection in primary care: a need for education. *British Journal of General Practice*, **51**, 52–56.

Matthews, P. and Macaulay, H. (2006) Sexually transmissible infections: a primary care perspective (eds T. Belfield, Y. Carter, P. Matthews, C. Moss and A. Weyman) *The Handbook of Sexual Health in Primary Care*. Family Planning Association, London, pp. 155–186, Chapter 6.

McAndrew, S. (2000) The process: acute care (eds H. Wilson, and S. McAndrew) *Sexual Health: Foundations for Practice*, Bailliere Tindall, London, pp. 219–230, Chapter 12.

Medical Foundation for Sexual Health (2004) *National Recommended Standards for Sexual Health Services (A Draft Document for Consultation)*, Medical Foundation for Sexual Health and the Department of Health, London.

Men's Health Forum (2006) *Men and Chlamydia: Putting Men to the Test*, MHF, London.

National AIDS Manual (2006) *GPs and Primary Care: Factsheet 62*, NAM, London.

Nursing and Midwifery Council (2004) *Code of Professional Conduct: Standards for Conduct, Performance and Ethics*, NMC, London.

Nusbaum, M.R.H. and Hamilton, C.D. (2002) The proactive sexual health history. *American Family Physician*, **66** (9), 1705–1712.

Peate, I. (2005a) *Manual of Sexually Transmitted Infections*, Whurr, London.

Peate, I. (2005b) Examining adult male genitalia: providing a guide for the nurse. *British Journal of Nursing*, **14** (1), 36–40.

Rogstad, K. (2003) *Intimate Examinations in Genitourinary Medicine Clinics*, Royal College of Physicians, London.

Royal College of Obstetricians and Gynaecologists (2002) *Gynaecological Examinations: Guidelines for Specialist Practice*, RCOG, London.

Royal College of Nursing (2003) *Chaperoning: The Role of the Nurse and the Rights of Patients*, RCN, London.

Royal College of Nursing (2005) *Good Practice in Infection Prevention and Control: Guidance for Nursing Staff*, RCN, London.

Skelton, J.R. and Matthews, P.M. (2001) Teaching sexual history taking to health professionals in primary care. *Medical Education*, **35**, 603–608.

Terence Higgins Trust (2004) *Blueprint for the future: modernising HIV and sexual health services: A Policy Report*, THT, London.

Tomlinson, J. (1998) The ABC of sexual health: taking a sexual history. *British Medical Journal*, **317**, 1573–1576.

Tomlinson, J.M. (2005) Taking a sexual health history (ed. J. M. Tomlinson) *ABC of Sexual Health*, 2nd edn, BMJ Books, London, pp. 13–16, Chapter 4.

Verhoeven, V., Bovijn, K., Helder, A. *et al.* (2003) Discussing STIs: doctors are from Mars, patients from Venus. *Family Practice*, **20** (1), 11–15.

Wakely, G. and Chambers, R. (2002) *Sexual Health Matters in Primary Care*, Radcliffe, Oxford.

Wakely, G., Cunnion, M. and Chambers, R. (2003) *Improving Sexual Health Advice*, Radcliffe, Oxford.

Wellings, K., Nanchalal, K., Macdowall, F W. *et al.* (2001) Sexual behaviour in Britain: early heterosexual experience. *Lancet*, **358**, 1843–1850.

Wilson, J. (2006) *Infection Control in Clinical Practice*, 3rd edn, Bailliere Tindall, London.

World Health Organization (2000) *Promotion of Sexual Health: Recommendations for Action*, WHO, Antigua, Guatemala.

8 Osteoporosis

INTRODUCTION

Traditionally osteoporosis is often associated with women. This, according to Lim and Fitzpatrick (2004), may be because of the higher prevalence in women. Many men and healthcare professionals view osteoporosis as a woman's disease. The risk of osteoporotic fracture of the hip, forearm or spine in men is 1 in 12 (Tuck and Francis, 2002).

The impact of fractures as a result of osteoporosis can have a devastating effect on the quality of life. A large number of men are unable to return to their former lifestyles and many require ongoing support after the event has occurred (Bilezikian, 1999). Brown (2006) suggests that the primary care team are in the best position to be able to identify and treat patients who have had a previous fracture to reduce the burden of further fractures. Proctor (2004) suggests that osteoporosis is a metabolic disease resulting in loss of bone mass, particularly in post-menopausal women. Khot and Polmear (2006) describe osteoporosis as a disorder of diminished bone density and degenerate microarchitecture, leading to increased fragility and risk of fracture. The skeleton is affected, the bones weaken and break, and bone breakdown occurs faster than bone is being built. See Figure 8.1 (below) for the bones of the skeleton. The skeleton provides support for the body, protects vital organs and stores active minerals, in particular calcium. The skeleton also acts as an anchor for the muscles.

This chapter aims to provide the practice nurse with an overview of male osteoporosis in a practical and informative manner based on available information. The condition is defined and a discussion is provided related to the measurement of bone mineral density, epidemiology, aetiology and the pathogenesis associated with osteoporosis. Risk factors are described and how a diagnosis is made is outlined. The importance of pain management in the acute and chronic stages is emphasized. The role of the practice nurse in relation to prevention and treatment, and non-pharmacological and pharmacological interventions, are considered.

DEFINING OSTEOPOROSIS

Literally, osteoporosis means porous bones and is characterized by a reduction in bone density. This is associated with skeletal fragility and an increased risk of fracture following minimal trauma (Tuck and Francis, 2002). Campion and Maricic (2003) suggest that osteoporosis is defined as a decrease in bone mass greater

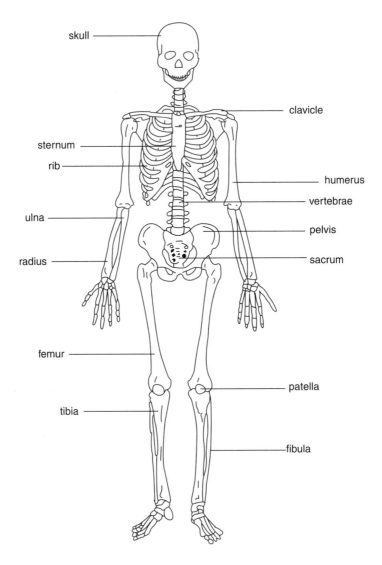

Figure 8.1. Bones of the human skeleton. (Source: http://www.learning-connections.co.uk/ curric/cur_pri/h_body/handson/answers/hands_1.html (accessed 30/01/07))

than would be anticipated for a person's sex, age and race. Working definitions of osteoporosis are usually based on the measurement of bone mineral density (National Osteoporosis Society, 2002). The World Health Organization (WHO; 1994) defines osteoporosis as based on bone mineral density of the spine, hip or forearm and is referred to as T-scores.

MEASURING BONE DENSITY

Prior to discussing the measurement of bone density it must be stated that the World Health Organization's definition of osteopenia and osteoporosis are bone mineral density measurements based on epidemiological studies of Caucasian women in their sixties (National Osteoporosis Society, 2002). This important fact should be borne in mind when considering the bone density measurements of men. Most available information regarding diagnosis and treatment is derived from research on the older female Caucasian population. Osteopenia is defined by the World Health Organization (WHO, 1994) as a state of reduced bone mineral density intermediate between normal bone density and osteoporosis.

There are many ways of measuring bone mineral density. Advances in technology now mean that the diagnosis of osteoporosis prior to fracture occurring is possible through dual energy X-ray absorptiometry (DXA) (Tuck and Francis, 2002). Several different techniques can be used to measure bone mineral density including quantitative computer tomography (QCT) and quantitative ultrasound (QUS). Bone mineral density is the most appropriate way of identifying osteoporosis. The examination – a scan – is non-intrusive and painless; the scan indicates bone strength. Bone mineral density demonstrates if there is a risk of fracture. As bone mineral density decreases, so the risk of fracture increases (Bates, 2001).

Calculation of T-score is carried out by taking the difference between a patient's measured bone mineral density and the mean bone mineral density of healthy young adults at the age of peak bone mass. This is matched for ethnicity and gender and is expressed by detailing the difference relative to the young adult population standard deviation (SD):

$$\text{T-score} = \frac{\text{Measured Bone Mineral Density} - \text{Young adult mean Bone Mineral Density}}{\text{Young adult standard deviation}}$$

The T-score indicates the difference between the patient's bone mineral density and ideal peak bone mass achieved by the young adult. Using bone mineral density allows diagnosis to be made, to identify those at risk and to monitor the effects of osteoporosis treatment.

Normal T-scores are expressed as within 1 SD (+1 or −1) of the young adult mean. T-scores that are below the norm are indicated by using negative numbers. A score of −1 to −2.5 SD indicates low bone mass or osteopenia. If a patient has a score that is less than −2.5 SD, this is considered as osteoporosis (see Table 8.1 below).

For the test the patient should be advised to wear clothes that do not have any metal buttons or buckles; jewellery, such as a bracelet (if the wrist is being scanned), should be removed. The patient lies on the couch in the X-ray department for approximately 10–20 minutes and the X-ray gantry passes over the area to be assessed, which can be the lower spine, hip or forearm. The test is usually painless; however, if they have back pain, the patient may experience discomfort while lying still on their back on the couch.

Table 8.1. Classification of DXA scan results

T-score	Fracture risk
Low bone mass (osetopenia) T-score = −1.0 to −2.5	Above average risk
Osteoporosis T-score ⩽ −2.5	High risk
Established osteoporosis T-score ⩽ −2.5 and one or more fractures	Very high risk

The Z-score is another score; this score expresses bone mineral density with patients of the same age; this score is useful in the evaluation of treatment. The age-matched score compares the patient's bone density to what would be expected in a person of the same age, sex, ethnic origin and size:

$$\text{Z-score} = \frac{\text{Measured Bone Mineral Density} - \text{Age-matched mean Bone Mineral Density}}{\text{Age-matched standard deviation}}$$

If a patient has a Z-score of less than −1, s/he is substantially at risk of fracture compared to a person of the same age, sex, ethnic origin and size who has a Z-score of 0 (National Osteoporosis Society, 2002). Z-scores are not as widely used as T-scores.

The prevalence of osteoporosis and incidence of fracture vary also by race/ethnicity. Racial differences in bone mass have been noted. African Americans have a higher bone mineral density than Caucasians; they also sustain fewer fractures (National Institute of Health, 2000).

EPIDEMIOLOGY

The numbers of men presenting with fractures as a result of osteoporosis or associated with osteoporosis is rising. This may be the result of increasing life expectancy and lifestyle changes – for example, reduced physical activity and an increase in male sedentary work styles (Francis, 2000). The number of men with osteoporosis is unknown. It is anticipated that the rates of hip fractures (for the whole population) will increase from 46 000 in 1985 to 117 000 in 2016 (Dennison, Cole and Cooper, 2005).

Lim and Fitzpatrick (2004) consider osteoporosis from an epidemiological perspective, stating that it can be seen as a disease that arises from the interaction of multiple aetiological factors in a genetically susceptible host (see Figure 8.2 below).

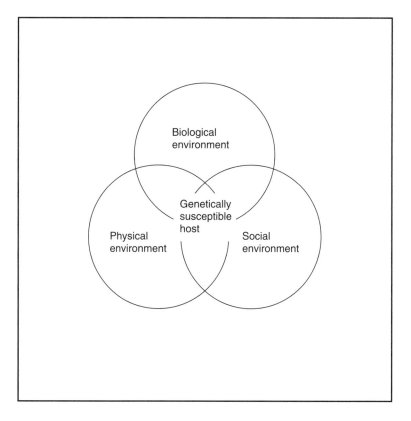

Figure 8.2. Multiple aetiological factors in a genetically susceptible host in relation to osetoporotic fractures. (Source: Lim and Fitzpatrick, 2004)

BIOLOGICAL ENVIRONMENT

- advancing age
- sex hormone deficiency
- low body mass index
- medications
- chronic disease.

PHYSICAL ENVIRONMENT

- immobility
- gait difficulty
- environmental hazards.

SOCIAL ENVIRONMENT

- smoking
- alcohol abuse
- physical inactivity.

Tuck, Raj and Summers (2002) suggest a man's lifetime risk of an osetoporotic fracture developing is 1 in 12; for women this is 1 in 3. The National Osteoporosis Society (2005a) suggests that in men over 50 years of age this is 1 in 5. The consequence of these fractures results in considerable morbidity, excess mortality and health and social services costs (Tuck and Francis, 2002); the importance of this disease cannot be underestimated.

It has been estimated that in the UK 50000 forearm fractures, 40000 vertebral fractures and 60000 hip fractures occur per year. Approximately 20% of all symptomatic vertebral fractures and 30% of all hip fractures occur in men (Eastell et al., 1998). Fractures of the forearm are lower in males than females; those men with a forearm fracture are at risk of vertebral and hip fracture (Cuddihy et al., 1999). While forearm fractures are less common in the male they can be associated with higher morbidity and mortality than in women (Center et al., 1999). Tuck, Raj and Summers (2002) demonstrate that men with distal forearm fractures have been shown to have lower bone mineral density than age-matched control subjects.

OSTEOPOROSIS PATHOGENESIS

In order to understand osteoporosis the nurse will need to learn and understand about bone. Most bone is made of collagen and is living tissue with the ability to regenerate; it is as hard as iron but as light as wood. Collagen provides a soft framework and is a protein; strength and hardness are provided for the framework in the form of calcium phosphate, which is a mineral. Bone, because of the combination of collagen and calcium phosphate, is strong yet flexible, which means that it has the ability to withstand stress. Bones and teeth account for over 99% of calcium, the remaining 1% is distributed between the extracellular fluid and intracellular compartment. Feedback mechanisms control the concentration of calcium ions in the blood; feedback is regulated by parathyroid gland activity: when blood calcium levels are decreased, parathyroid hormone is secreted, promoting bone resorption and reabsorption of calcium at the renal tubule (Tanna, 2005; Waugh and Grant, 2006).

Cortical and trabecular bone are found in the body. These two types of bone have particular properties. Cortical bone is dense and compact and forms the outer shell of the bone. The inner aspect of the bone is made up of trabecular bone, which is spongy and porous and has a honeycomb appearance. Trabecular bone can also be known as cancellous bone. It has a network of thin bars or plates of bone – the trabeculae – which are interspaced with marrow (see Figures 8.3 and 8.4 below).

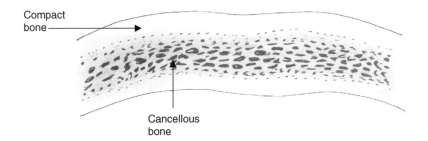

Compact
bone

Cancellous
bone

Figure 8.3. Structure of a flat bone

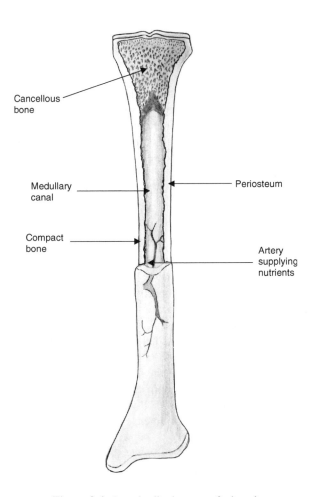

Cancellous
bone

Medullary
canal

Periosteum

Compact
bone

Artery
supplying
nutrients

Figure 8.4. Longitudinal aspect of a long bone

BONE REMODELLING

The networks of bone described above are being continually renewed throughout life. This is a continuous, two-part process known as remodelling. It is estimated that each year the healthy skeleton undergoes 10% of remodelling, which occurs when bone is resorbed and then replaced with new bone – resorption and formation. During the resorption phase, the old bone tissue is broken down and removed by cells known as osteoclasts. When new bone is being formed to replace the old bone, it is the osteoblasts that are responsible for new bone formation. Osteoblast and osteoclast activity (bone homoeostasis), degrading and replenishing bone, is regulated by a number of hormones:

- calcitonin
- parathyroid hormone
- vitamin D
- testosterone
- oestrogen.

This remodelling activity is usually perfectly matched; however, when this homeostatic mechanism is disrupted – for example, when more bone is destroyed faster than it is formed – osteoporosis occurs, increasing the risk of fractures.

Over a man's lifetime approximately half of the bone mass achieved during growth to young adulthood is lost. The same amount is lost by women but men compensate better by laying down more bone on the outer surface of the bones during natural bone remodelling (Seeman, 1995); however, the compensatory mechanisms at play fail to counteract the loss of bone on the inside surface.

AETIOLOGY

For approximately half the number of men who have been diagnosed with osteoporosis the cause is unknown (National Osteoporosis Society, 2005a). Osteoporosis can be either primary (idiopathic) or secondary to several identifiable causes. There are a number of factors that cause osteoporosis.

Primary osteoporosis is also known and defined as age-related or idiopathic reduction in bone mass (Lim and Fitzpatrick, 2004). Idiopathic osteoporosis is different from age-related osteoporosis in so far as the former occurs more in younger men.

Men are at increased risk of osteoporosis from secondary causes (Scottish Intercollegiate Guidelines Network, 2003). Bilezikian (1999) notes that the three main causes of secondary osteoporosis in men accounting for 40–50% of all cases of osteoporosis are:

- long-term glucocorticosteroid use
- hypogonadism
- chronic alcohol use.

In men and women peak bone mass occurs around their early 20s (Bonjour *et al.*, 1991). Bilezikian (1999) states that peak bone mass is a major determinant of osteoporosis as it is the reservoir that will be drawn upon as the skeleton begins to erode. Tuck and Francis (2002) and Campion and Maricic (2003) suggest that this is influenced by:

- hereditary factors
- nutrition
- hormones
- environment
- exercise.

Campion and Maricic (2003) point out that age-related bone loss can be influenced by:

- low body mass index
- smoking
- alcohol consumption
- physical inactivity
- impaired vitamin D production and metabolism
- secondary hyperparathyroidism.

Sex steroids play an important part in the maintenance of bone density in men; rapid bone loss occurs, for example, after orchidectomy for prostate cancer (Campion and Maricic, 2003). In men with hip fractures, Anderson *et al.* (1998) note that approximately 50 % of those men are hypogonadal. Falahati-Nini *et al.* (2000) point out that oestradiol appears to be the most dominant sex hormone regulating bone resorption.

RISK FACTORS

The risk of osteoporotic fracture is determined by skeletal and non-skeletal factors (Francis, 2001). It is difficult to provide an evidence base with regards to risk factors that justify further investigation as the evidence is lacking; there are a number of risk factors and the more of these that are present the more at risk is the patient (Lydick *et al.*, 1998).

It has already been discussed above that lack of male hormone is a risk factor for osteoporosis in men. Table 8.2 (below) provides details of more factors that can be considered by the practice nurse to identify those men at risk.

Seeman (2004) has produced an osteoporosis risk test for men. The practice nurse can adapt the test and use it when assessing the male patient (see Table 8.3 below).

After the patient completes the test the nurse can then begin to engage with the patient discussing lifestyle changes and suggesting further investigations should they be needed. The opportunity can then arise where current medications can be reviewed and an in-depth assessment can be made.

Table 8.2. Factors to be considered in order to identify those men at risk of osteoporosis

High-risk causes

- History of non-traumatic fracture (hip, vertebrae or wrist)
- Osteopenia seen on plain radiograph
- Glucocorticoid use of 5 mg or more per day for longer than six months
- Hypogonadism (glucocorticoid-induced or following orchidectomy)
- Hyperparathyroidism

Medium-risk causes

- Anticonvulsant drug use (phenytoin or phenobarbital)
- Excessive alcohol consumption
- Tobacco use
- Rheumatoid or other inflammatory arthritis
- Multiple myeloma or lymphoma
- Hypothyroidism or hyperthyroidism
- Conditions associated with increased risk of falling (i.e. hemiparesis, dementia)
- Family history of osteoporosis

Infrequent causes

- Cushing's syndrome
- Chronic liver or kidney disease
- Low body mass index
- Pernicious anaemia
- Gastric resection
- Gastrointestinal disorders

(Source: Adapted from Tuck and Francis, 2002; Campion and Maricic, 2003)

Table 8.3. Osteoporosis risk test for men

1. Have either of your parents broken a hip after a minor bump of fall? Yes No	5. Do you regularly drink heavily (in excess of safe drinking limits)? Yes No
2. Have you broken a bone after a minor bump or fall? Yes No	6. Do you smoke more than 20 cigarettes a day? Yes No
3. Have you taken corticosteroid tablets (cortisone, prednisone) for more than 3 months? Yes No	7. Do you suffer frequently from diarrhoea (caused by problems such as coeliac disease or Crohn's disease)? Yes No
4. Have you lost more than 3 cm (just over one inch) in height? Yes No	8. Have you ever suffered from impotence, lack of libido or other symptoms related to low testosterone levels? Yes No

(Source: Seeman, 2004)

It is generally considered that bone loss and the resulting osteoporosis are the major causes of fractures after minimal trauma in the older person (Francis, 2001). Genetics and age increase an individual's risk of experiencing fracture, and parental history of fracture is a major risk factor. A large genetic component has been identified as a significant factor in risk; genetic predisposition is said to account for 80 % of variance in peak bone mass in males and females (Sutcliffe, 2001). There is a bimodal age distribution associated with the incidence of osteoporotic fractures with peaks in youth and old age (Seeman, 2004).

The practice nurse needs to be aware that, despite advances in identifying those men at risk of osteoporosis in order to target treatment more cost-effectively, the patient must also be encouraged to take their treatment and for the recommended duration. Compston and Seeman (2006) describe this as compliance and persistence; both compliance and persistence are poor in at least 50 % of patients during the first year of treatment for osteoporosis and in 80 % after three years (Caro *et al.*, 2004; Huybrechts, Ishak and Caro, 2006). Patient education provided by the practice nurse may improve compliance and persistence in relation to the effective management of osteoporosis.

OSTEOPOROSIS AND EATING DISORDERS

Anorexia nervosa is an eating disorder that can affect men (Chelvanayagam, 2006). Paterson (2004) estimates that approximately a third of people with an eating disorder are male. The condition is associated with low body weight, an intense fear of weight gain and an inaccurate perception of body size; bulimia nervosa has similarities, although there is not always such severe weight loss (National Osteoporosis Society, 2005b).

Those men who suffer with anorexia nervosa, and to a lesser degree bulimia nervosa, will have a bone mineral density that is lower than the average. The outcome may result in fractures occurring at young age. Bone loss in anorexia nervosa is related to several factors, for example, low levels of the hormone oestrogen, lack of adequate nourishment of the body and high levels of cortisol production.

An awareness of eating disorders in men and the possible relationship with anorexia nervosa and osteoporosis may help the nurse identify those men with eating disorders who may also be at risk of developing osteoporosis. Having identified those at risk the nurse, working with the patient and other healthcare professionals, can develop a plan of treatment that addresses the issues the patient presents with. The National Institute for Health and Clinical Excellence (NICE; 2004) has advocated that the use of hormones should not be used in children and adolescents who have eating disorders.

DIAGNOSIS

Often diagnosis is made after the patient has sustained a fracture, and sometimes diagnosis as a result of osteoporosis can be overlooked. In the past the only way to

Table 8.4. Some common diagnostic tests used in the investigation of osteoporosis

---

- History and physical examination
- Blood cell count
  - Erythrocyte sedimentation rate
  - Serum calcium, albumin, phosphate
  - Serum creatinine
  - Serum TSH
  - Alkaline phosphatase and liver transaminases
- Radiograph of lumbar and/or thoracic spinal column
- Bone mass measurement (i.e. DXA)
- 24-hour urine test

(Source: Adapted from Lim and Fitzpatrick, 2004)

diagnose osteoporosis in men was based on fractures that had occurred after minimal trauma. Diagnosis of osteoporosis in the male is usually made by bone densitometry in the context of signs or symptoms; a full clinical appraisal is required if the results of bone densitometry are to be interpreted accurately. Table 8.4 outlines some of the common diagnostic procedures that may be used in the investigation of osteoporosis (this is not exhaustive).

In men who present with fracture it is important that pathologics fractures are ruled out and to establish a differential diagnosis. Bone biopsy, suggests Bilezikian (1999), may be required in order to arrive at a differential diagnosis. Suspected pathologic fractures could be related to:

- osteomalacia
- osteomyelitis
- Paget's disease
- cancer (in particular lung and prostate disease)
- multiple myeloma.

Bone mineral density is a useful tool in determining risk of fracture as well as identifying those men who may benefit from intervention. Lim and Fitzpatrick (2004) state that currently there is no consensus regarding the optimal frequency of bone mineral density testing or the value of bone mineral density measurements for monitoring treatment.

The patient may complain of back pain and this may be accompanied by loss in height and kyphosis (All Party Parliamentary Osteoporosis Group, 2004). The effects of vertebral fractures and kyphosis can cause difficulties with the patient's ability to carry out the activities of living (Roper, Logan and Tierney, 1996), for example, eating and drinking, washing and dressing. The pain associated with fractures varies widely, and can have a debilitating effect on the person's quality of life and can result in severe physical dysfunction. The nurse must be aware of the many causes of back pain and should also have osteoporosis in mind. The patient may become shorter with a hunchback condition. Fracture occurs after minimal trauma and as a result of a trivial accident, for example, tripping over a kerb edge or an uneven paving stone.

PREVENTION AND TREATMENT

The burden of fractures, according to Seeman (2004), will grow as life expectancy increases; there will be more elderly people in the population who are predisposed to sustaining a fracture. The patient may experience immobility and an increase in dependence on others and for some men the result may be death. With respect to the personal distress described, pressures will also be placed on the finances of already overstretched healthcare budgets. It is estimated that £1.7 billion is spent on the consequences of osteoporotic fractures in the UK each year (Torgerson, Iglesias and Reid, 2001). Increasing awareness and instigating activities to reduce risk can prevent the issues described above from occurring.

Osteoporosis, according to Campion and Maricic (2003), is a clinically silent disease until fractures occur. Those men who are at risk of developing the disease and those who have the disease need to be identified early so that treatment can be instigated and the deleterious effects of the condition be reduced or eliminated. The National Osteoporosis Society (2006a) terms osteoporosis the 'silent epidemic'.

Currently prevention and early identification are the best forms of management (Wright, 2006). The treatment plan for a man with osteoporosis or who is at risk of developing it should include issues associated with nutrition, exercise and lifestyle. The practice nurse is ideally placed to prevent and identify those at risk as s/he provides primary care and has the ability to initiate measures to prevent fractures or further fractures occurring. Osteoporosis can be diagnosed and treatment is available. The Royal College of Physicians and the Bone and Tooth Society of Great Britain (2000) have produced guidance with respect to the management of osteoporosis. The results of the investigations (i.e. DEX) will determine what treatment is appropriate.

ANALGESIA

Pain is a feature of osteoporosis either immediately when a bone fractures or in the long term in association with hip, wrist or vertebral fractures; the pain of osteoporotic fractures can therefore be both acute and chronic. Over-the-counter analgesia may help some patients, and the pharmacist may be able to provide the patient with advice; some patients, however, require stronger analgesia. The use of the World Health Organization's analgesic ladder may be of value in helping to achieve optimum analgesia (WHO, 1996) (see Figure 8.5 below). Acute pain can be debilitating and the nurse may need to liaise with pain services; opiates may be required.

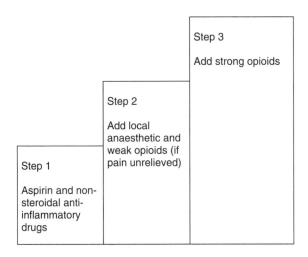

Figure 8.5. The World Health Organization's analgesic ladder (Source: WHO, 1996)

The use of the analgesic ladder is discussed by Khot and Polmear (2006). They recommend the following drugs:

Step 1   Non-opioid analgesia, for example, paracetamol and/or a non-steroidal anti-inflammatory drug

Step 2   Opioid for mild to moderate pain, for example, codeine or dihydrocodeine and/or paracetamol and a non-steroidal anti-inflammatory drug

Step 3   Opioid for moderate to severe pain, for example, morphine and/or paracetamol and a non-steroidal anti-inflammatory drug.

In the acute phase, rest and elevation of the affected limb is advocated; for some, relief can be found when using a hot-water bottle or ice packs; analgesia should be used regularly as opposed to on demand in order to prevent pain breakthrough. Fractures may need to be immobilized; plaster may be necessary as well as reduction of the fracture and use of splints. Admission to hospital may be needed and the practice nurse may be required to liaise with colleagues in the acute care sector to organize immobilization of the fracture and the management of acute pain.

Management of chronic pain can be a challenge; the use of non-steroidal anti-inflammatory drugs, physiotherapy and physical activity programmes may be of value. Transcutaneous Electrical Nerve Stimulation (TENS), a device that uses electrical signals to block or reduce pain impulses from getting to the brain, is used by many patients for many types of pain (Chartered Society of Physiotherapy, 2002). The apparatus can be applied to painful areas, for example, the hip or spine; often the patient will need help with this. The nurse may need to refer the patient to a physiotherapist for his/her advice. Complementary medicines, for example, aromatherapy, homeopathy and acupuncture may help to relieve pain and increase well-being (National Osteoporosis Society, 2001).

While it is vital that the physical effects associated with osteoporosis are managed effectively, it is also important to consider the impact the disease may have on the patient's psychological status (Scottish Intercollegiate Guidelines Network, 2003). The nurse must be aware that pain and lack of sleep, for example, have the potential to make the patient depressed. There may be a need for the nurse to refer the patient for clinical psychological assessment and interventions, and to consider the use of adjunctive therapies, for example, the use of antidepressants.

NON-PHARMACOLOGICAL APPROACHES

The practice nurse should aim to address issues associated with lifestyle change and the prescribing and monitoring of medications. The patient should be encouraged to reduce and, if possible, stop smoking. Issues associated with alcohol intake should also be addressed and if this is excessive it should be reduced. Regular physical activity should be encouraged and vitamin D and/or calcium supplements may be required (Lane, Russell and Khan, 2000).

The bone mass attained early in life is the most important determinant of lifelong skeletal health. Those who have the highest bone mass after adolescence have the greatest protective advantage when the unavoidable decline in bone density related with increasing age, illness and diminished sex hormone production take their toll (National Institute of Health, 2000). Armstrong (2001) suggests that fractures as a result of osteoporosis, due to an increasing sedentary lifestyle, in children (as well as adults) will grow. The practice nurse may therefore need to consider providing children and young boys with health promotion activities, such as the importance of an adequate diet and regular exercise in relation to their bones, at an early age so as to prevent potential complications later in life. A prevention strategy of building up bone mass when young may help to prevent osteoporosis in later life (Department of Health (DH), 2001). If exercise has been suggested to those patients with compression vertebral fractures, this should be appropriate to the setting, and the assistance of the physiotherapist may be required (Bilezikian, 1999).

The risk of falls should also be addressed and the practice nurse may need to instigate a multidisciplinary/integrated approach referring the patient to the most appropriate agency when needed. Brown (2006) advocates an approach that manages the osteoporosis as well as identifying and managing patients at increased risk of falls. A coordinated approach across the primary, community and secondary sectors of health and social care is required. Standard 6 of the *National Service Framework for Older People* (NSF) (DH, 2001) has set out a programme of action and reform to deliver fully integrated falls and osteoporosis services. The National Institute for Health and Clinical Excellence is producing guidance in relation to the assessment of fracture risk and the prevention of osteoporotic fractures in those individuals at high risk; this guidance is to build upon and improve the services that the NSF is already establishing.

The patient must also be given further advice about the implications and risks associated with osteoporosis; lifestyle advice should include information concerning lifting and handling as well as posture. The nurse needs to ask the man to consider risk assessment in conjunction with his occupational health nurse, if appropriate.

PHARMACOLOGICAL INTERVENTIONS

Recent advances in bringing osteoporosis to the public's attention, along with a deeper understanding of its pathogenesis and diagnostic methods, follow the development of new and improved prospects in drug treatment of this disease. Medications that worsen osteoporosis – for example, psychotropic drugs, aluminium-containing antacids, and anticoagulants – should be stopped if possible. The nurse should also review any medications the patient is taking that may make him drowsy or cause him to fall.

The fundamental nature of a pharmacological approach is to decrease turnover of bone or increase bone mass and as a result increase bone strength. Antiresorptive and anabolic agents are used: antiresorptives reduce bone loss while anabolic agents stimulate new bone formation. There is a lack of comparative data to make it possible to recommend specific treatments based on a sound evidence base, and there are fewer approved treatments for men than women. Table 8.5 is based on Royal College of Physicians and Bone and Tooth Society of Great Britain (2000) recommendations for men and women. The various modalities of treatment have been subjected to review ensuring that there is, where possible, sound evidence to support their use.

The grade of evidence regarding efficacy of treatments in Table 8.5 has also been included. Levels of evidence are defined as follows:

Ia　　from meta-analysis of randomized controlled trials (RCTs)
Ib　　from at least one RCT
IIa　　from at least one well-designed controlled study without randomization

Table 8.5. Treatment approaches

Intervention	Bone mineral density	Vertebral fracture	Hip fracture
Calcium (+/− vitamin D)	A	A	B
Oestrogen	A	A	B
Alendronate	A	A	A
Etidronate	A	A	B
Calcitonin	A	A	B
Fluoride[a]	A	A[b]	—
Anabolic steroids	A	—	B
Calcitriol	A	A[b]	C

(Source: Royal College of Physicians and Bone and Tooth Society of Great Britain, 2000)
[a]This agent is licensed in the UK for use in osteoporosis but can only be used in specialist centres.
[b]Data is inconsistent.

III   from well-designed non-experimental descriptive studies, e.g. comparative studies, correlation studies, case-control studies

IV   from expert committee reports or opinions and/or clinical experience of authorities

I   from meta-analysis of observational studies

The quality of guideline recommendation is also graded to indicate the levels of evidence on which they are based:

Grade A   evidence levels Ia and Ib
Grade B   evidence levels IIa, IIb and III
Grade C   evidence level IV

TESTOSTERONE REPLACEMENT THERAPY

The first step to prevent further bone loss in hypogonadal men is to replace sex steroids; testosterone has been demonstrated to prevent bone loss in elderly hypogonadal men (Kamel, Perry and Morley, 2001). Seeman (2004) suggests that the two most important hormones associated with skeletal maintenance are testosterone and oestrogen. As the man ages, the levels of these hormones fall; bone is lost and becomes brittle just as it does in females.

Testosterone replacement can be given by tablets, patches, injection or implants. Some men experience an increase in general well-being, sexual interest and there may be aggression. There is also a possibility that prostate problems and heart disease can be exacerbated. The patient needs to be told about these potential side effects in order to make an informed decision (National Osteoporosis Society, 2001). Further clinical trials are required in order to assess the risk-to-benefit ratio of hormone replacement therapy.

CALCIUM/VITAMIN D

For older men, those who are at risk and those who have established osteoporosis should be given routine calcium and vitamin D. The recommended calcium intake in elderly men should be approximately 1200 mg daily. There are queries about optimal vitamin intake, and it has been suggested that 400–800 IU is appropriate. Gillespie (2001) is of the opinion that vitamin D or vitamin D analogues without concurrent calcium supplementation do not reduce fracture risk. The evidence relating to calcium and vitamin D supplementation is inconsistent.

CALCITRIOL

This is an active form of vitamin D and improves calcium absorption from the gut as well as its metabolism into bone. Usually it is prescribed for post-menopausal women but may be used for men.

BISPHOSPHONATES

Bisphosphonates are antiresorptive drugs and include alendronate and etidronate; they are non-hormonal drugs whose prime action is to slow down osteoclast activity, thus enabling osteoblasts to work more effectively in order to increase bone density. Campion and Maricic (2003) suggest that treatment with bisphosphonates should be considered as soon as osteoporosis has been diagnosed. Alendronate when used for treatment in male osteoporosis has been shown to increase bone mineral density (Orwoll et al., 2003). When the patient is prescribed alendronate, he should be advised that the drug may cause abdominal pain as well as oesophagitis (Quantock and Beynon, 1997).

Etidronate is taken in a three-monthly cycle and is usually prescribed with calcium supplement. The drug can cause gastrointestinal disturbances, nausea and diarrhoea.

CALCITONIN

Calcitonin is a useful drug if the patient is unable to tolerate bisphosphonates or if they are contraindicated. Calcitonin is a hormone produced by the thyroid gland and acts by interfering with osteoclast activity providing the osteoblasts with an opportunity to build bone more effectively. Calcitonin has had much success in the treatment of vertebral fractures in osteoporitic post-menopausal women (Lim and Fitzpatrick, 2004). There have been insufficient controlled trials with respect to the use of calcitonin in men; however, when used nasally, calcitonin has effective analgesic properties when controlling acute pain associated with fractured vertebrae.

ANABOLIC AGENTS

Teriparatide, an anabolic agent, is prescribed for patients who are at high risk of fracture. The safety and efficacy of teriparatide is yet to be determined and, therefore, sustained used (no longer than two years) is not recommended (National Osteoporosis Society, 2006b).

CONCLUSION

Bone is a living tissue. Osteoclasts and osteoblasts are the primary cells involved in bone formation and resorption. At approximately 25 years of age bone loss begins. Risk factors such as age, smoking, physical activity and some medical conditions are associated with osteoporosis. Osteoporosis is a preventable and treatable condition.

Osteoporosis is not a disease that only affects women; osteoporosis in men is not rare, nor are the consequences of this disease. The osteoporosis spotlight has been on women in the past as it is more likely to occur in the female than the male. The principal focus on females has been to the detriment of men, in so far as this has delayed an understanding of the condition in men. What is known about osteoporosis in females should not be applied, without caution, to the male: the female skeleton differs from the male. A similar error was made many years ago concerning heart disease and the belief that what was learnt about male heart disease could be applied to females. Osteoporosis is different in males than it is in women, but there are similarities.

There are non-pharmacological and pharmacological interventions associated with the disease. The non-pharmacological interventions encompass issues associated with nutrition, exercise and lifestyle. The practice nurse is ideally suited to provide the patient with advice and understanding. It is advocated that early intervention – that is, interventions taking place during childhood – be instigated in an attempt to reduce the morbidity and mortality associated with osteoporosis at a later age. A number of pharmacological approaches are available; however, with some there is limited evidence available to support efficacy in the male patient.

More research is required into osteoporosis and the male in order to determine what brings about this disease in those men where there is no identifiable cause. Osteoporosis in men should be seen as an important public health issue and the practice nurse needs to develop an increased awareness of the risk factors; this will, it is anticipated, lead to faster diagnosis and earlier treatment if the morbidity and mortality resulting in osetoporotic fractures are to be reduced. Our understanding of this condition in men is growing but a great deal more needs to be understood.

REFERENCES

All Party Parliamentary Osteoporosis Group (2004) *Falling Short: Delivering Integrated Falls and Osteoporosis Services in England*, All Party Parliamentary Osteoporosis Group, Bath.

Anderson, F.H., Francis, R.M., Selby, P.L. and Cooper, C. (1998) Sex hormones and osteoporosis in men. *Calcified Tissue International*, **62**, 185–188.

Armstrong, E. (2001) *Health in Scotland*, Scottish Executive, Edinburgh.

Bates, V. (2001) Preventing osteoporosis: the practice nurse's role. *Practice Nursing*, **12** (3), 102–105.

Bilezikian, J.P. (1999) Osteoporosis in men. *Journal of Clinical Endocrinology and Metabolism*, **84** (10), 3431–3434.

Bonjour, J.P., Thienz, G., Buchs, B. *et al.* (1991) Critical years and stages of puberty for spinal and femoral bone mass accumulation during adolescence. *Journal of Clinical Endocrinology and Metabolism*, **73**, 555–563.

Brown, P. (2006) Osteoporosis. In (eds S. Chambers, G. Kassianos and J. Morrell) *Improving Practice in Primary Care: Practical Advice from Practising Doctors*, CSF Medical Communications, Long Hanborough, pp. 287–299, Chapter 26.

Campion, J.M. and Maricic, M.J. (2003) Osteoporosis in men. *American Family Physician*, **67** (7), 1521–1526.

Caro, J.J., Ishak, K.J., Huybrechts, K.F. *et al.* (2004) The impact of compliance with osteoporosis therapy fracture rates in actual practice. *Osteoporosis International*, **15**, 1003–1008.

Center, J.R., Nguyen, T.V., Schneider, D. *et al.* (1999) Mortality after all major types of osteoporotic fracture in men and women: an observational study. *Lancet*, **353**, 878–882.

Chartered Society of Physiotherapy (2002) *Physiotherapy Guidelines for the Management of Osteoporosis*, CSP, London.

Chelvanayagam, S. (2006) Eating disorders (eds I. Peate and S. Chelvanayagam) *Caring for Adults with Mental Health Problems*, John Wiley & Sons Ltd, Chichester, pp. 117–129, Chapter 9.

Compston, J.E. and Seeman, E. (2006) Compliance with osteoporosis therapy is the weakest link. *Lancet*, **368**, 973–974.

Cuddihy, M.T., Gabriel, S.E., Crowson, C.S. *et al.* (1999) Forearm fractures as predictors of subsequent osetoporotic fracture. *Osteoporosis International*, **9** (6), 469–475.

Dennison, E., Cole, Z. and Cooper, C. (2005) Diagnosis and epidemiology of osteoporosis. *Current Opinion in Rheumatology*, **17**, 456–461.

Department of Health (2001) *National Service Framework for Older People*, DH, London.

Eastell, R., Boyle, I.T., Compston, J. *et al.* (1998) Management of male osteoporosis: report of the UK consensus group. *Quarterly Journal of Medicine*, **91** (2), 71–92.

Falahati-Nini, A., Riggs, B.L., Atkinson, E.J *et al.* (2000) Relative contributions of testosterone and oestrogen in regulating bone resorption and formation in normal men. *Journal of Clinical Investigation*, **106**, 1553–1560.

Francis, R.M. (2000) Male Osteoporosis. *Rheumatology*, **39**, 1055–1059.

Francis, R.M. (2001) Falls and fractures. *Age and Ageing*, **30** (Suppl. 4), 25–28.

Gillespie, W.J. (2001) Extracts from 'Clinical Evidence': hip fracture. *British Medical Journal*, **322**, 968–975.

Huybrechts, K.F., Ishak, K.J. and Caro, J.J. (2006) Assessment of compliance with osteoporosis and its consequences in a managed care population. *Bone*, **38**, 922–928.

Kamel, H.K., Perry, H.M. and Morley, J.E. (2001) Hormone replacement therapy and fractures in older adults. *Journal of the American Geriatric Society*, **49** (2), 179–187.

Khot, A. and Polmear, A. (2006) *Practical General Practice: Guidelines for Effective Clinical Management*, Butterworth-Heinemann, Edinburgh.

Lane, J.M., Russell, L. and Khan, S.N. (2000) Osteoporosis: pathogenesis, diagnosis and treatment in older adults. *Rheumatic Diseases Clinics of North America*, **26** (3), 569–591.

Lim, L.S. and Fitzpatrick, L.A. (2004) Osteoporosis in men (eds R.S. Kirby, C.C. Carson, M.G. Kirby and R.N. Farah) *Men's Health*, 2nd edn, Taylor & Francis, London, pp. 203–221, Chapter 15.

Lydick, E., Cook, K., Turpin, J. *et al.* (1998) Development and validation of a simple questionnaire to facilitate identification of women likely to have low bone density. *American Journal of Managing Care*, **4** (1), 37–48.

National Institute of Health (2000) Osteoporosis: prevention, diagnosis and therapy. *NIH Consensus Statement*, **17** (1), 1–45.

National Institute for Health and Clinical Excellence (2004) *Eating Disorders:Core Interventions in the Treatment and Management of Anorexia Nervosa, Bulimia Nervosa and Related Eating Disorders*, NICE, London.

National Osteoporosis Society (2001) *Osteoporosis: Causes, Prevention and Treatment*, NOS, Bath.

National Osteoporosis Society (2002) *Position statement on the reporting of dual energy X-ray absorptiometry (DXA) bone mineral density scans*, NOS, Bath.

National Osteoporosis Society (2005a) *Osteoporosis in Men*, NOS, Bath.

National Osteoporosis Society (2005b) *Anorexia Nervosa and Osteoporosis*, NOS, Bath.

National Osteoporosis Society (2006a) *Osteoporosis Facts and Figures:* Volume 1, NOS, Bath.

National Osteoporosis Society (2006b) *Information Sheet: Teriparatide (Forsteo)*, NOS, Bath.

Orwoll, E.S., Scheele, W.H., Paul, S. *et al.* (2003) The effect of teriparatide (human parathyroid hormone (1–34)) therapy on bone density in men with osteoporosis. *Journal of Bone Mineral Research*, **18** (1), 9–17.

Paterson, A. (2004) *Fit to Die: Men and Eating Disorders*, Lucky Duck Publishing Ltd, Bristol.

Proctor, J. (2004) Arthritis (eds J. Martin and J. Lucas), *Handbook of Practice Nursing*, 3rd edn, Churchill Livingstone, Edinburgh, pp. 233–249, Chapter 13.

Quantock, C. and Beynon, J. (1997) Evaluating an osteoporosis service using a focus group. *Nursing Standard*, **11** (42), 45– 47.

Roper, N., Logan, W. and Tierney, A.J. (1996) *The Elements of Nursing*, 2nd edn, Churchill Livingstone, Edinburgh.

Royal College of Physicians and Bone and Tooth Society of Great Britain (2000) *Osteoporosis: Clinical Guidelines for Prevention and Treatment*, RCP, London.

Scottish Intercollegiate Guidelines Network (2003) *71: Management of Osteoporosis: A National Clinical Guideline*, SIGN, Edinburgh.

Seeman, E. (1995) The dilemma of osteoporosis in men. *American Journal of Medicine*, **98** (Suppl. 1A), 75S–87S.

Seeman, E. (2004) *Invest In Your Bones: Osteoporosis in Men: The 'Silent Epidemic' Strikes Men Too*, International Osteoporosis Foundation, Nyon, Switzerland.

Sutcliffe, A.M. (2001) Osteoporosis in men. *Journal of Orthopaedic Nursing*, **5**, 73–75.

Tanna, N. (2005) Osteoporosis and its prevention. *The Pharmaceutical Journal*, **275**, 521–524.

Torgerson, D.J., Iglesias, C.P. and Reid, D.M. (2001) The economics of fracture: The effective management of osteoporosis (eds D.H. Barlow, R.M. Francis, A. Miles, and R.N. Farah), *The Effective Management of Osteoporosis. Key Advances in Clinical Practice Series*. National Osteoporosis Society, London, pp. 111–121.

Tuck, S.P. and Francis, R. (2002) Osteoporosis: recognition of the problem in men. *Men's Health Journal*, **4**, 102–106.

Tuck, S.P. and Francis, R.M. (2002) Osteoporosis. *Postgraduate Medical Journal*, **78**, 526–532.

Tuck, S.P., Raj, N. and Summers, G.D. (2002) Is distal forearm fracture in men due to osteoporosis? *Osteoporosis International*, **18** (8), 630–636.

Waugh, A. and Grant, A. (2006) *Ross and Wilson: Anatomy and Physiology in Health and Illness*, 10th edn, Churchill Livingstone, Edinburgh.

World Health Organization (1994) *Technical Report Series 843: Assessment of Fracture Risk and its Application to Screening for Post Menopausal Osteoporosis*, WHO, Geneva.

World Health Organization (1996) *World Health Organization Guidelines: Cancer Pain Relief*, 2nd edn, WHO, Geneva.

Wright, V.J. (2006) Osteoporosis in men. *Journal of the American Academy of Orthopaedic Surgeons*, **14** (7), 347–353.

9 Obesity

INTRODUCTION

Despite the variations in the incidence of obesity and overweight with sex, age, socioeconomic status and ethnicity, the problems of obesity and overweight affect the whole of our society. It is estimated that approximately three-quarters of people in England are obese and current trends mean that today's children will have a shorter life expectancy than their parents (Jotangla *et al.*, 2005). Men have a higher prevalence of overweight and obesity; despite this they are grossly under-represented in weight management programmes in primary care settings. Men are also much less likely to have their weight routinely recorded in the primary care setting (Men's Health Forum, 2005).

Weight management should become an integral aspect of the practice nurse's work, not an optional extra (Campbell, 2004). The practice nurse should not wait for the patient to raise the question of weight-related issues. As men become more aware of the consequences of overweight and obesity, the more likely they will be to seek advice from the practice nurse.

This chapter will provide the reader with a definition of obesity as well as overweight. The role of the practice nurse in preventing and helping men to lose weight is discussed. In order to provide effective care, the practice nurse must be able to assess the needs of the patient effectively in relation to obesity; this will entail measuring and recording body mass index (BMI). A plan of care is then necessary and this will require the nurse, after assessing needs, to plan, implement and evaluate. Prevention and management are the two approaches that will help to halt the year-on-year increase in overweight and obesity.

Treatment modalities are discussed, concentrating on preventative activities – for example, healthy-eating options, continuing with pharmacological interventions and surgical options.

PRIMARY CARE AND OBESITY

Primary care is ideally placed to tackle the increasing burden of obesity. Campbell (2006) suggests that much of the clinical burden of the condition falls upon the entire primary healthcare team to manage. More than 90 % of patient contact with the NHS is in primary care, which has an important role to play in the prevention and management of obesity.

The White Paper *Choosing Health* (Department of Health (DH), 2004) is committed to developing a care pathway for obesity, stating that trends in diet and lifestyle over the last 30 years have united to bring about an obesity epidemic. The National Obesity Forum (2005) suggests that primary care is ideally placed to tackle the increasing burden of obesity. The National Audit Office (2001) estimates that projected costs for obesity for 2010 would be £2.5 billion. The Clerk's Department (Scrutiny Unit) (House of Commons Health Select Committee, 2004) has now revised that estimate and suggests it is closer to £3.3–3.7 billion.

'OBESE' AND 'OVERWEIGHT'

The terms obese and overweight are used to describe increasing degrees of excess body fatness that may lead to increasingly adverse effects on the health and well-being of the individual (Swanton and Frost, 2006).

Obesity is a complex disease of multiple causes, leading to an imbalance between energy intake and output and to the accumulation of large amounts of body fat (see Figure 9.1). The causes, just like the disease, are complex and multifactoral. It is doubtful that the cause is a result of genetic changes, as the exponential rate at which the disease has grown has occurred in too short a time period (National Audit Office, 2001). Genes do, however, appear to influence metabolism and the distribution of body fat and are thought to play a 25–40 % role in relation to the causes of obesity and overweight (Maffeis, 2000). The more probable result of overweight and obesity is likely to be a combination of factors caused by behavioural and environmental changes in our society, for example, less active lifestyles and changes in eating patterns (DH, 2004).

The prime cause of obesity and overweight is closely related to a high-calorie diet and more sedentary lifestyle (National Audit Office, 2001). Calorie intake in the home increased from the late 1950s and peaked in 1970, declining by approximately

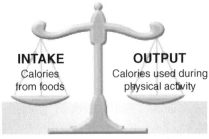

THE ENERGY BALANCE

Figure 9.1. The energy balance. (Source: Department of Health and Human Services Centers for Disease Control and Prevention (www.cdc.gov/nccdphp/dnpa/nutrition/images/scale_energy_balance.gif))

9 % by 2004 (Department for Environment, Food and Rural Affairs, 2005). That data refers only to food consumed within the home and fails to take account of food consumed outside the home. Eating outside of the home is becoming increasingly popular, with these foods being higher in fats and added sugars than the food that is eaten at home (National Audit Office, 2001).

The Department for Transport (2002) suggests that over the last 25 years in the UK there has been a significant decrease in the amount of physical activity undertaken by the population as part of their daily routine. The average number of miles travelled per year between 1975/76 and 2002 on foot has fallen by a quarter and by bicycle by approximately a third, with the average number of miles travelled by car increasing by just under 70 %.

Only 35 % of men have met the Government's recommended target of achieving at least 30 minutes of moderately intense physical activity at least five times per week. This target falls steadily with age from 56 % for those men aged between 16 and 24 years to 9 % at age 75 years and above (NHS Health and Social Care Information Centre, 2005).

Social and psychological factors influence eating, drinking and exercise habits. Kennedy (2001) points out that there is a noticeable socioeconomic dimension to being overweight and obese: those who have low income find it difficult to adopt healthy lifestyles including healthy eating habits. Mercola (2002) suggests that men were more likely to eat when stressed if they were single, divorced or frequently unemployed. Many men, according to Campbell (2004), become overweight after a significant life event has occurred, leading to the man experiencing an intense period of excessive calorie intake possibly with a reduction in energy expenditure. The occurrence of these life events may culminate in the man comfort-eating, having irregular and unhealthy dietary patterns and usually excessive alcohol intake. Redundancy, unemployment and the effects of sports injury, for example, may also result in a more sedentary lifestyle leading to rapid weight gain. The practice nurse needs to understand these behavioural determinants if they are to engage with men in a meaningful manner; understanding can help to provide treatment plans that are realistic and appropriate.

There are other issues the practice nurse needs to consider when providing healthcare; these are the wider determinants of health. These determinants are made up of a wide range of factors that contribute to the health of the individual. Dahlgren and Whitehead (1991) provide a diagrammatic representation of these determinants (see Figure 2.3, p. 36). Determinants of health are defined by the World Health Organization (1998) as a variety of personal, social, economic and environmental issues which determine the health status of individuals or populations.

A number of the determinants of health have the potential to impact on the prevalence of overweight and obesity. Personal choice is related to individual lifestyle factors, habits and customs. Social networks can also determine the diet the person eats. The environment where a person lives can discourage a person from engaging in physical activity as s/he may fear crime. Swanton and Frost (2006) suggest that the accessibility of fresh, affordable fruits can also influence intake.

The causes of obesity and overweight are complex and the practice nurse must ensure that all the determinants of health are considered when working with the patient/community in tackling overweight and obesity. Preventative and weight management interventions are two broad approaches that are advocated. Operating in partnership and working in a variety of settings in a coordinated manner will result in a more effective way of achieving lifestyle change (Maryon-Davis, 2005).

ASSESSING OVERWEIGHT AND OBESITY

There is a need to ensure that the ranges of weight at which health risks to men increase are identified. BMI is one method that can be used to identify increases. The possibility of developing life-threatening conditions such as type 2 diabetes rises sharply as body fatness increases.

Clinical examination of the man should include the physiological measurements mentioned below, along with blood pressure and urinalysis. Blood tests are required and the National Obesity Forum (2001) suggests that biochemical investigation should include:

- urea and electrolytes
- liver function tests
- fasting blood sugar
- fasting lipids
- thyroid function tests
- full blood count.

Campbell (2004) suggests that the reason for performing these tests is to provide a baseline to monitor future progress as well as excluding the existence of co-morbid conditions such as type 2 diabetes. The nurse can also inform the patient that there are no other underlying physical reasons why he is unable to lose weight.

The most common method of assessing overweight and obesity is by using BMI, which is defined as the man's weight in kilograms divided by the square of his height in metres – kg/m^2; this measurement correlates with the proportion of body fat. For example, the BMI of a man weighing 105 kg and 180 cm tall is calculated thus:

$$BMI = \frac{105}{(1.80 \times 1.80)} = \frac{105}{3.24} = 32.40 \, kg/m^2$$

The World Health Organization (2000) suggests that in adults a BMI of 25–29.9 kg/m^2 is defined as overweight while obesity is said to be when the BMI is over 30 kg/m^2 (see Table 9.1).

The degree of overweight and obesity in adult Asian[1] men in the UK is classified in a different manner. Asian men have a higher proportion of body fat in comparison

[1] The populations included in the review for expert consultation were from China, Hong Kong, India, Indonesia, Japan, Republic of Korea, Malaysia, Philippines, Singapore, Taiwan and Thailand.

Table 9.1. WHO classifications of overweight and obesity (adults)

Classification	BMI (kg/m^2)
Underweight	Less than 18.5
Healthy weight	18.5–24.9
Overweight	25–29.9
Obese	30 or more
Obesity I	30–34.9
Obesity II	35–39.9
Obesity III (severely or morbidly obese)	40 or more

(Source: WHO, 2000)

with men of the same age and BMI in the general UK population. The outcome of this is higher risk for cardiovascular disease and type 2 diabetes (Swanton and Frost, 2006) (see Table 9.2).

Two other methods of measurement that may be used to determine the proportion and distribution of body fat are waist circumference and waist–hip ratio. These methods, as opposed to BMI, allow assessment of mass due to body fat and mass as a result of muscular physique.

WAIST CIRCUMFERENCE

Abdominal fat content or 'central' fat distribution is measured using waist circumference. DeVille-Almond (2006) suggests that there are two general body shapes in relation to the distribution of body fat – apple and pear shapes. Those who are said to be pear-shaped (predominantly women) carry excess weight around their hips, thighs and buttocks, whereas those who are said to be apple-shaped (usually men) are said to carry the excess weight around their middle part of the body; this is known as central obesity and is closely linked to a higher risk of type 2 diabetes and coronary heart disease. Central obesity is associated with metabolic syndrome. Those with central obesity provide the nurse with a more sensitive indicator of risk

Table 9.2. Classification of overweight and obesity in Asian adult populations

Classification	BMI (kg/m^2)
Underweight	Less than 18.5
Healthy weight	18.5–22.9
Overweight	23 or more
At risk	23–24.9
Obesity I	25–29.9
Obesity II	30 or more

(Source: National Institute for Health and Clinical Excellence, 2006)

Table 9.3. Waist circumference thresholds, general and Asian male adult populations

General male population	Asian male population
102 cm (40 in. or more)	90 cm (35 in. or more)

(Source: Adapted from National Institute for Health and Clinical Excellence, 2006)

in relation to metabolic syndrome than BMI does (DeVille-Almond, 2006). The National Institute for Health and Clinical Excellence (2006) recognizes that there are thresholds in the general population (see Table 9.3).

Waist circumference measurements should never be used in isolation as there may be a number of patients who require weight measurements (National Health and Medical Research Council, 2003). The World Health Organization (2000) advocates that both BMI and waist circumference be used when assessing the man's relative health risk. Table 9.4 provides classifications that combine both BMI and waist circumference and risk of co-morbidities for the general male population, and Table 9.5 relates to the Asian male population.

Table 9.4. BMI and waist measurement combination to assess obesity and the risk of type 2 diabetes and cardiovascular disease in the general male adult population

		Waist circumference and risk of co-morbidities	
Classification	BMI (kg/m^2)	94–102 cm	More than 102 cm
Underweight	Less than 18.5	—	—
Healthy weight	18.5–24.9	—	Increased
Overweight	25–29.9	Increased	High
Obesity	30 or more	High	Very high

(Source: WHO, 2000; National Institute for Health and Clinical Excellence, 2006; National Health and Medical Research Council, 2003)

Table 9.5. BMI and waist measurement combination to assess obesity and the risk of type 2 diabetes and cardiovascular disease in the Asian male adult population

		Waist circumference and risk of co-morbidities	
Classification	BMI (kg/m^2)	Less than 90 cm	90 cm or more
Underweight	Less than 18.5	Low (but increased risk of other clinical problems)	Average
Healthy weight	18.5–22.9	Average	Increased
Overweight	23 or more	—	—
At risk	23–24.9	Increased	Moderate
Obese I	25–29.9	Moderate	Severe
Obese II	30 or more	Severe	Very severe

(Source: National Institute for Health and Clinical Excellence, 2006)

WAIST–HIP RATIO

This measure also assesses body fat distribution. The waist–hip measurement is defined as waist circumference divided by hip circumference – waist girth/hip girth. There is no consensus regarding exact thresholds associated with waist–hip ratio; however, it is commonly accepted that raised waist–hip ratio in men is 0.95 or more (Sproston and Primatesta, 2004).

The practice nurse must ensure that assessment of the patient is conducted using a holistic approach. The determinants of health, for example, psychological, social and environmental factors, must be taken into account. It is vital that a sensitive approach is used. The Department of Health (2006) would suggest that assessment of BMI and other parameters be routinely measured, providing the nurse with the best possible indicator of obesity and related health risks.

THE SCALE OF THE PROBLEM

There are two main sources of information regarding routine data on the prevalence of obesity – the Health Survey for England and the National Diet and Nutrition Survey. Recording of BMI among adult men in general practice is ad hoc. While data refers predominantly (although not exclusively) to England, similar data may be found for the rest of the UK.

PREVALENCE

The International Council of Nurses (2002) states that obesity is spreading at an alarming rate in both industrialized and developing countries. Obesity coexists in some countries alongside malnutrition. The World Health Organization (2002) considers obesity to be a global epidemic as well as a serious public health problem with over 1 billion adults who are overweight and at least 300 million who are obese (World Health Organization 2003). Obesity over the last 25 years has increased by approximately 400% (House of Commons Health Select Committee, 2004).

Obesity is now the second leading cause of preventable death after smoking and is predicted to have an effect on the health of the population equivalent to tobacco smoking (Gnani and Majeed, 2006). By 2020 the Government estimates that at least one-third of adults, a third of girls and a fifth of boys will be obese (DH, 2004). Since the 1980s the prevalence of obesity has trebled (DH, 2004). In 2004 22.7% of men were identified as obese; over 31 million adults were said to be either obese or overweight; furthermore, the proportion of men who were severely (morbidly) obese, with a BMI of over 40 kg/m^2, was 0.9% (NHS Health and Social Care Information Centre, 2005).

AGE

Generally, mean BMI increases as the man ages; the exception to this is in men aged 75 years and over. Approximately three-quarters (73.2%) of men are classified as overweight or obese, with 2.0% of men aged between 55 and 64 years said to be severely overweight (those with a BMI of 40 kg/m^2) (NHS Health and Social Care Information Centre, 2005). The prevalence of expanded waist circumference increases more with age in those men aged between 16 and 74 years (Sproston and Primatesta, 2004).

GENDER

Men and women have similar mean BMI levels. For the man this is 27.1 kg/m^2 and the woman 26.8 kg/m^2. A greater proportion of men (43.9%) are overweight than women (34.7%) (NHS Health and Social Care Information Centre, 2005).

SOCIOECONOMIC FACTORS

Those who belong to lower socioeconomic and socially disadvantaged groups are more likely to be overweight and obese (Working Party of the Royal College of Physicians of London, Royal College of Paediatrics and Child Health and Faculty of Public Health, 2004). Sproston and Primatesta (2004) point out that obesity prevalence is much lower in managerial and professional households as opposed to those in routine or semi-routine occupations.

ETHNICITY

The mean BMI of male Chinese is 24.1 kg/m^2, for Bangladeshi men this is 24.7 kg/m^2 and is significantly lower than that of the general male population, which is 27.1 kg/m^2. For all ethnic groups waist circumference increases with age (NHS Health and Social Care Information Centre, 2005). Table 9.6 (below) demonstrates the prevalence of male obesity by ethnic group in England.

Zaninotto *et al.* (2006) have produced a great deal of data that makes assumptions, predictions and projected prevalence of obesity and overweight in 2010. The assumptions about future changes in obesity are based on past patterns of change. Being aware of the predictions may help the practice nurse plan strategically, acting in a proactive way as opposed to a reactive manner.

HEALTH IMPLICATIONS

Obesity is not a cosmetic issue; it is a serious life-threatening medical condition and is the major contributor to the global burden of chronic disease and disability (World Health Organization, 2003; Gray, 2005). Being obese can reduce life expectancy on

Table 9.6. Prevalence of obesity and overweight amongst adult males aged 16 years and over in England, by ethnic group (2003/2004)

	Black Caribbean	Black African	Indian	Pakistani	Bangladeshi	Chinese	General population
Overweight (including obese)	67.4%	61.8%	53.2%	55.5%	44.4%	36.8%	66.5%
Obese (including severely obese)	25.2%	17.1%	13.8%	15.1%	5.8%	6.0%	22.7%
Severely obese	0.2%	0.3%	0.4%	1.0%	0.3%	0.3%	0.9%
Raise waist–hip ratio	25.0%	16.0%	36.0%	37.0%	32.0%	17.0%	33.0%
Raised waist circumference	22.0%	19.0%	20.0%	30.0%	12.0%	8.0%	31.0%

(Source: NHS Health and Social Care Information Centre, 2005; Sproston and Primatesta, 2004)

average by approximately nine years. Obesity is responsible for 9000 premature deaths yearly (DH, 2004). As well as the substantial human costs that accompany obesity and overweight there are also financial costs incurred by the NHS and the economy of the nation. Costs to the NHS are reflected in the illnesses associated with overweight and obesity, directly and indirectly. Direct costs are the result of consultations, diagnostic tests, drugs and other treatments of the diseases that are associated with obesity and overweight. Indirect costs come in the form of lost output in the economy that may be due to sickness or death of workers. The House of Commons Health Select Committee (2004) states that in 2002 there were approximately 15.5–16 million lost days of certified incapacity as a result of obesity and other co-morbidities. These estimations do not take into account the impact of undiagnosed obesity. Currently obesity is not treated as a disease or illness: instead the medical complications are addressed (Swanton and Frost, 2006). The next challenge for health services will be to do something about obesity and to see it as an issue in its own right (DH, 2004). The House of Commons Health Select Committee (2004) suggests that between £3.3 billion and £3.7 billion per year is spent on obesity alone; this coupled with overweight rises to between £6.6 billion and £7.4 billion per year.

Adolfsson *et al.* (2005) state that being overweight or obese will increase the risk of a wide range of diseases and illnesses including, for example, coronary heart disease and the possibility of developing type 2 diabetes. Obesity affects almost every organ of the body (see Figure 9.2 below).

Table 9.7 (below) outlines the relative risks of health problems that are associated with obesity.

TYPE 2 DIABETES

Type 2 diabetes is the most common obesity-related co-morbidity and is most likely to cause the greatest health burden. Approximately 70 % of those with a BMI of 35 kg/m^2 or above are expected to experience type 2 diabetes: as weight increases, the risk of developing type 2 diabetes rises exponentially (Avenell *et al.*, 2004).

Van Dam *et al.* (2002), in a study conducted in the United States, point out that those men consuming a Western diet (defined as one that consists of a high consumption of red meat, processed meat, high-fat dairy products, chips, refined grains and sweets and desserts), combined with a lack of physical activity, have a dramatically increased risk of developing type 2 diabetes.

CORONARY HEART DISEASE

Men with a BMI of over 26 kg/m^2 are two times more likely to develop coronary heart disease compared with those men with a BMI of 21 kg/m^2 or less. The relationship between weight gain, obesity and coronary heart disease is well established. Women with an elevated BMI are more likely to develop coronary heart disease than men (Swanton and Frost, 2006).

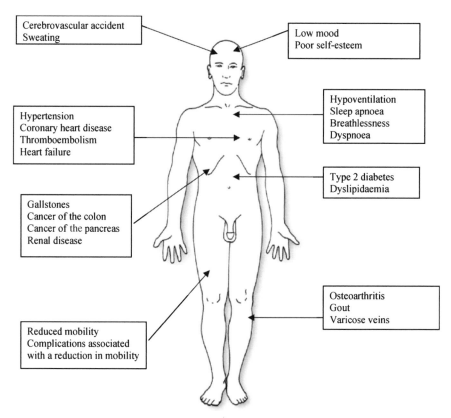

Figure 9.2. Obesity and its effects on the male body

Table 9.7. Relative risks of health problems associated with obesity

Greatly increased risk (relative risk much greater than 3)[a]	Moderately increased risk (relative risk 2–3)[a]	Slightly increased risk (relative risk 1–2)[a]
• Type 2 diabetes	• Coronary heart disease	• Cancer
• Insulin resistance	• Hypertension	• Impaired fertility
• Gallbladder disease	• Cerebrovascular accident	• Low back pain
• Dyslipidaemia	• Osteoarthritis	• Anaesthetic risk
• Breathlessness	• Hyperuricaemia	
• Sleep apnoea	• Gout	
	• Psychological factors	

(Source: Adapted from Swanton and Frost, 2006; World Health Organization, 2000)

[a]All relative risk estimations are approximate. The relative risk indicates the risk measured against that of a non-obese person of the same sex.

HYPERTENSION AND CVA

Three-quarters of cases of hypertension in men are the result of overweight and/or obesity (Garrison, Kannel and Stokes, 1987). Increasing BMI is said to be a risk factor for cerebrovascular accident (CVA). The evidence, however, is inconclusive; Jood et al. (2004) suggest that the key factor is associated with those men who have 'central obesity' as opposed to those who are 'generally obese'. Those men who have a BMI of between 20 kg/m^2 and 22.49 kg/m^2 were significantly less likely to suffer a CVA than those who had a BMI of above 30 kg/m^2 (Jood et al., 2004).

METABOLIC SYNDROME

Swanton and Frost (2006) describe metabolic syndrome as a cluster of risk factors related to a state of insulin resistance, in which the body becomes less able to respond to insulin. An increased risk of developing coronary heart disease, CVA and type 2 diabetes are associated with those who have metabolic syndrome (DH, 2004). Tonkin (2003) suggests that approximately 25 % of the adult population show signs of metabolic syndrome.

There are certain ethnic groups that have a higher incidence of metabolic syndrome. Nugent (2004) identifies these groups as Asian and African Caribbean. Metabolic syndrome increases with age and is higher in men than women (Isomaa et al., 2001).

DYSLIPIDAEMIA

Dyslipidaemia is defined as an increase in triglycerides, elevated LDL cholesterol and decrease in concentrations of HDL cholesterol (Lakasing, 2006). The more fat, the more likely the man is to be dyslipidaemic. The outcome of this (among other things) is that he will be prone to metabolic syndrome (Swanton and Frost, 2006). The location of fat combined with age and gender are important modifiers of the impact of obesity on blood lipids. Fat cells that are centrally located cause most damage as central fat (as opposed to peripheral fat) is resistant to insulin as well as having the ability to recycle fatty acids. Younger people, regardless of the level of obesity, have larger changes in blood lipids.

CANCER

There is convincing evidence that being overweight or obese increases the risk of cancer (World Health Organization and Food and Agricultural Organization, 2002). Obesity in men increases the risk of colorectal and prostate cancers. Cancer of the colon is most clearly associated with obesity; obesity increases the risk by nearly three times (National Audit Office, 2001).

PSYCHOLOGICAL ISSUES

The psychological effects of obesity during childhood can have a significant impact on the well-being of the child, resulting in the development of a negative self-image, lowered self-esteem and a substantial risk of depression. The adult male can also suffer from psychological damage as a result of overweight/obesity. Depression and anxiety in obese men is three to four times higher than the general population (Wadden and Stunkard, 1985). The physical consequences of overweight and obesity are complex; so too are the psychological effects. They, too, are associated with culture, societal values and norms.

REDUCING OVERWEIGHT AND OBESITY

Any advice the nurse offers the man in attempting to make changes to lifestyle associated with weight loss, for example, dietary changes and increasing physical activity, need to be practical, taking into consideration his home and work circumstances. Drummond (2002) recommends that advice given to obese individuals must be perceived as achievable, for example, advocating small changes to dietary habits.

Two broad approaches to tackling obesity and overweight have been suggested by Maryon-Davis (2005): prevention and weight management, using a holistic approach. Preventative approaches incorporate interventions that are aimed at preventing overweight developing in the first place, starting at childhood and onwards. Weight management is aimed at weight reduction or weight control in those men who have already become overweight or obese. The three Es model is outlined below (see Figure 9.3) as an example of using a holistic approach.

The key objective in the primary care setting is to manage obesity and overweight by achieving and maintaining weight loss through the promotion of sustainable

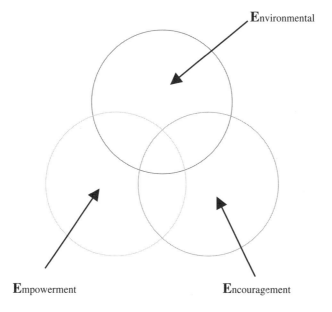

Figure 9.3. The three Es model. (Source: Maryon-Davis, 2005)

lifestyle changes. Within the primary care setting the nurse may only be concerned with encouraging the individual and promoting empowerment; however, s/he should also be concerned with aiming to create a less 'obesogenic' environment. Approximately 75 % of the population consult with their GP in the course of one year and 90 % in five years (House of Commons Health Select Committee, 2004). The nurse is ideally situated to detect and manage obesity in high-risk patients; they are also able to influence the whole family, beginning with preventative activities early on in life and continuing as the family/individual ages. Primary care is potentially an ideal setting for weight management interventions for adults (Maryon-Davis, 2005). Weight management must be seen by the practice nurse as a part of their everyday practice. Dr Foster (a service that provides information to help inform decision-making in health and social care) points out that in a study undertaken with staff in the primary care setting 55 % of respondents believed that obesity was one of their top priorities but less than half had been involved in setting up weight measurement clinics, with the majority of general practices (69 %) failing to establish such clinics. Further guidance for the prevention and management of obese and overweight is provided by the Department of Health (2006) and the National Obesity Forum (2006). The practice nurse must adopt a multidisciplinary approach to prevention and management activities. Working with health trainers as described in the Department of Health's *Choosing Health: Making Healthier Choices Easier* (DH, 2004) is one way of drawing on the expertise of others. Resources (both human and material) in the public and private sector can be combined to provide advice on diet and physical activity with behavioural strategies to help the patient (Steptoe and Doherty, 1999).

MEDICAL AND SURGICAL INTERVENTIONS

DRUG THERAPY

Prior to prescribing drugs, it is vital that every effort has been made to encourage the patient to attempt to diet, engage in physical activity and to change lifestyle behaviour. Drugs should be prescribed only as part of an overall treatment plan for the management of nutritional obesity. Sibutramine and orlistat are licensed for use in England for the treatment of obesity in adults, and healthcare professionals should adhere to the guidance provided by the National Institute for Health and Clinical Excellence (2001a and b) as well as any local policy and protocols that may be in place. Table 9.8 (below) provides details of the criteria that must be met prior to prescribing sibutramine and orlistat.

SURGERY

Surgical intervention should only be seen as a last resort in those men who are obese after all other interventions have been tried and exhausted. Availability of surgery is dependent on local policy and strategy. Bariatric surgery (surgery that forces a

Table 9.8. Criteria for the prescription of Sibutramine and orlistat

Sibutramine	Orlistat
• Those aged between 18 and 65 years	• Those aged between 18 and 75 years
• A BMI of 27 kg/m^2 or more in the presence of co-morbidities	• A BMI of 28 kg/m^2 or more in the presence of co-morbidities
• A BMI of 30 kg/m^2 or more without associated co-morbidities	• A BMI of 30 kg/m^2 or more without associated co-morbidities
• Have controlled blood pressure (145/95 mm/Hg or below)	
• Have no history of coronary artery disease, arrhythmias, congestive heart failure or stroke	

(Source: Department of Health, 2006)

restriction in capacity by reducing gastric size) is recommended as a treatment option for people with morbid obesity providing all of the following criteria (provided by the National Institute for Health and Clinical Excellence, 2002) have been met:

• a BMI of above 35 kg/m^2 with evidence of co-morbidity
• a BMI of above 40 kg/m^2 with no co-morbidity
• the patient is assessed as suitable by a multidisciplinary team
• the patient must be well informed (the patient must be able to comprehend)
• the patient must be motivated
• the patient must have an acceptable level of surgical risk.

Surgical intervention can include those procedures that are performed either as open procedures or those preformed via the laparoscope. The procedures include restrictive procedures such as gastroplasty (vertically banded or silicone ring) or gastric banding and malabsorptive procedures, for example, biliopancreatic diversion, Roux-en-Y gastric bypass or jejunoileal bypass (Clegg *et al.*, 2002).

RECOMMENDATIONS

The practice nurse must seek help, advice and guidance from the myriad publications provided by various statutory and non-statutory organizations, for example, the National Institute for Health and Clinical Excellence, the Department of Health and the National Obesity Forum. From a macro perspective, strategic health authorities and primary care trusts should ensure that they set realistic objectives; and targets for improving nutrition and diet and for promoting physical activity, local overweight and obesity strategies must be formulated. The suggested structure for the development of a local overweight and obesity strategy should reflect the contents of Table 9.9 (below).

Table 9.9. Suggested structure for the development of a local overweight and obesity strategy

Structure	Activity
Making the case for a local overweight and obesity strategy	The proposed strategy should outline the key essentials – prevention and management – providing a rationale for why local action is necessary (i.e. why focus on men)
Partnership working	Outline in this section the key partners who will help to plan, implement and evaluate the strategy. Provide an outline of the establishment of an overweight and obesity action team – who will it include? The patient must not be forgotten in this section
Resource mapping: reviewing current activity and identifying gaps	Consider in this section what is currently happening in the practice and within the locale in relation to prevention and management of overweight and obesity. An audit may be necessary to map activity and as a result identify gaps and the actions that are needed and by whom
Identifying priorities and target groups	This section should consider how resources will be targeted and where to focus efforts
Aims, objectives, standards, targets and milestones	The broad aims of the strategy are required in this section along with specific objectives and standards. A timescale should also be provided reflecting the targets and milestones
Interventions to prevent and manage overweight and obesity	Focusing on the setting, this section should outline interventions that will be required in order to prevent and manage overweight and obesity
Understanding barriers and facilitating change	Provide information in this section that will enable you to outline the obstacles that prevent the men in your care from adopting a healthier lifestyle or adhering to treatment; describe ways in which these may be overcome and explain the roles of those who you expect to contribute to the strategy
Infrastructure support	What structures need to be in place at a local level to implement an obesity and overweight strategy, consider, for example, IT support, funding and public and patient involvement
Monitoring and evaluation	Describe in this section the methods to be used to monitor progress, assess performance and evaluate the strategy
Mainstreaming and sustainability	The overall strategy should have plans on how to ensure that local action to prevent and manage overweight and obesity is mainstreamed and sustained

(Source: Adapted from Swanton and Frost, 2006)

Detailed delivery plans have been produced in several guises, for example, those in *Delivering Choosing Health: Making Healthier Choices Easier* (DH, 2005). The plans include advice about diet – choosing better diets and a food health action plan as well as a physical activity action plan. The aim is to inform the patient to make informed choices about his health so that he can be empowered to make his own choices.

CONCLUSION

Obesity is a potentially curable medical condition. Research and a solid evidence base are emerging, providing a deeper understanding that the practice nurse can utilize in order to provide high-quality nursing care. A gendered approach to the management and prevention of overweight and obesity is needed if the nurse is to provide the male patient with information and advice that he will find useful. It is acknowledged that obesity is not an easy problem to tackle; however, even modest weight loss can bring about significant medical benefits.

While much of the nurse's work will involve dealing with men who are already overweight or obese, a large part of the solution to this epidemic lies with preventing men from becoming overweight or obese in the first place. Within the NHS most contact with overweight and obese men occurs in general practice. The practice nurse, with the rest of the primary care team, can do much to identify those at risk from weight gain, offering them support and advice. Much advice and guidance is available to the primary care team in their endeavours to address this problem in the population in general, and with men in particular. This guidance and advice will help to direct the work of the practice nurse, providing information about the most effective interventions. Joint working is essential in attempting to provide care that is holistic and, above all, effective.

The practice nurse, along with all other members of the primary care team (private and independent), has a key role to play in assessing risk, planning interventions, implementing care pathways and evaluating interventions. They are ideally placed to refer the patient to other appropriate agencies who may be able to produce interventions than can help the male patient avoid overweight or obesity or help him manage his health concerns.

Encouraging men to attend the practice is known to be problematic; the practice nurse needs to be proactive, innovative and creative in the methods used to entice men into the practice. When men do avail themselves of the services offered by the practice nurse, then it is important that the response made is sensitive and custom-built.

REFERENCES

Adolfsson, B., Andersson, I., Elofsson, S. *et al.* (2005) Locus of control and weight reduction. *Patient Education and Counselling*, **56** (1), 55–61.

Avenell, A., Broom, J., Brown, T.J. *et al.* (2004) Systematic review of the long-term effects and economic consequences of treatments for obesity and implications for health improvement. *Health Technology Assessment*, **8** (21), 1–473.

Campbell, I.W. (2004) Obesity and men's health. In (eds R.S. Kirby, C.C. Carson, M.G. Kirby and R.N. Farah) *Men's Health*, 2nd edn, Taylor & Francis, London, pp. 55–62, Chapter 5.

Campbell, I.W. (2006) Obesity, in *Improving Practice in Primary Care: Practical Advice from Practising Doctors* (eds S. Chambers, G. Kassianos and J. Morrell), CSF Medical Communications, Long Hanborough, pp. 263–273, Chapter 24.

Clegg, A.J., Colquitt, J., Sidhu, M.K. *et al.* (2002) The clinical effectiveness and cost effectiveness of surgery for people with morbid obesity: a systematic review and economic evaluation. *Health and Technology Assessment*, **6** (12).

Dahlgren, G. and Whitehead, M. (1991) *Policies and Strategies to Promote Social Equity in Health*, Institute for Future Studies, Stockholm.

Department for Environment, Food and Rural Affairs (2005) *Family Food in 2003–2004: A National Statistics Publication by Defra*, The Stationery Office, London.

Department for Transport (2002) *National Travel Survey*, DT, London.

Department of Health (2004) *Choosing Health: Making Healthier Choices Easier*, DH, London.

Department of Health (2005) *Delivering Choosing Health: Making Healthier Choices Easier*, DH, London.

Department of Health (2006) *Care Pathway for the Management of Overweight and Obesity*, DH, London.

DeVille-Almond, J. (2006) Apples and pears: targeting abdominal obesity. *British Journal of Primary Care Nursing*, **3** (4), 168–172.

Drummond, S. (2002) The management of obesity. *Nursing Standard*, **16** (48), 47–52.

Garrison, R.J., Kannel, W.B. and Stokes, J. (1987) Incidence and precursors of hypertension in young adults: the Framingham offspring study. *Preventative Medicine*, **16**, 235–251.

Gnani, S. and Majeed, A. (2006) *A User's Guide to Data Collected in Primary Care in England*, Eastern Region Public Health Observatory, Cambridge.

Gray, M. (2005) *Fundamental Aspects of Men's Health*, Quay Books, London.

House of Commons Health Select Committee (2004) *Obesity: Third Report of Session 2003–2004, vol. 1*, HCHC, London.

International Council of Nurses (2002) *Fact Sheet: ICN on Obesity*, ICN, Geneva.

Isomaa, B., Almgren, P., Tuomi, T. *et al.* (2001) Cardiovascular morbidity and mortality associated with the metabolic syndrome. *Diabetes Care*, **24**, 683–689.

Jood, K., Jern, C., Wilhelmsen, L. and Rosengren, A. (2004) Body mass index in mid-life is associated with a first stroke in men: a prospective population study over 28 years. *Stroke*, **35**, 2764.

Jotangla, D., Moody, A., Stamatakis, E. and Wardle, H. (2005) *Obesity Among Children Under 11*, National Center for Social Research, Department of Epidemiology and Public Health at the Royal Free and University College Medical School, London.

Kennedy, L.A. (2001) Community involvement at what cost? – local appraisal of a pan-European nutrition promotion programme in low-income neighbourhoods. *Health Promotion International*, **16** (1), 35–45.

Lakasing, E. (2006) Metabolic syndrome. *Practice Nurse*, **31** (9), 57–61.

Maffeis, C. (2000) Aetiology of overweight and obesity in children and adults. *European Journal of Paediatrics*, **159** (Suppl. 1), S35–S44.

Maryon-Davis, A. (2005) Weight management in primary care: how can it be made more effective? *Proceedings of the Nutrition Society*, **64**, 97–103.

Men's Health Forum (2005) *Hazardous Waist? Tackling the Epidemic of Excess Weight in Men*, Men's Health Forum, London.

Mercola, J. (2002) Stress often leads to overeating and extra weight. *Preventative Medicine*, **34**, 29–39.

National Audit Office (2001) *Tackling Obesity in England*, NAO, London.

National Health and Medical Research Council (2003) *Clinical Practice Guidelines for the Management of Overweight and Obesity in Adults*, National Health and Medical Research Council, Canberra.

NHS Health and Social Care Information Centre (2005) *Health Survey for England 2004: Updating of Trend Tables to Include 2004 Data*, NHSHSCIC, London.

National Institute for Health and Clinical Excellence (2001a) *Orlistat for the Treatment of Obesity in Adults: Guidance 22*, NICE, London.

National Institute for Health and Clinical Excellence (2001b) *Guidance on the Use of Sibutramine for the Treatment of Obesity in Adults: Guidance 31*, NICE, London.

National Institute for Health and Clinical Excellence (2002) *Guidance on the Use of Surgery to Aid Weight Reduction for People with Morbid Obesity: Guidance 46*, NICE, London.

National Institute for Health and Clinical Excellence (2006) *Obesity: The Prevention, Identification, Assessment and Management of Overweight and Obesity in Adults and Children, NICE Guidance: First Draft for Consultation*, NICE, London.

National Obesity Forum (2001) *Guidelines for Management of Adult Obesity*, NOF, London.

National Obesity Forum (2005) *General Medical Services Contract*, NOF, London.

National Obesity Forum (2006) *National Obesity Forum Guidelines on Management of Adult Obesity and Overweight in Primary Care*, NOF, London.

Nugent, A.P. (2004) Review: The metabolic syndrome. *Nutrition Bulletin*, **29**, 36–43.

Sproston, K. and Primatesta, P. (2004) *Health Survey for England 2003: Risk Factors for Cardiovascular Disease*, The Stationery Office, London.

Steptoe, A. and Doherty, S. (1999) Behavioural counselling in general practice for the promotion of healthy behaviour among adults at increased risk of coronary heart disease: randomised trial. *British Medical Journal*, **319**, 943–948.

Swanton, K. and Frost, F. (2006) *Lightening the Load: Tackling Obesity and Overweight*, National Heart Forum and Faculty of Public Health, London.

Tonkin, R. (2003) *The X Factor: Obesity and the Metabolic Syndrome*, The Science and Public Health Affairs Forum, London.

Van Dam, R.M., Rimm, E.B., Willett, W.C. *et al.* (2002) Dietary patterns and risk for type 2 diabetes mellitus in US men. *Annals of Internal Medicine*, **136**, 210–209.

Wadden, T.A., and Stunkard, A.J. (1985) Social and psychological consequences of obesity. *Annals of Internal Medicine*, **103**, 1062–1067.

Working Party of the Royal College of Physicians of London, Royal College of Paediatrics and Child Health and Faculty of Public Health (2004) *Storing up Problems: the Medical Case for a Slimmer Nation*, Royal College of Physicians, London.

World Health Organization (1998) *Health Promotion Glossary*, WHO, Geneva.

World Health Organization (2000) Obesity: Preventing and Managing the Global Epidemic, Report of a WHO Consultation, Technical Report Series, vol. 894 no. 3, WHO, Geneva, pp. 1–253.

World Health Organization (2002) Secretariat of the 1st International Conference and World Forum on Technology Transfer of Obesity and Nutrition, Cairo, Egypt, 25–28 June 2002.

World Health Organization (2003) *Global Strategy on Diet, Physical Activity and Health: Obesity and Overweight*, WHO, Geneva.

World Health Organization and Food and Agricultural Organization (2002) Diet, Nutrition and Prevention of Chronic Disease: Report of a Joint WHO/FAO Expert Consultation in WHO Technical Report Series, WHO/FAO, Geneva.

Zaninotto, P., Wardle, H., Stamatakis, E. *et al.* (2006) *Forecasting Obesity to 2010*, National Centre for Social Research, Department of Epidemiology and Public Health at the Royal Free and University College Medical School, London.

10 Erectile dysfunction

INTRODUCTION

Erectile dysfunction is also known by many men and healthcare workers as impotence; some people use the term erectile failure; however, these terms have largely been replaced by erectile dysfunction. Nearly every chapter in this text alludes to the fact that men often find it difficult (for whatever reason) to approach healthcare providers with issues relating to their health. They are, in general, notoriously reticent about seeking help for their health problems (Kirby, 2005). This is confounded even further when it comes to discussing issues of a sexual nature. Many patients (and nurses) find it difficult to discuss erectile dysfunction with their partners let alone with the practice nurse. As a result of this the practice nurse should be proactive and not wait for the patient to present with the condition already established.

When discussing the treatment or conditions that are commonly associated with erectile dysfunction – for example, hypertension – a proactive approach by the nurse is advocated in speaking with the patient about his sexual relations. Erectile dysfunction might be the last subject a male patient may wish to bring up with a female (or male) practice nurse (Weeks and Ficorelli, 2006).

Being aware of the psychological and physical impact erectile dysfunction may have on the patient (and his partner) will help provide a service that affects a large number of men (Watson, 2003). By understanding the events that may occur and result in erectile dysfunction the nurse can help to explain to the patient what might be the cause of his problem (Grover, 2006). While men may present with physical symptoms, bear in mind that they may also have emotional feelings related to concerns about inadequacy as well as a feeling of emasculation. To understand erectile dysfunction in more depth, the nurse should appreciate the pathophysiology associated with the instigation and maintenance of an erection; not until this is achieved can the nurse appreciate how the disease can interfere with erection.

PATHOPHYSIOLOGY OF ERECTILE FUNCTION

A number of pathophysiological mechanisms need to be active to initiate and maintain penile erection. Penile erection is a complex physiological process that occurs as a result of a coordinated combination of neurological, vascular and hormonal events.

Anatomically the penis is highly vascular, with a plentiful supply of rich, smooth, erectile muscular tissue, and has three cylindrical erectile columns of tissue. The structure of erectile tissue (vascular and muscular) is vital for erection to occur. Dorsally the two corpora cavernosa communicate with each other for three-quarters of their length through the medial septum which separates them (Grover, 2006). Ventrally the corpus spongiosum surrounds the penile portion of urethra; this is the third column and extends to form the sensitive glans penis (Carson, Holmes and Kirby, 2002). The base of the penis is attached to the pelvis and consists of the bulb (within this is the urethra) and the cura, which are attached to the ischial and pubic rami (Astbury-Ward, 2000).

The outer layer of the corpora cavernosa is known as the tunica albuginea; this is a tough and fibrous tissue that is relatively indistensible and is made of collagen and elastin. Within the tunica albuginea is the erectile tissue; this is high vascular and is known as the trabeculae. There are a number of sinusoids allowing enhanced perfusion of the penis within the trabeculae.

The sinusoids are lined by vascular endothelium and supplied by the helicine branches of the penile artery – lying deep within the penis. The internal pudendal artery is where the penile artery originates. The helicine arterioles supply the sinusoidal spaces. When erection occurs, the spaces expand and fill with blood; venous drainage occurs via the subtunical venous plexus with most of the venous drainage occurring via the deep dorsal and circumflex veins. Figure 10.1 illustrates the anatomy of a penis.

Kirby (2003) states that an erection occurs as a result of a combination of changes associated with:

- vascular system
- endocrine system
- psychological changes.

When alteration in any of the pathways above occurs, there is a potential for erectile failure to take place.

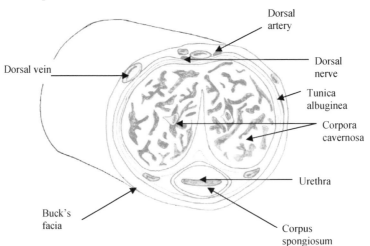

Figure 10.1. The anatomy of the penis

Table 10.1. The six vascular phases associated with penile erection

- Flaccidity
- Filling phase
- Tumescence
- Full erection
- Rigidity
- Detumescence

(Source: Dorey, 2000)

Vascular activity to initiate and sustain an erection occurs following a series of integrated vascular processes ending with a collection of blood under pressure and end organ rigidity (Moncada-Iribarren and Sáenz de Tejada, 1999). Dorey (2000) notes that the vascular process can be divided into six phases (see Table 10.1).

Christ (1995) suggests that penile erection and detumescence are primarily vascular events relying on a fine balance of arterial and venous outflow. When arterial inflow is low and is balanced by venous outflow, the penis is in a flaccid state; tumescence occurs when inflow increases and outflow falls.

FLACCIDITY

Within the penis there is low blood flow accompanied by low pressure. Muscular activity is within the pelvis, for example, the cavernosus and bulbocavernosus muscles are relaxed. The sympathetic nervous system is dominant at this stage, ensuring that arterioles are constricted and smooth muscle relaxed. Sexual stimulation promotes parasympathetic nervous system activity, resulting in vasodilation (Astbury-Ward, 2000).

FILLING PHASE

Excitatory input to the penis is initiated during the erection stage by parasympathetic nerve stimulus from segments 2–4 of the sacral spinal cord. A number of stimuli can lead to the penis becoming erect, for example, tactile stimuli to the penis and genitalia that result in a reflex erection; erotic stimuli such as visual, auditory, olfactory or imaginative stimuli can also produce penile erection (Eardley, 2003). The result is relaxation of the smooth penile arterial muscle with cavernosal and helicine arterial dilation, allowing blood to flow into the lacunar spaces.

One other mechanism associated with the filling phase is the production of nocturnal erections. Nocturnal erections occur in men during rapid eye movement (REM) sleep. The exact process associated with nocturnal erections remain unclear. Eardley (2003) suggests that there is hypothalamic involvement with increased parasympathetic and decreased sympathetic nervous activity.

TUMESCENCE

Compression of the subtunical venules against the tunica albuginea causes venous outflow to become reduced, with the penis expanding and elongating. There is little increase at this stage of intercavernosal pressure.

FULL ERECTION

At this stage intracavernous pressure rapidly increases.

RIGIDITY

Intracavernous pressure rises above diastolic pressure and blood outflow takes place with the systolic phase of the pulse allowing complete rigidity to happen. Intracavernous pressure is further enhanced by the contraction or reflex contraction of the ischiocavernosus and bulbocavernosus muscles. At this point no arterial flow takes place.

DETUMESCENCE

A reversal of events that have occurred above happens during the detumescence stage, often after erotic stimuli have been removed or ejaculation has occurred (Astbury-Ward, 2000). Detumescence occurs as a result of sympathetic nervous system activity via the thoracic segments (T10–T12) as well as lumbar segments (L1–2) in the spinal cord. A decrease of blood in the lacunar spaces happens as a result of contraction of the penile smooth muscles of the penis and the penile arteries. Contraction of the smooth trabecular muscle leads to a collapse of the lacunar spaces.

A variety of neurotransmitters contribute to erectile function such as acetylcholine (ACh); the most important neurotransmitter is nitric oxide (NO). NO functions via the cyclic guanosine monophosphate (cGMP) system and is produced from the precursor L-arginine by the enzyme nitric oxide synthase (NOS). cGMP the secondary transmitter is ultimately responsible for smooth muscle relaxation in the corpus cavernosum, resulting in erection. The process is very complex and requires an intricate coordination of various neurotransmitters and enzymes, for example, phosphodiesterase (PDE). The hormone-like fatty acid prostaglandin E1 (PGE-1) and papaverine help with the cGMP system. Carson (2004) provides an in-depth discussion of the physiological process associated with erection.

When sexual activity is concluded, the physical and psychological stimuli responsible for initiating erection fade away, smooth muscle tone increases along with vasoconstriction, cGMP is broken down by PDE-5 and detumescence occurs.

DEFINITION AND EPIDEMIOLOGY

The most common definition of erectile dysfunction is provided by the National Institutes of Health (National Institutes of Health Consensus Development Panel on Impotence, 1993), an American Government organization. Erectile dysfunction is defined as the man's inability to achieve and maintain an erection sufficient for sexual activity. There is insufficient rigidity within the penis to allow satisfactory sexual performance. Sexual performance or sexual activities are preferred terms as opposed to sexual intercourse. Sexual activity means many different things to many different people. The practice nurse must not make the assumption that penetrative intercourse with a penis will always take place during sexual activity and as a result of this assumption the measurement of successful treatment should not be measured by the ability of the man to penetrate during sexual activity. Some men (in a relationship or not) require an erect penis to engage in masturbation; the ability to instigate and maintain an erection may be part of that man's sense of masculinity. Those men who wish to start or maintain a current relationship may be fearful that they will jeopardize sexual situations if they are unable to initiate or maintain an erection for sexual activity – whatever that may be (Grover, 2006).

As men are known to be unwilling to seek help or advice for erectile dysfunction (Kirby, 2004), this makes it difficult to obtain precise data in relation to prevalence; therefore the data cited are under-representations of true numbers. McKinley (2001) suggests that approximately 150 million men worldwide are unable to achieve and maintain an erection sufficient for sexual intercourse. It is estimated that 30–50 % of men aged 40–70 years of age, globally, report some form of erectile dysfunction (Mak *et al.*, 2002; McKinley, 2001; Moreira, Lisboa and Glaser, 2000; Feldman *et al.*, 1994). In the UK it is estimated that there are 2.3 million men with the condition, representing 1 in every 10 men (Lilly ICOS, 2006).

Feldman *et al.* (1994) demonstrate that age is an important variable in relation to erectile dysfunction. In those men aged 40–70 years the incidence of moderate erectile dysfunction doubles from 17 to 34 % and severe erectile dysfunction triples from 5 to 15 %. Erectile dysfunction, it must be remembered, is not an inevitable consequence of ageing (Wakely, 2006). Weeks and Ficorelli (2006) suggest that most men at some point in their lives will have erection problems that may be stress-related, a result of smoking or alcohol ingestion, associated with a psychological or emotional disorder or the consequence of disease.

The practice nurse should be aware that the numbers of men currently presenting with erectile dysfunction will rise, and there are several reasons for this. There is a global trend for an ageing population; screening and diagnostic techniques have become more accurate and more men are having more confidence to come forward for help. Kirby (2004) suggests that by 2025 there will be over 300 million worldwide, double the current number.

ERECTILE DYSFUNCTION

Theories related to the pathophysiology of erectile dysfunction over the years have changed and developed. Early theories determined that most cases of erectile dysfunction had a psychogenic cause (Eardley, 2003) and, indeed, the patient's psychological status can have an impact on penile erection. For over a decade now it has been known that erectile dysfunction is closely associated and interrelated with a number of chronic conditions that involve compromised vascular function (Feldman *et al.*, 1994), for example:

- coronary artery disease
- hypertension
- diabetes mellitus
- hypercholesterolaemia.

As technology progresses and more data becomes available the close association and interconnectedness are becoming clearer. Some of the central mechanisms that are involved in the control of erection are related to vascular, endocrine, cellular and neural mechanisms (Eardley, 2003). The advances in science and improved clinical acumen mean that the nurse and other healthcare professionals can improve the patient's quality of life and save lives.

Erectile dysfunction may therefore serve as an early warning or wake-up call of potential heart disease upon the horizon. Those nurses caring for men with heart-related conditions should also consider the treatment of erectile dysfunction and vice versa: treating both the cardiac condition and ensuing erectile problems is truly practising holistic nursing care; it can also help to enhance the patient's quality of life. Erectile dysfunction can cause or exacerbate depression. Hence, identification and treatment can improve a couple's sexual and psychological well-being as well as facilitating the management of other important chronic diseases earlier in their development (Kirby, 2004).

For many men with erectile dysfunction there may be a variety of aetiological factors that impinge on his ability to instigate and maintain an erection. Erectile dysfunction that accompanies ageing, for example, may be the result of vascular, endocrine, psychological and neural factors – multiple aetiologies.

Eardley (2003) suggests that there are several ways of classifying the pathophysiological causes of erectile dysfunction. Table 10.2 provides an outline of the pathophysiological causes of erectile dysfunction.

Table 10.2. Six pathophysiological causes of erectile dysfunction

Psychogenic
Neural
Endocrine
Vascular
Cellular
Iatrogenic

(Source: Eardley, 2003)

ERECTILE DYSFUNCTION – RISK FACTORS

The causes of erectile dysfunction can be related to organic and/or inorganic disorders (a combination of both factors). Current thinking has shifted from attributing the cause to mainly inorganic causes to both organic and inorganic (Weeks and Ficorelli, 2006). According to Williams and Pickup (2004), organic causes are associated with physiological disorders; inorganic causes are psychological in nature and may be more common in the younger man. Dorey (2006) and Paterson (2006) provide a list of the organic causes (risks) of erectile dysfunction (see Table 10.3 below).

Psychogenic factors are involved in nearly all cases of men with erectile dysfunction (Eardley, 2003) despite the fact that in the majority of men with erectile dysfunction the dominant pathophysiology is organic (see Figure 10.2 below).

Sex is an important aspect of many people's lives. Penile erection in most men is an important facet of the male psyche and is linked to their social functioning, self-esteem, and social and familial roles (Fugl-Meyer *et al.*, 1997), hence even when the smallest of malfunction occurs affecting a man's ability to initiate or sustain an erection, this can have immense psychological consequences. Embarrassment and shame may ensue as a result of so-called performance-related anxiety. Eardley (2003) suggests that a variety of factors can contribute to psychogenic erectile dysfunction (see Table 10.4 below); he divides them into three groups:

- predisposing factors
- precipitating factors
- maintaining factors.

If the man is able to inform the nurse that he experiences nocturnal erections then it is likely that the neural, vascular and endocrine mechanisms are still intact and intrinsic to normal penile erection. The assumption to be made (until proven otherwise) is that there is a predominant psychogenic component to his condition. The relationship between psychiatric disorders such as depression and erectile dysfunction is complex. Depression can result in erectile dysfunction and erectile dysfunction can result in depression.

Men who have suffered spinal cord injury may, dependent on the level at which injury has occurred, experience erectile dysfunction. Higher level lesions may generally result in men being able to experience erections that are the result of reflex activity via intact reflex pathways. Those men who have had a lower spinal cord level injury can also enjoy erection as a result of an intact sympathetic pathway – a psychogenic erection (Eardley, 2003).

A reduction in testosterone – testosterone is central to male sexual functioning and is the principal androgen (Jenkins, Kemnitz and Tortora, 2007) – can impinge on libido. Men who are hypogonadal, according to Eardley (2003), do not automatically lose psychogenic and reflex erection. These men may experience a reduction in nocturnal erections, accompanied by reduced duration and rigidity of erection.

Table 10.3. Some potential organic causes of erectile dysfunction

Factor	Potential components
Vasculogenic	• Hypertension • Atherosclerosis • Ischaemia
Neurogenic	• Spinal injury • Multiple sclerosis • Dementia • Spinal tumour • Parkinson's disease • Cerebrovascular disease • Cauda equina compression • Prolapsed intravertebral disc

Endocrinologic	• Hormone deficiency
	  – Hypogonadism
	  – Thyroid disease
	• Hyperprolactinaemia

Drug-related	• Certain antihypertensives • Some psychotropics • Some hormonal agents
Systemic	• Diabetes mellitus • Malignancy • Chronic renal failure
Surgical	• Transurethral and radical prostatectomy • Cystectomy • Pelvic surgery (abdominal perineal resection) • Radiotherapy
Lifestyle	• Smoking • Alcohol • Recreational drugs • Trauma to the perineum • Bicycling • Horse riding
Other	• Arthritis • Aetiology unknown

(Source: Adapted from Dorey, 2006; Paterson, 2006; Carson, 2004; Eardley, 2003)

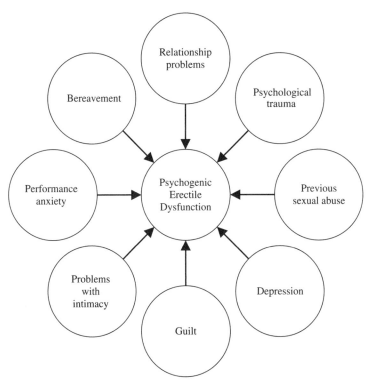

Figure 10.2. Some psychogenic causes of erectile dysfunction

Table 10.4. Predisposing, precipitating and maintaining factors

Predisposing factors	Educational issues such as poor sexual education
	Cultural issues, for example, restricted upbringing
	Traumatic sexual experience
	Lifestyle issues such as marital (partnership), financial stress
Precipitating factors	Organic disorders
	Extramarital (partnership) affairs
	Unreasonable expectations
	Depression and anxiety
	Loss of partner
Maintaining factors	Performance-related anxiety
	Diminishing attraction to partner
	Educational issues such as poor sexual education
	Fear of intimacy

(Source: Adapted from Eardley, 2003)

The most common cause of erectile dysfunction is vascular disease, with atherosclerosis being the most common of all vascular causes (Carson, 2004). The risk factors related to atherosclerosis – for example, hyperlipidaemia and diabetes mellitus – are associated with the development of erectile dysfunction (Paterson, 2006). Erectile dysfunction can be an independent marker for other serious life-threatening conditions, for example, hypertension and hypercholesterolaemia (Edwards, 2005). The British Heart Foundation (2005) suggests that:

• erectile dysfunction in a patient with no cardiac symptoms may be a marker of occult vascular disease
• all men over the age of 25 years with erectile dysfunction should be screened for cardiac risk factors and symptoms of vascular disease.

Kirby (2004) points out that men who present with erectile dysfunction provide the practice nurse with an opportunity to detect if the patient has, or is at risk of, cardiovascular disease as well as other concurrent conditions, for example, diabetes mellitus, benign prostatic hypertrophy, depression and hypogonadism.

The restriction of blood flow into the penis may be the first sign of impending damage to the vessels of the heart as the narrower blood vessels of the penis are more susceptible to occlusion than the larger vessels of the heart in the early stages of atherosclerotic disease. Erectile dysfunction as a result of penile atherosclerosis may indicate arterial disease elsewhere in the body.

Any antihypertensive medication has the potential to cause erectile dysfunction by lowering the pressure in the arteriosclerotic vessels. There are some, however, that have a greater effect than would be expected from this alone (Wakely, 2002). Iatrogenic erectile dysfunction occurs as a result of prescribed medication. It should be noted that the older the patient becomes the more medications he is likely to be prescribed (DH, 2001). The effects of the man's sexual competence in relation to the use of recreational drugs (non-prescribed) is also significant (see Table 10.5).

Most of the medication listed in Table 10.5 can result in:

• erectile dysfunction
• loss of libido
• ejaculatory dysfunction
• orgasmic dysfunction.

DIAGNOSING ERECTILE DYSFUNCTION

Kirby (2005) suggests that most cases of erectile dysfunction are treated in the primary care setting. Edwards (2005) points out that the management of erectile dysfunction can be treated successfully within the general practice setting without the need to refer the patient to specialist secondary care. Patients are becoming more aware that simple, effective treatments are becoming available

Table 10.5. Commonly used therapeutic (and non-prescribed) medications associated with erectile dysfunction

Psychotropics
- Benzodiazepines
- Amphetamines
- Barbiturates
- Opiates
- Tranquilizers
  - Phenothiazines
  - Butyrophenones
  - Thioxanthenes
- Antidepressants
  - Monoamine oxidase inhibitors
  - Tricylics
  - Serotonin re-uptake inhibitors

Antihypertensives
- Diuretics
- Vasodilators
- Sympatholytics
- β Blockers
- Ganglion blockers

Anticholinergics
  - Atropine
  - Diphenhydramine

Androgenic agents
- Luteinising Hormone-Replacement Hormone
- Anti-androgens
- Oestrogen

Recreational (non-prescribed) drugs
- Alcohol
- Marijuana
- Amphetamine
- Opiates
- Cocaine
- Anabolic steroids
- Nicotine

Others
- Cimetidine
- Digoxin
- Metoclopramide
- Phenytoin
- Carbamazepine
- Clofibrate
- Indomethacin

(Source: Paterson, 2006; Carson, 2004; Eardley, 2003)

Table 10.6. Summary of the psychogenic and organic causes of erectile dysfunction

Psychogenic origin	Organic origin
Sudden onset	Gradual onset
Good-quality or better spontaneous/self-stimulated/nocturnal erections/waking erections	Lack of tumescence
Premature ejaculation or inability to ejaculate	Normal libido (except in hypogonadal men) and ejaculation
Relationship problems or changes	Risk factor in current or past history in particular with reference to cardiovascular, endocrine and neurological systems
Major life events	Operations, radiotherapy or trauma to the pelvis or scrotum
Psychological problems	Use of medications recognized as being associated with erectile dysfunction
Specific situation	All circumstances
	Lifestyle factors such as smoking, high use of alcohol, use of recreational drugs or body-building drugs

(Source: Erectile Dysfunction Alliance, 1999; Carson, Holmes and Kirby, 2002)

for the treatment of erectile dysfunction, and as a result are demanding more access to the various treatments available (Carson, Holmes and Kirby, 2002).

Prior to providing treatment and offering the patient choice with respect to his treatment options, a diagnosis will need to be made, as this will guide the treatment options available to the patient. The practice nurse is a highly skilled and competent member of the primary healthcare team who comes into contact with many patients during the course of his/her duty. The men s/he works with present with a multitude of healthcare needs; s/he is often the first point of contact for the patient, including men who may be experiencing problems associated with erectile dysfunction and, as such, is ideally placed to assess, plan, implement and evaluate care.

Table 10.6 summarizes the differences associated with psychogenic and organic origins of erectile dysfunction.

THE CONSULTATION – HISTORY-TAKING

Prior to undertaking the consultation the practice nurse must appreciate that consultations of this type will take more time than the average consultation (Ralf and McNicholas, 2000) and as such the practice nurse needs to factor this into his/her workload. The first part of the process of identifying those men who may have or may be at risk of erectile dysfunction is to ask questions; this allows the man to tell his story. The nurse should assume a proactive approach to identifying such men. The patient's partner may also be part of the history-taking exercise, if the patient feels this is appropriate.

Weeks and Gambescia (2000) have determined that a number of men with erectile dysfunction have delayed seeking help and advice for up to five years after the onset of the problem. Often these men hope and think that the problem will cure itself or go away. Many men report that they felt they were the only one it happened to. As most men will be reluctant to talk about the issue of erectile dysfunction (and some nurses as well), the nurse should make assessment of erectile dysfunction a routine aspect of taking a patient history. Explain to the patient that the questions you are asking are routine and you ask them of all male patients. Once the patient (and the nurse) has made the first step to seeking help and advice, according to Laumann, Paik and Rosen. (1999), they are relieved.

All aspects of clinical assessment demand that the nurse is knowledgeable; this is also true when assessing men with erectile dysfunction. An in-depth nursing, medical, psychosocial, sexual history as well as a physical examination is needed to help elucidate the cause of erectile dysfunction. Determine if the source of the problem is psychogenic, organic or both in origin and identify any clinical signs of the known risk factors. At all stages of the assessment, if required, the nurse should refer the patient to a GP or another appropriate healthcare worker. During history-taking, the nurse should ensure privacy at all times in order to encourage the man to explain more about his condition. History-taking, according to Carson, Holmes and Kirby (2002), has many functions:

- to confirm that the patient is suffering from erectile dysfunction;
- to assess the severity of the condition;
- to identify a possible underlying aetiology;
- to assess the fitness of the patient for resuming sexual activity.

It is vital that the language used is one that the patient and the nurse understand and can clarify the meaning of technical and slang terms that might be used. At all times the nurse should aim to correct any misunderstanding by either party as the terminology associated with erectile dysfunction can be confusing. The tactful use of simple questions can help to eradicate confusion. Hallam-Jones and Birch (2002) suggest that the nurse broach the subject by asking the patient non-threatening open-ended questions. The nurse might bring up the issue when working with a diabetic patient by asking him, 'Did you know that some men with diabetes can develop erection problems and when this happens there are treatments available to help?' Paterson (2006) raises the issue with her diabetic patients by saying, 'Diabetes can cause problems with your sex life. Do you ever have this problem?' Such approaches provide the patient with permission to raise the issue or to leave it. The patient may not wish to discuss the issues during this consultation but it may encourage him to raise them at subsequent consultations. Carson, Holmes and Kirby (2002) suggest that the following points should be covered during the consultation, providing the nurse with more insight and understanding of the issues the man is experiencing:

- the patient's sexual development and the onset of puberty;
- the patient's and his partner's attitude to the problem;
- the presence of any obvious stress factors, such as marital problems, financial concerns, sexual inhibitions;
- medical and drug history, in particular smoking, chronic medical illness, pelvic, perineal or penile surgery, pelvic radiotherapy, recreational drug use or psychiatric illness.

PHYSICAL EXAMINATION

The knowledge gained during the history-taking aspect of the consultation will more or less guide the physical examination. Ralf and McNicholas (2000) suggest that in the majority of patients who require examination this should be limited to the basic minimum. Weeks and Ficorelli (2006) suggest:

- blood pressure measurements
- examination of the abdomen
- examination of the genitalia
- assessment of secondary sexual characteristics
- assessment of peripheral pulses
- digital rectal examination to evaluate prostate size

See Figure 10.3.

CLINICAL INVESTIGATIONS

As with the physical examination, investigations will vary depending on the findings from the history and the physical examination as well as the willingness of the patient. Carson, Holmes and Kirby (2002) suggest that clinical investigations can be divided into three sections: essential, possible and specialized (see Table 10.7 below).

TREATMENT OPTIONS

Effective treatment can enhance a man's sense of self-esteem, his relationships and his quality of life. Once an in-depth evaluation has been undertaken and a diagnosis of erectile dysfunction has been made, there are a number of treatment options available to the patient. The patient must be closely involved with choosing the options on offer to him and a bespoke or tailor-made treatment plan should be devised. The treatment plan may include issues associated with lifestyle adjustments such as reduction in smoking and alcohol consumption and taking up exercise

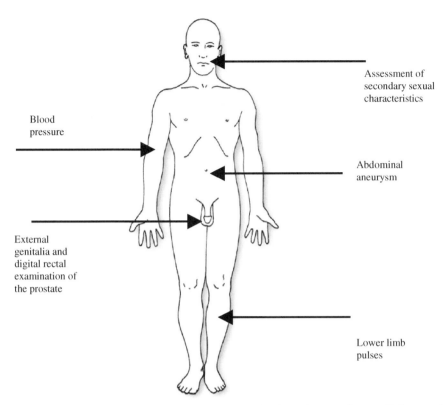

Figure 10.3. Essential aspects of the physical examination. (Source: Carson, Holmes and Kirby, 2002; Weeks and Ficorelli, 2006)

Table 10.7. Potential clinical investigations for erectile dysfunction

Essential	Possible	Specialized
• Urine dipstick • Serum glucose	• Serum testosterone • Sex-hormone-binding globulin • Prolactin • Creatinine • Thyroid hormones • Fasting lipid profile • Prostate-specific antigen • Follicle-stimulating hormone/ luteinizing hormone	• Nocturnal penile tumescence testing • Colour Doppler imaging • Pharmacocavernosography • Pharmacoarteriography • Psychiatric evaluation • Vascular evaluation • Cardiac evaluation

(Source: Carson, Holmes and Kirby, 2002)

(Wakely, 2006). The nurse must aim, in the first instance, to address any reversible conditions that are contributing to erectile dysfunction. When lifestyle changes and medication adjustments do not improve erectile function, effective treatments are available. There are over ten different types of treatments (Lilly ICOS, 2006). The introduction of oral agents such as sildenafil have, according to Kirby (2004), revolutionized the treatment of erectile dysfunction, providing men with a success-ful and safe method of restoring sexual function with minimal side effects. There is a common myth that the use of oral treatments gives an instant and prolonged erection. Oral treatments need to be used in conjunction with mental and physical sexual stimulation to work effectively. The nurse must inform the patient of this (Tomlinson and Evans, 2005). Three key oral treatments are discussed here as well as penile injections, intraurethral pellets and vacuum pumps. Other treatments include:

- counselling (psychosexual therapy)
- hormone treatment
- surgery.

Astbury-Ward (2000) points out that treatment not only affects the patient but also, if the patient has one, his partner. The issue of including the partner in the consulta-tion will have already been addressed earlier on in the consultation and the nurse may also need to offer him/her support. Time must be spent with the patient (and if appropriate his partner) in discussing the pros and cons of the various treatment options available. It may be that the patient needs to experience several treatments prior to deciding on the most appropriate one for him. Other conditions, such as dia-betes mellitus, must be well controlled and treated accordingly (Romeo *et al.*, 2000). See Table 10.8 (below) outlining three oral treatments.

INTRACAVERNOSAL AND INTRAURETHRAL THERAPY

The use of self-injection with vasoactive drugs has increased over the years. The first effective drug for intracavernosal use, papaverine, was introduced in the 1980s. Papaverine is a powerful, direct, smooth muscle relaxant, acting on trabecular muscle as well as the erectile tissues. The erection, as a result of its use, can last for several hours. Alprostadil, a prostaglandin, has a success rate of 95 % (Tomlinson and Evans, 2005); despite the success rate of intracavernosal injections (ICIs) there are not many men who are prepared to self-inject their penis.

There is another method of using alprostadil and that is as an intraurethral pellet – the Medicated Urethral System for Erection (MUSE), the rate of success with this therapy according to Tomlinson and Evans (2005) is 50 %. Carson, Holmes and Kirby (2002) suggest that alprostadil is the first drug of choice for intracavernosal pharmacotherapy, with several preparations

Table 10.8. Three types of oral treatment for erectile dysfunction

Treatment	What it is	Time of action	Cautions	Contraindications	Side effects
Sildenafil (Viagara)	Sildenafil is a selective inhibitor of PDE 5, enhancing normal vasodilatory erectile mechanisms. A blue tablet available in the following strengths 25 mg, 50 mg and 100 mg. Should be swallowed approximately one hour prior to desired sexual activity. Sexual stimulation is required to enhance effectiveness. Sildenafil is metabolized in the liver.	Time of action varies approximately 25 minutes to four hours after ingestion depending on the individual. Effectiveness can be reduced if taken with food.	• Cardiovascular disease • Peyronie's disease • Predisposition to priapism	Contraindicated in those men who are receiving nitrates or in those in whom vasodilation or sexual activity are inadvisable. Also contraindicated in those men with unstable angina, recent stroke, hypotension and myocardial infarction without full history. This drug should not be taken with other erectile dysfunction medication.	Side effects can include dyspepsia, vomiting, flushing, headaches, dizziness, blocked nose, visual disturbance, backache, raised intraocular pressure and rash. Rarely may cause painful red eyes and priapism. The side effects are usually mild and transient.

(continued)

Table 10.8. (*Continued*)

Treatment	What it is	Time of action	Cautions	Contraindications	Side effects
Vardenafil (Levita)	Vardenafil is also a PDE 5 inhibitor. The tablet is orange in colour and is available in the following strengths: 5 mg, 10 mg and 20 mg. Should be swallowed 25 to 60 minutes prior to the desired sexual activity. Sexual stimulation is required to enhance effectiveness. Vardenafil is metabolized in the liver.	Time of action varies approximately 15 minutes to five hours after ingestion depending on the individual. Not usually affected by food intake but effectiveness can be reduced where fat content is high.	• Cardiovascular disease	Contraindicated in those men who are receiving nitrates or in those in whom vasodilation or sexual activity are inadvisable. Also contraindicated in those men with unstable angina, recent stroke, hypotension and myocardial infarction without full history. This drug should not be taken with other erectile dysfunction medication.	Side effects can include dyspepsia, vomiting, flushing, headaches, dizziness, blocked nose, visual disturbance, backache, raised intraoccular pressure and rash. May cause painful red eyes and priapism.
			• Peyronie's disease		The side effects are usually mild and transient.
			• Predisposition to priapism		

(*continued*)

Table 10.8. (*Continued*)

Treatment	What it is	Time of action	Cautions	Contraindications	Side effects
Tadalafil (Cialis)	Tadalafil is a light-yellow tablet and should be swallowed between 30 minutes and 12 hours before desired sexual activity. This drug only comes in 20mg strength. Sexual stimulation is required to enhance effectiveness.	Time of action varies from approximately 30 minutes to 24 hours after ingestion depending on the individual. Not affected by food intake.	• Cardiovascular disease	Contraindicated in those men who are receiving nitrates or in those in whom vasodilation or sexual activity are inadvisable. Also contraindicated in those men with unstable angina, recent stroke, hypotension and myocardial infarction without full history. This drug should not be taken with other erectile dysfunction medication.	Side effects can include dyspepsia, vomiting, flushing, headaches, dizziness, blocked nose, visual disturbance, backache, raised intraocular pressure and rash. May cause painful red eyes and priapism.
	Like sildenafil and vardenafil, tadalafil is also a PDE 5 inhibitor and is also metabolized in the liver.		• Peyronie's disease		The side effects are usually mild and transient.
			• Predisposition to priapism		

(Source: Adapted from Paterson, 2006; British Medical Association and Royal Pharmaceutical Society of Great Britain, 2005; Carson, Holmes and Kirby, 2002)

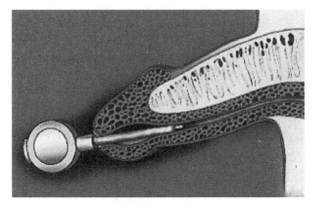

Figure 10.4. Medicated Urethral System for Erection (reproduced by permission of Media Pharmaceuticals Ltd)

licensed for treatment. The patient is required to use an applicator to insert the pellet into the urethra (see Figure 10.4). When the pellet is *in situ* the preparation dissolves and is absorbed by the urethral mucosa and from there enters the corpora.

VACUUM ERECTION DEVICES

The use of a vacuum erection device is another mode of treatment. The prime action of the vacuum pump is to draw blood into the penis by creating a vacuum, when the blood is trapped in the intra- and extra-corporal compartments of the penis. It is kept there by the use of constriction ring(s) (see Figure 10.5 below). Table 10.9 (below) provides an overview of three further treatments.

PRIAPISM

Priapism is persistent erection that is usually painful. A man who has endured an erection for over four hours must be seen by a medical practitioner as this is deemed a medical emergency (Tomlinson and Evans 2005). Priapism, according to Carson, Holmes and Kirby (2002), is a troublesome side effect related to some treatments for erectile dysfunction. The nurse should provide the patient with information about the possibility of priapism occurring and what to do if it does occur. Failure to achieve detumescence after 6–8 hours may result in irreversible damage to the corpora cavernosa as well as scarring caused by fibrosis. Priapism can be relieved by the aspiration of blood by placing a needle in the corpora cavernosa.

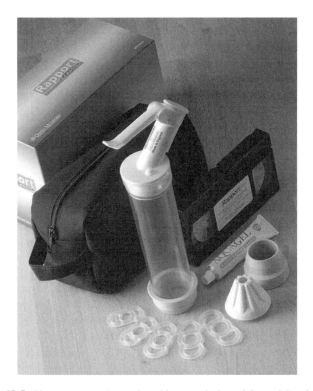

Figure 10.5. Vacuum pump (reproduced by permission of Owen Mumford Ltd)

TEACHING

The nurse will have to engage with the patient and teach him (and if appropriate his partner) first how to handle the needles and syringes and the drawing up of the drug; some drugs may require reconstituting from powder prior to injection. Once the drug has been made up, the skin over the penis is drawn taut and the needle and syringe are held at right angles to the penis.

The nurse should advise the patient to give the injection as far to the base of the penis as possible on either side and avoiding any visible veins; the sites for injection should be alternated. Reinforcement of technique can be given by providing the patient with supplementary materials, such as written instructions, DVDs and videos to take away.

The patient must be given information about how to dispose safely of sharps outside of the clinical setting. It is also important to explain about the possibility of the development of the formation of fibroid nodules around the injection site after repeated use that may lead to penile curvature, haematoma formation and pain along the shaft of the penis after injection.

Prior to inserting a pellet using the MUSE, the patient should be advised to urinate as this may aid the insertion of the applicator as well as facilitating the

Table 10.9. Treatment options available to treat erectile dysfunction

Treatment	What it is	Time of action	Cautions	Contraindications	Side effects
Alprostadil (Caverject)	Intracavernosal injection. The medication is injected into the intracavernosa at the base of the penis. The products are prostaglandins-prostaglandin E_1 available in strengths of 10 and 20 microgram cartridges. The first dose should be 2.5 micrograms followed by 5 micrograms (if some response to the first dose), and 7.5 micrograms if no response to first dose. The dose should be titrated to response. The first dose must be given by medically trained personnel and self-administration only after patient education has occurred.	The injection should be taken 5–15 minutes prior to the desired time of the erection. The erection can last up to approximately one hour. The patient should be advised that there must be 24 hours between injections.	If an erection lasts for longer than 4 hours, then the patient must seek medical advice as this is deemed priapism. The penis may take on anatomical deformity as a result of penile fibrosis (e.g. Peyronie's disease). Should not be taken in conjunction with other erectile dysfunction medication.	There is a predisposition to prolonged erection in those with leukaemia and multiple myeloma. In those men who have penile implants or when sexual activity is not advised then intracavernosal medicines should not be used.	Priaprism, penile bruising and pain, penile rash and oedema. Haemorrhage, rash and infection may occur but are rare.

(continued)

Table 10.9. (*Continued*)

Treatment	What it is	Time of action	Cautions	Contraindications	Side effects
Alprostadil (MUSE) (Medicated Urethral System for Erection)	MUSE is produced in single application applicators. Initially 250 mg and adjusted according to response with a range of 0.125 micrograms to 1 mg. A maximum of 2 doses in 24 hours and 7 doses in 7 days. The first dose must be given by medically trained personnel and self-administration only after patient education has occurred.	Within 5–10 minutes of insertion of the pellet erection is usually achieved and this lasts approximately 30–60 minutes. May be used twice in a 24 period.	If an erection lasts for longer than 4 hours, then the patient must seek medical advice as this is deemed priapism. The penis may take on anatomical deformity as a result of penile fibrosis (e.g., Peyronie's disease). Should not be taken in conjunction with erectile dysfunction medication.	There is a predisposition to prolonged erection in those with leukaemia and multiple myeloma. In those men who have penile implants or when sexual activity is not advised, then intracavernosal medicines should not be used.	Priaprism, penile bruising and pain, penile rash and oedema. Haemorrhage, rash and infection may occur but are rare.

(continued)

Table 10.9. (*Continued*)

Treatment	What it is	Time of action	Cautions	Contraindications	Side effects
Vacuum pump	A vacuum is created around the penis resulting in increased arterial inflow leading to an erection. A constriction ring is applied around the base of the penis to sustain erection.	An erection with the constriction ring in place (or until it is removed) can sustain an erection for up to 30 minutes. The ring can be left in place safely for up to 30 minutes.	Not to be left *in situ* for longer than 30 minutes.	Peyronie's disease, corporal fibrosis bleeding or clotting disorders, such as, sickle-cell anaemia, leukaemia. Inappropriate for those who have poor manual dexterity.	Priapism. Numbness and discomfort on orgasm. Cold feeling penis.

(Source: Paterson, 2006; British Medical Association and Royal Pharmaceutical Society of Great Britain, 2005; Carson, Holmes and Kirby, 2002)

intraurethral dispersion of the drug (Carson, Holmes and Kirby, 2002). The patient should be in the sitting position; when the application is inserted into the urethra, the button that releases the pellet is depressed. After insertion the penis is held upright and gently rolled to disperse the drug.

RESTRICTIONS ON NHS TREATMENT FOR ERECTILE DYSFUNCTION

The Department of Health has placed restrictions on the prescribing of NHS treatments for erectile dysfunction. This was reviewed in 2001 and the restrictions put in place by the Department of Health in 1999 were upheld (DH, 1999). Unless a man has been receiving treatment prior to 14 September 1998 only those signified in specific groups can be given treatment paid for by the NHS. Table 10.10 outlines these conditions. Kirby (2005) reports that the restrictions mean that those men whose erectile dysfunction is caused by diabetes or severe pelvic injury can be treated on the NHS; however, those whose erectile dysfunction is a result of cardiovascular disease or depression cannot. There are exceptional circumstances where the patient who is experiencing severe distress from the condition can be treated after specialist assessment in a hospital.

SURGICAL TREATMENT

When conservative methods for treating erectile dysfunction have been unsuccessful, surgical treatment may be an option. Carson, Holmes and Kirby (2002) suggest

Table 10.10. Conditions associated with erectile dysfunction where treatment will be paid for by the NHS

Diabetes
Multiple sclerosis
Parkinson's disease
Poliomyelitis
Prostate cancer
Prostatectomy (including transurethral prostatectomy)
Radical pelvic surgery
Renal failure treated by dialysis or transplant
Severe pelvic injury
Single gene neurological disease
Spinal cord injury
Spina bifida

(Source: DH, 1999)

that the incidence of morbidity and complications is significantly greater than with medical treatment.

There are several surgical procedures that are available and the correct procedure will need to be decided upon after careful assessment with the patient and, if appropriate, his partner. Penile prosthetic implants provide penile rigidity and erectile size that satisfactorily simulates the normal physiological erectile state necessary for sexual intercourse (Woodworth, Carson and Webster, 1991). Semi-rigid rod prostheses are implanted into the corpora cavernosa. The two rods or cylinders vary in length and are trimmed to the patient's measurements. Inflatable penile prostheses come as self-contained two-piece and three-piece designs with pumps and reservoirs. The reservoirs are embedded within the scrotal sac and are used to inflate and deflate the device (Carson, 2004). There is, however, an infection risk at insertion and the potential for mechanical failure.

CONCLUSION

Erectile dysfunction is a common condition and is easily treated. The nurse is ideally placed to use a proactive approach to the identification of erectile dysfunction. Nurses in the practice setting have often developed a role that incorporates health promotion, they usually have longer consultation sessions with patients as well as being multi-skilled and competent practitioners and they are also often the first point of contact for the patient.

It has been stated that erectile dysfunction can be a marker for the patient's overall vascular health and occult cardiovascular disease; this means that the nurse has a unique opportunity to engage in primary prevention of vascular disease. The link between erectile dysfunction and cardiovascular disease is the vascular endothelium. This has an essential role in the regulation of circulation.

A detailed history is vital if a correct diagnosis is be to made. Diagnosis will also require a physical examination. The outcome of the consultation will be a tailor-made care pathway. The nurse needs to ask personal and often intimate questions of the patient in a tactful and sensitive manner in order to ellicit the patient's history and the problems he is presenting with. If appropriate, the consultation may take place with the patient's partner present; again, tact and diplomacy are needed by the nurse when this issue is introduced.

The patient must be given an opportunity to be informed of the most appropriate type of treatment. He should also be told about the advantages and disadvantages of the various treatments in order to make an informed decision. There are several treatment modalities available and it may be that the patient tries more than one if others fail or are unacceptable. Patient education is vital during assessment and prior to treatment and at follow-up sessions when the treatment modalities are being reviewed and evaluated. Referral to specialists in the secondary care sector may be required.

REFERENCES

Astbury-Ward, E. (2000) The erectile dysfunction revolution. *Nursing Standard*, **15** (1), 34–40.

British Heart Foundation (2005) *Drugs for Erectile Dysfunction*, BHF, London.

British Medical Association and Royal Pharmaceutical Society of Great Britain (2005) *Nurse Prescribers' Formulary for Community Practitioners 2005–2007*, British Medical Association and Royal Pharmaceutical Society of Great Britain, London.

Carson, C.C. (2004) Erectile dysfunction: diagnosis and treatment. In (eds R.S. Kirky, C.C. Carson, M.G. Kirby and R.N. Farah) *Men's Health*, 2nd edn, Taylor & Francis, London, pp. 343–357, Chapter 27.

Carson, C., Holmes, S. and Kirby, R.S. (2002) *Fast Facts Erectile Dysfunction*, 3rd edn, Health Press Ltd, Abingdon.

Christ, G.J. (1995) The penis as a vascular organ. *Urological Clinics of North America*, **22** (4), 727–745.

Department of Health (1999) *HSC/1999/148: Treatment for Impotence*, DH, London.

Department of Health (2001) *Medicines and Older People: Implementing Medicines: Related Aspects of the NSF for Older People*, DH, London.

Dorey, G. (2000) Conservative treatment of erectile dysfunction 1: anatomy/physiology. *British Journal of Nursing*, **9** (11), 691–694.

Dorey, G. (2006) *Pelvic Dysfunction in Men: Diagnosis and Treatment of Male Incontinence and Erectile Dysfunction*, John Wiley & Sons Ltd, Chichester.

Eardley, I. (2003) Pathophysiology of erectile dysfunction. *British Journal of Diabetes and Vascular Disease*, **2**, 272–276.

Edwards, D. (2005) Erectile dysfunction. In (eds S. Chambers, G. Kassianos and J. Morrell) *Improving Practice in Primary Care: Practical Advice from Practising Doctors*, CSF Medical Communications, Long Hanborough, pp. 143–153, Chapter 14.

Erectile Dysfunction Association (1999) *UK Management Guidelines for Erectile Dysfunction*, Royal Society of Medicine, London.

Feldman, H.A., Goldstein, I., Hatzichristou, D.G. *et al.* (1994) Impotence and its medical and psychological correlates: results of the Massachusetts aging study. *Journal of Urology*, **151**, 54–61.

Fugl-Meyer, A.R., Lodnett, G., Brandholm, I.B. and Fugl-Meyer, K.S. (1997) On life satisfaction in male erectile dysfunction. *International Journal of Impotence*, **9** (3), 141–148.

Grover, L. (2006) Erectile dysfunction. *Primary Health Care*, **16** (6), 43–50.

Hallam-Jones, R. and Birch, P. (2002) Erectile dysfunction: identification and advice. *Practice Nursing*, **13** (7), 292–297.

Jenkins, G.W., Kemnitz, C.P. and Tortora, G.J. (2007) *Anatomy and Physiology from Science to Life*, John Wiley & Sons Inc., New Jersey.

Kirby, M. (2003) *Erectile Dysfunction and Vascular Disease*, Blackwell, Oxford.

Kirby, M. (2004) Erectile dysfunction. *Primary Care Nursing*, **1** (2), 92–95.

Kirby, M. (2005) Look beneath the surface of ED. *Independent Nurse*, 9th May 2005.

Laumann, E.O., Paik, A. and Rosen, R.C. (1999) Sexual dysfunction in the United States: prevalence and predictors. *Journal of the American Medical Association*, **281** (6), 537–544.

Lilly, ICOS. (2006) Man Matters: Helping You to Find the Right Answer, Lilly Pharmaceuticals, Basingstoke.

Mak, R., De Backer, G., Kornitzer, M. and DeMeyer, J.M. (2002) Prevalence and correlates of erectile dysfunction in a population based study in Belgium. *European Urology*, **41** (2), 132–138.

McKinley, J.B. (2001) The worldwide prevalence and epidemiology of erectile dysfunction. *International Journal of Impotence Research*, **12**(suppl.), S6–S11.

Moncada-Iribarren, I. and Sáenz de Tejada, I. (1999) Vascular physiology of penile erection. In (eds C.C. Carson, R.S. Kirby and I. Goldstein) *Textbook of Erectile Dysfunction*, Isis Medical Media, Oxford, pp. 51–57, Chapter 2.

Moreira, E.D., Lisboa, C.C.F. and Glaser, D.B. (2000) A cross sectional population based study of erectile dysfunction epidemiology in North Eastern Brazil. *Journal of Urology*, **163**(Suppl. 15).

National Institutes of Health Consensus Development Panel on Impotence (1993) 'Impotence'.

Paterson, C. (2006) Erectile dysfunction in men with diabetes. *Practice Nurse*, **5** (31), 41–48.

Ralf, D. and McNicholas, T. (2000) UK management guidelines for erectile dysfunction. *British Medical Journal*, **321**, 499–503.

Romeo, J.H., Seftel, A.D., Madhun, Z.T. and Aron, D.C. (2000) Sexual function in men with type two diabetes: association with glycemic control. *Journal of Urology*, **163** (3), 788–791.

Tomlinson, J.M. and Evans, C. (2005) Erectile dysfunction. In (ed. J.M. Tomlinson) *ABC of Sexual Health*, 2nd edn, BMJ Books, London, pp. 43–47, Chapter 12.

Wakely, G. (2006) Sexual dysfunction in primary care. In (eds T. Belfield, Y. Carter , P. Matthews, C. Moss and A. Weyman) *The Handbook of Sexual Health in Primary Care*, Family Planning Association, London, pp. 209–222, Chapter 8.

Watson, P. (2003) Primary care and sex: too close for comfort? *Journal of Family Planning and Reproductive Health Care*, **29** (2), 43.

Weeks B. and Ficorelli, C.T. (2006) How new drugs help treat erectile dysfunction. *Nursing*, **36** (1), 18–19.

Weeks, G.R. and Gambescia, N. (2000) *Erectile Dysfunction: Integrating Couple Therapy, Sex and Therapy, and Medical Treatment*, Norton and Company, New York.

Williams, G. and Pickup, J.C. (2004) *Handbook of Diabetes*, 3rd edn, Blackwell, Oxford.

Woodworth, B.E., Carson, C.C. and Webster, G.D. (1991) Inflatable penile prosthesis: effect on functional longevity. *Urology*, **38** (6), 533–536.

11 Smoking and the male reproductive tract

INTRODUCTION

Smoking is bad for your health; this must be one of the most profound understatements ever made. Smoking is known to be the principal avoidable cause of premature deaths in the United Kingdom (Department of Health (DH), 2004). Smoking can also make men infertile (Tengs and Osgood, 2001) and impact on their reproductive abilities in many ways; a number of men may defer consultation as they perceive infertility to be a threat to their masculinity (Hirsh, 2003). The effects of cigarette smoking can impinge not only on the health and fertility of men but also on:

- the fertility of women
- sexual function in men
- pregnant women's health
- the health of an unborn child
- the health of young children.

Chapter 10 has already discussed the impact cigarette smoking can have on man's erectile function. This chapter provides a general discussion of the effects of smoking on the male; the male reproductive tract is discussed and described followed by an examination of the impact smoking has on male reproductive health. The role and function of the nurse in smoking cessation is briefly discussed. Figure 11.1 (below) provides an overview of data associated with cigarette smoking in the UK.

THE EFFECTS OF SMOKING

A HISTORICAL PERSPECTIVE

The inhalation and burning of dried herbs and incense in order to provide pharmacological and psychoactive effects go back at least 3000 years when smoking was used in magical, ceremonial and religious practices by the Maya Indians in South America and the Egyptians. The use and spread of tobacco by Europeans following the importation by Spanish explorers after the fifteenth century became a commonplace habit. In contemporary society, it has become a killer.

Mackaness (1985) states that two factors favoured the rapid spread of tobacco smoking: the ease of technique combined with the quick onset of the effects on the central nervous

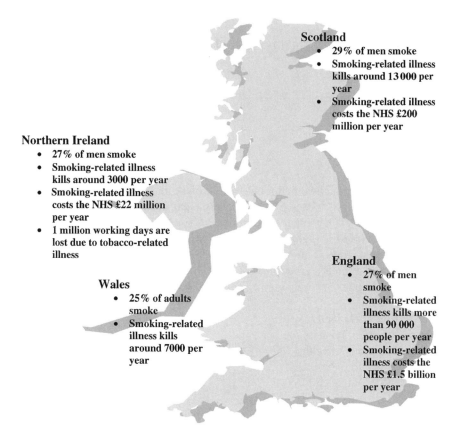

Scotland
- 29% of men smoke
- Smoking-related illness kills around 13 000 per year
- Smoking-related illness costs the NHS £200 million per year

Northern Ireland
- 27% of men smoke
- Smoking-related illness kills around 3000 per year
- Smoking-related illness costs the NHS £22 million per year
- 1 million working days are lost due to tobacco-related illness

Wales
- 25% of adults smoke
- Smoking-related illness kills around 7000 per year

England
- 27% of men smoke
- Smoking-related illness kills more than 90 000 people per year
- Smoking-related illness costs the NHS £1.5 billion per year

Figure 11.1. Data associated with smoking in the UK. (Source: Adapted from British Medical Association, 2004)

system. These effects include stimulation, sedation and a combination of both, depending on the dose and the individual's rate of absorption of the nicotine inhaled.

THE COMPOSITION OF A CIGARETTE

Over 600 additives can be added to cigarettes – legally (DH, 2000). Nicotine is the addictive substance of tobacco, and cigarettes are designed to deliver a steady dose of nicotine. In addition to the two types of blended leaves in cigarette tobacco there are filters that are made up from the stems and other bits of tobacco which otherwise would be waste products. Additives are used to make tobacco products more acceptable to the consumer. A range of additives are present (see Figure 11.2 below).

Over 50 of the chemicals in cigarettes are carcinogenic; see Table 11.1 below for an outline of some components used in cigarettes (Action on Smoking and Health (ASH), 2001).

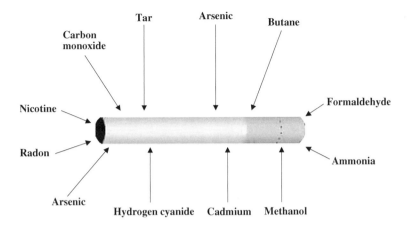

Figure 11.2. Some cigarette additives

Table 11.1. Some additives used in cigarettes and their potential effects

Component	Potential effects
Acetaldehyde	Used in glues and resins, may increase the absorption of other chemicals in the bronchial tree
Acetone	Used in solvent, irritating to the throat, nose and eyes. Long-term exposure can cause hepatic and renal damage
Ammonia	Causes asthma and hypertension, used in cleaning products
Benzene	Found in pesticide, gasoline and solvents. Can cause leukaemia and other chemicals
Cadmium	Used in corrosive metal coatings as well as storage batteries. Can cause cancer. May cause renal, cerebral and hepatic damage
Carbon monoxide	The main poisonous gas in car exhausts, binds to haemoglobin much more readily than oxygen resulting in the blood having a reduced oxygen carrying content. Decreases heart and muscle function. Causes fatigue and dizziness
Cocoa	While in its natural form this component is harmless; when used in conjunction with other substances and burned can be toxic
Creosol	Used in solvents, disinfectants and wood preservatives. Highly irritating to the skin. Can cause upper respiratory, nasal and throat irritation
Hydrogen cyanide	Used in the production of resins and acrylic plastics. Impedes effective lung function. Causes nausea, headaches and fatigue
Lead	Causes damage to the central nervous, renal and reproductive systems. May cause anaemia and gastric problems
Nicotine	This is an alkaloid and is an extremely powerful drug. Used as a highly controlled insecticide. Stimulates the central nervous system, increases heart rate and blood pressure. Exposure can result in seizures and vomiting
Tar	Associated with an increase in lung cancer – adenocarcinoma

(Source: ASH and Imperial Cancer Research Fund, 1999; DH, 2000; ASH, 2001)

Table 11.2. Statistical data associated with smoking

- In Great Britain in 2005, 72 % of current smokers aged 16 years and over reported that they wished to give up smoking
- Health reasons were given as the most popular reason for wishing to give up smoking
- In England and Wales in 2004, there were a total of 500 755 of deaths of adults aged 35 years and over. Eighteen percent (88 800) of these deaths were the result of smoking with a larger proportion of men (23 %) estimated to die than women (13 %) from smoking related diseases
- In the UK the total household expenditure on tobacco was £15.7 billion
- In England in 2004/5, there were approximately 1.4 million NHS hospital admissions with a primary diagnosis of a disease that can be related to smoking. This figure has increased from approximately 1.1 million admissions in 1995/6
- The proportion of adults who smoke hand-rolled cigarettes has increased from 10 % in 1984 to 24 % in 2004

(Source: Adapted from Information Centre Lifestyle Statistics, 2006)

SMOKING AND POOR HEALTH

Smoking harms sexual and reproductive health. In the UK approximately 106 000 people die as a result of cigarette-smoking-related disease every year, with most cigarette-related deaths being associated with cancer and cardiovascular disease. The difference in smoking rates across socioeconomic groups explains nearly half of the inequalities across these groups. Smoking has become a public health priority as a result of the devastation it has the potential to cause (DH, 2005). Table 11.2 provides statistical data concerning smoking.

In general smokers endure poorer health than non-smokers; they also face a higher risk from a variety of illnesses; many of these illnesses are lethal (see Figure 11.3 below). While there are a number of illnesses that are not fatal, they can result in debilitation. Table 11.3 (below) considers some of these debilitating illnesses.

The non-lethal illnesses caused by cigarette smoking have a profound affect on an individual's economy and also on the economy of the nation. The same is true for the deaths attributed to smoking (see Table 11.4 below).

The Government has set a target to reduce the cancer death rate in people under 75 years by 20 % by 2010 (DH, 1999). This attempt at reducing death rates associated with cancer attributed to smoking will also have an impact on those lethal and non-lethal diseases outlined above.

SMOKING AND HEALTH INEQUALITIES

Smoking rates increase with every marker of social disadvantage; the same is true of smoking-related ill health. Those who are from the poorer social classes are more likely to die early owing to an assortment of factors. The dominant factor among

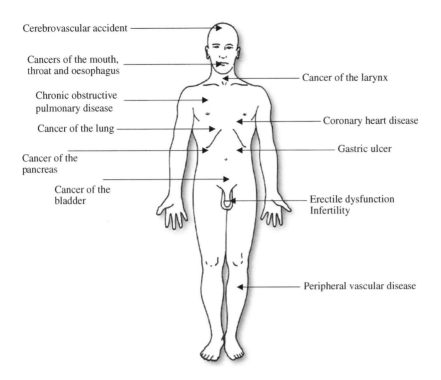

Figure 11.3. Some of the health effects as a consequence of smoking

Table 11.3. Some of the non-lethal illnesses caused by smoking

Increased risk for smokers
- Angina
- Duodenal ulcer
- Depression
- Erectile dysfunction
- Optic neuropathy

- Osteoporosis
- Osteoarthritis
- Peripheral vascular disease
- Pneumonia
- Tuberculosis

Function impaired in smokers
- Impaired immune system
- Sperm count reduced
- Sperm motility impaired
- Sperm less able to penetrate the ovum

- Sperm shape abnormalities increased
- Volume of ejaculate reduced

Symptoms worse in smokers
- Asthma
- Chronic rhinitis

- Multiple sclerosis

Diseases more severe in smokers
- Common cold
- Crohn's disease
- Influenza

- Pneumonia
- Tuberculosis

(Source: Adapted from American Council on Science and Health, 2003)

Table 11.4. Causes of death attributable to smoking

Cancer
- Lung
- Upper respiratory
- Oesophagus
- Bladder
- Kidney
- Stomach
- Pancreas

Respiratory
- Chronic obstructive pulmonary disease
- Pneumonia

Circulatory/vascular
- Ischaemic heart disease
- Cerebrovascular disease
- Aortic aneurysm
- Myocardial degeneration
- Atherosclerosis

Digestive
- Gastric ulcer
- Duodenal ulcer

(Source: Information Centre Lifestyle Statistics, 2006)

men is smoking; this accounts for over half the difference in risk of premature death between the social classes (Jarvis and Wardle, 1999). Those men in manual and service industries are most likely to be exposed to second-hand smoke. In men, smoking is responsible for over half the excess risk of premature death between the social classes (Action on Smoking and Health and Health Development Agency (ASH and HDA), 2001).

Most people who die of a smoking-related illness will die as a result of cancer, chronic obstructive pulmonary disease and coronary heart disease. Premature deaths from lung cancer are five times higher among men in unskilled manual work compared with those in professional work (DH, 1998).

MENTAL HEALTH

In those men who have mental health problems – and it has been estimated that in the United Kingdom approximately 1 in 6 adults experiences mental distress at any one time (Collishaw *et al.*, 2004) – such as schizophrenia, smoking rates are as high as 50%. Men who are depressed are more likely to smoke and experience difficulties when they attempt to stop (McNeil, 2001).

Table 11.5. Smoking rates in penal institutions

Smoking behaviour among men in penal institutions	Remand (%)	Sentenced (%)
Heavy smoker	31	24
Moderate smoker	36	34
Light smoker	18	19
All smokers	85	77
Ex- or non-smokers	15	23

(Source: Adapted from Marshall, Simpson and Stevens, 2000)

PRISONS AND SMOKING

A high proportion of the prison population come from socially excluded sections of the population (ASH and HDA, 2001). Smoking rates in prisons are particularly high, in both inmates and prison staff (Hek, Condon and Harris, 2005). Over 75% of all prisoners smoke and half of them are moderate or heavy smokers (see Table 11.5).

MINORITY ETHNIC COMMUNITIES

The use of tobacco among some minority ethnic communities living in the UK is a cause for concern (ASH and HDA, 2001). Smoking prevalence is highest among Bangladeshi men, followed by Irish men and lowest prevalence is among men of Chinese origin (Erens, Primatesta and Prior, 2001). In some communities cigarette smoking may not be the most popular way of using tobacco; some make use of oral tobacco products (Erens, Primatesta and Prior, 2001).

Smoking presents a challenge for all; it is particularly challenging among those men from the poorest social classes. Identifying those men from those communities who may be at risk allows the nurse to develop strategies to decrease smoking among men in those groups.

REPRODUCTIVE HEALTH

Smoking can compromise the capacity to have a family; parental smoking has the potential to cause long-term and serious consequences for child health. Jenkins, Corrigan and Chambers (2003) point out that a smoker's sperm concentration is, on average, 13–17% lower than a non-smoker. Giving up smoking can reduce or eliminate many of the risks to reproductive life and health. The practice nurse is encouraged to develop strategies that tackle the burden of smoking on reproductive life not only among the older man but also with younger men, as well as protecting all from second-hand smoking. The burden of smoking on reproductive life falls most heavily on the least privileged social classes.

The World Health Organization (WHO; 1998) provides a definition of reproductive health as:

> A state of physical, mental and social well-being in all matters relating to the reproductive system at all stages of life. Reproductive health implies that people are able to have a satisfying and safe sex life and that they have the capability to reproduce...

Key reports associated with male reproductive diseases include the 1990 US Surgeon General's report (US Department of Health and Human Services, 1990), which notes that men who smoke had altered levels of male sex hormones. The British Medical Association (BMA) and ASH determined that smoking is a cause of male impotence (BMA and ASH, 1999). The most recent report produced by the British Medical Association and the Board of Science and Education and Tobacco Control Resource Centre (2004) presents the first focused overview of the impact of smoking on sexual, reproductive and child health in the UK. An understanding of the male reproductive tract is necessary if the practice nurse is to provide a competent and confident service to the male patient and, if appropriate, his partner.

The male reproductive system consists of two testes. Sperm is produced in the testes and stored in the epididymis, where they mature; the epididymis is connected to the vas deferens leading to the ejaculatory ducts. There are two seminal vesicles where the glands therein produce most of the fluid in semen. The seminal fluid contains fructose that provides nourishment and energy for the sperm cells and other substances that sperm requires once they enter the vagina; the prostate gland adds important chemicals to the semen. The bulbourethral glands secrete fluid that lubricates and prepares the urethra where semen is ejaculated (Schover and Thomas, 2000). Chapter 14 provides more detail about the testes.

SPERMATOGENESIS

The production of sperm is a very complex process. When the male foetus develops spermatogonia (specialist cells that have migrated to the scrotum), these cells (parent cells) have the potential to form sperm. The male begins to produce mature sperm cells at the time of a boy's puberty and in a healthy male he will continue until his death. The most easily damaged cells in the testes are the spermatogonia, which are easily damaged by:

- irradiation
- excessive alcohol intake
- dietary deficiencies
- local inflammation.

While the production of sperm begins in the testes, it is controlled by various hormones released from the pituitary gland; hormonal production is controlled by the hypothalamus, starting the process of sperm maturation. Heffner and Schust (2006) report that spermatogenesis can be divided into three phases:

- mitotic proliferation to produce large numbers of cells;
- meiotic division to produce genetic diversity;
- maturation, preparing sperm for transit and penetration of the oocyte in the female tract.

Hypothalamic regulation of hormonal activity occurs when the pituitary gland secretes gonadotropin-releasing hormone (GnRH), GnRH controls the production of gonadotropins, follicle-stimulating hormone (FSH) and luteinzing hormone (LH) that are released from the pituitary gland in the brain and travel to the testes via the bloodstream. LH has the ability to trigger the production of testosterone in the Leydig cells, these cells contain large amounts of androgen, testosterone is crucial for sperm production. FSH activates the Sertoli cells and can also trigger other important hormones required to aid sperm production. Sertoli cells are responsible for the metabolic and structural support of the developing spermatozoa (Heffner and Schust, 2006). The actions of testosterone on the male can be seen in Figure 11.4.

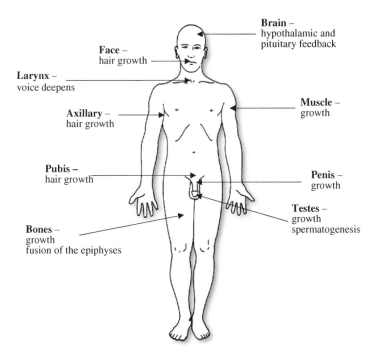

Figure 11.4. The action of testosterone on the male. (Source: Adapted from Meszaros and Sanders, 2006)

It is estimated that it takes approximately 72–74 days to form, mature and release sperm. For the first 50 days sperm spend their lives in the testes and the latter 22–24 days are in the epididymis. In the epididymis the sperm matures and gains motility. On average several hundred million sperm are produced on a daily basis. Spermatogenesis is most effective at a temperature of 34 °C; excess heat can induce degenerative changes in spermatogonia. The testes are suspended within the scrotal sac providing optimal spermatogenesis that occurs in temperatures that are 2–3 °C below the body's core temperature (Coad and Dunstall, 2005).

SEMEN

Prior to ejaculation a mixture of sperm and semen emerge through the ejaculatory ducts through the prostate gland and out through the urethra. Semen is a white/grey fluid; it contains both sperm and secretions from the various glands in the male reproductive tract. Table 11.6 (below) indicates where semen is made.

Semen has an important role in protecting the sperm from the hostile, external and internal influences they will face as they travel through the female reproductive tract. A healthy female vaginal environment is a slightly acidic environment. If sperm comes into contact with vaginal fluid without the semen acting as protection, they would be quickly immobilized. The woman's cervix at the time of ovulation is alkaline, a more affable environment for sperm.

Semen clots almost immediately after ejaculation: it becomes a jellylike sticky liquid and liquefies. The average amount of semen produced at ejaculation is in the region of 2–5 ml. Hypospermia is said to occur when the man produces less than 1.5 ml, with hyperspermia occurring when he produces more than 5.5 ml. Lower volumes occur after frequent ejaculation and conversely more is produced after a period of abstinence.

SPERM

The male gamete – the spermatozoon or sperm cells – are developed in the seminiferous tubules of the testes. They are among the smallest human cells at approximately

Table 11.6. Where semen comes from

Contributing gland	Percentage of the whole ejaculate
Testes and epididymis	5%
Seminal vesicles	46–80%
Prostate gland	13–33%
Bulbourethral glands	2–5%

17–20 μm long. The sperm maintains its ability to fertilize for 2–5 days on average, post coitus in the female reproductive tract (the upper vagina). There are common abnormalities related to some sperm, for example, having no tail or head, two heads, a small head or a coiled tail. Coad and Dunstall (2005) provide a summary of some abnormalities of sperm (see Table 11.7 below).

MALE INFERTILITY

Normal fertility has been defined as achieving pregnancy within two years by regular sexual intercourse (European Society for Human Reproduction and Embryology, 1996); however, Laws (2006) suggests it is a non-pregnancy in a couple who have tried (unprotected intercourse) for a child for one year. There has been an increase in the incidence of male reproductive problems (Iammarrone *et al.*, 2003) and it has been estimated (BMA, 2004) that in the region of 120 000 men aged between 35 and 50 years are infertile as a result of smoking.

The quality of sexual relations and the ability to father a child for some men are key concerns (Laws, 2006). Other key issues regarding reproduction have already

Table 11.7. Some abnormalities of sperm

Type of abnormality	Description	Possible cause
Azoospermia	No sperm present within the ejaculate	Primary testicular failure; blockage to the vas deferens as a result of infection or trauma, for example. Often these patients have small testes and a raised FSH level
Oligozoospermia	Reduced numbers of sperm in the ejaculate, sometimes called low sperm count	Gonadotrophin insufficiency; iatrogenic, use of non-prescribed medications, toxins as found in cigarettes and alcohol, for example
Idiopathic oligospermia	Low sperm count but physiological parameters normal	Idiopathic – unknown, unexplained
Teratozoospermia	Abnormal morphology, for example, small heads, double tails	Genetic, toxins, viral infection
Asthenospermia	Sperm that have a reduced mobility or those that are immobile	Toxins, infection
Sperm agglutination	Sperm clump together in groups	Infection autoimmune response

(Source: Adapted from Coad and Dunstall, 2005; Briggs, 2004)

been discussed in this text, for example, the effects of erectile dysfunction and contraception. Infertility (sometimes known as sub-fertility) is different from erectile dysfunction. Many men who experience erectile dysfunction often have normal sperm function. McQueen (2006) divides male fertility problems into three therapeutic groups:

- untreatable sterility
- treatable conditions
- subfertility.

The causes of infertility can be varied and some causes are unknown. Alam, Niederberger and Meacham (2004) suggest that 25 % of cases of infertility in men are unknown. Over 75 % of male infertility difficulties are associated with sperm problems; men who smoke have a lower sperm count as well as a higher proportion of malformed sperm (BMA, 2004). Hirsh (2003) reports that less common types of infertility are the result of testicular or genital infection (for example, chlamydia), disease or abnormality. Male fertility depends on the man's ability to produce viable sperm in the testes and to transport that sperm. As well as being able to produce sperm the man has to be able to initiate and also maintain an erection. Problems may arise at any stage of the process rendering the man infertile (Briggs, 2004). Hirsh (2003) points out that one-third of infertilities arise from a problem with the male reproductive physiology, with an estimate of 1 : 20 men affected by some form of infertility.

CLINICAL ASSESSMENT

While it may be the nurse that the patient first turns to for help and advice, he should be referred to an infertility specialist, urologist or endocrinologist. Laws (2006) suggests that assessment should be made by a clinical andrologist in a reproduction medical clinic. Diagnosis may be made in the primary care setting by taking a detailed history from the patient and the performance of a physical examination. Hirsh (2003) considers semen analysis as the cornerstone of male infertility assessment. Analysis of semen is often the trigger to referring the patient for a specialist opinion.

HISTORY-TAKING

History-taking should aim to elicit the information required in Table 11.8. Extensive history-taking is required in order to identify possible causes in infertile men. Burrows, Schrepferman and Lipshultz (2002) suggest that detailed history allows an efficient work-up of the problem. As with all consultations with the patient, the way the nurse approaches the situation, with tact and sensitivity, will enhance the quality of information the patient wishes to impart. Alam,

Table 11.8. Information required from the patient when taking a history

---

Male reproductive history
- Duration of unprotected intercourse
- Previous infertility evaluations

Female reproductive history
- Age
- Gravida/para
- Current status of female infertility evaluation
- Number of successful, previous pregnancies

Family history
- Cystic fibrosis
- Androgen receptor deficiency
- Hypogonadism

Endocrine history
- Headaches, visual disturbances, anosmia
- Excessive growth of hands, feet, jaw
- Retardation of hair growth (facial, body)
- Breast changes (i.e. gynaecomastia)
- Vasomotor symptoms

Personal history
- Developmental (i.e., history of cryptorchidism, mumps, testicular torsion)
- Surgical procedures (i.e., pelvic surgery, transurethral surgery, herniorrhaphy)
- Exposure to certain medicines (i.e. androgenic steroids, H2 blockers, antihypertensives), non-prescribed drugs (i.e. heroin, marijuana), chemicals (i.e. anaesthetic gases, lead), toxins (i.e. tobacco)
- Thermal exposure (i.e., use of sauna, hot baths, briefs as opposed to boxer shorts)
- Sexual history, libido, timing and frequency of intercourse, use of lubricants, sexually transmitted infections

---

(Source: Adapted from Christmas, Dinneen and Lipshultz, 1999; Hirsh, 2003; Alam, Niederberger and Meacham, 2004)

Niederberger and Meacham (2004) suggest that the history should focus on three key areas:

- general fertility history
- childhood history
- past medical or surgical history.

The nurse will also require information about his partner's reproductive history and a decision will need to be made to determine if the man's partner should attend. The Royal College of Obstetricians and Gynaecologists (RCOG; 1998) recommends that both partners are involved in the management of infertility, with both the male and female partner being assessed for infertility (Jenkins, Corrigan and Chambers, 2003).

PHYSICAL ASSESSMENT

During the physical examinations, the nurse must examine the whole body. The assessment will include assessment of overall appearance, bodily proportions, body hair distribution and general masculine traits. The physical examination is crucial as it may reveal information regarding the cause of the man's infertility (Christmas, Dinneen and Lipshultz, 1999); for example, gynecomastia could be the result of primary testicular failure or secondary hypothalamic pituitary abnormality. There may be signs of hypogonadism, for example, small testes. This can be objectively assessed by the use of an orchidometer. Testicular size is assessed and measured by length in centimetres and volume in millilitres. As 85 % of testicular tissue produces sperm cells, small testes may indicate a fertility problem (Schover and Thomas, 2000).

Palpation of the epididymis is required as irregularities could indicate infection or obstruction; confirmation that the vasa exist is also required as 2 % of infertile men have congenital absence of the vas and seminal vesicles; it has also been determined that these men may also be carriers of cystic fibrosis (Christmas, Dinneen and Lipshultz, 1999). The presence of varicocele should also be excluded by palpating the testicular cord and if required confirmation by ultrasonography (Hirsh, 2003). Varicocele is found in approximately 25 % of male partners who seek help for infertility (Hargreave and Mills, 1998). The prostate gland should be carefully assessed. Christmas, Dinneen and Lipshultz (1999) suggest that in men with androgen deficiency it is often small and in those men who are experiencing prostatitis the gland is described as tender and boggy to the touch. The penis is assessed, noting any abnormalities associated with hypospadias.

SEMEN ANALYSIS

The patient will be required to produce and provide two semen specimens, and these specimens are best collected for immediate assessment in laboratories linked within fertility services (Christmas, Dinneen and Lipshultz, 1999; Hirsh, 2003). Table 11.9 provides terminology used in semen analysis.

Hormonal investigation and assessment are also required to consider endocrine defects in infertile men (Christmas, Dinneen and Lipshultz, 1999). Semen should be collected for analysis after 48–72 hours of abstinence from sexual intercourse; the specimen must be kept at body temperature and analysis has to take place within one hour of collection. Two specimens of semen are required after similar periods of abstinence. The patient and his partner must be advised to use lubricants only if essential, and if lubrication is required then only small amounts should be used. Some lubricants such as KY Jelly are spermatotoxic and therefore must be avoided; the evidence regarding alternative types of lubricant is undecided (Christmas, Dinneen and Lipshultz, 1999; Schover and Thomas, 2000). Christmas et al. suggest the avoidance of saliva yet Schover and Thomas (2000) advocate its use. The most advantageous condition would be to use no lubricant; if lubricant is needed then it may be

Table 11.9. Terminology used in semen analysis

Term	Meaning
Normozoospermia	All semen parameters are normal
Oligozoospermia	Reduced sperm numbers
	• Mild to moderate: 5–20 million/ml of semen
	• Severe: less than 5 million/ml of semen
Asthenozoospermia	Reduced sperm motility
Teratozoospermia	Increased abnormal forms of sperm
Oligoasthenoteratozoospermia	Sperm variables all subnormal
Azoospermia	No sperm in semen
Aspermia (anejaculation)	No ejaculate (ejaculation failure)
Leucocytospermia	Increased white cells in sperm
Necrozoospermia	All sperm are non-viable or non-motile

(Source: Hirsh, 1999)

advisable to encourage the couple to spend some time during foreplay increasing sexual arousal and, hence, natural lubricant.

Analysis of semen includes assessment of volume, density, sperm motility, forward progression, sperm morphology and the presence of leucocytes. Normal values of semen variables are provided in Table 11.10 (below).

The semen specimens are produced by masturbation. The nurse must bear in mind that there may be some men who may have difficulty with masturbation or have religious objections to masturbation (see Table 11.11 below). If condoms are used to collect semen, advice must be sought as to the best type: avoid using condoms and lubricants that are spermatotoxic.

After history-taking, physical examination and semen analysis have taken place referral to a specialist may be required who can then advise the patient on the most appropriate form of treatment. Laws (2006) outlines some treatment options that the practice nurse needs to be aware of in order to provide the patient with information he (and his partner) may require in order to make an informed decision (see Table 11.12 below). A conservative approach to treatment for infertility would, according to Hirsh (2003), include:

Table 11.10. Normal values – semen analysis

Volume	Over 2 ml
Sperm concentration	Over 20 million/ml
Sperm motility	Over 50 % progressive or over 25 % rapidly progressive
Morphology	Over 15 % normal forms
White blood cells	Below 1 million/ml
Immunobead or mixed antiglobulin reaction tests	Below 10 % coated

(Source: World Health Organization, 2000)

Table 11.11. Some world religions and their views on semen collection for infertility

Religion	Views on collection	Notes
Orthodox Judaism	Masturbation is only acceptable as a last resort. Semen should be collected during intercourse using a collection condom (some Rabbis specify that the condom should be perforated to allow the possibility of ejaculation into the vagina). Laws that restrict intercourse to the times in a woman's cycle when she has been free of bleeding for the last seven days and has visited the ritual bath for purification should be observed	Jewish law forbids 'spilling one's seed' outside of the vagina and considers this a form of adultery. In general, however, conceiving a child is a duty and a blessing that supersedes most other laws governing sexuality
Conservative or Reform Judaism	Masturbation is acceptable as part of infertility treatment	Conceiving a mutual genetic child for a married couple supersedes other religious concerns about masturbation
Islam	Masturbation is not allowed as a sexual practice, but may be acceptable as a medical procedure for infertility treatment	Procreation is a very important value. Infertility treatment is allowed, so long as it occurs within a marriage whose contact remains valid and preserves the mutual genetic heritage of the two parents
Catholicism	Masturbation is not acceptable. Collecting sperm cells from the vas deferens or epididymis through a needle may be acceptable. Collecting semen through intercourse is acceptable if the condom is perforated, allowing the possibility of natural conception	All conception should occur through sexual intercourse between spouses, uniting two fleshes into one in an act that symbolizes the sacred aspect of marriage and leaves open the possibility of conception.
Protestant denominations	Most sanction masturbation to obtain semen for infertility treatment	Evangelical churches may ban masturbation based on direct biblical sources such as those used by Orthodox Judaism or Roman Catholic scholars

(Source: Schover and Thomas, 2000)

Table 11.12. Some treatment options for infertility

Treatment option	Explanation
Drug treatments	Drug treatments are unlikely to improve sperm quality
Gonadotrophin	May help to produce more sperm for those men who have a deficiency of this hormone; however, fertility rates are not increased
Artificial insemination (AI)	The partner's semen is washed and concentrated and directly inserted into the uterus
In vitro fertilization and embryo transfer (IVF-ET)	A selection of strong sperm is isolated and put in contact with the ovum in a test tube. The patient and partner must be told that there is a 90 % failure rate with this technique
Gamete intrafallopian transfer (GIFT)	Sperm is placed directly into the fallopian tube and has a better chance of fertilizing an ovum than the IVF-ET method
Pronuclear stage transfer (PROST)	The IVF-ET method precedes placement of fertilized ovum into the fallopian tube
Intra-cytoplasmic sperm injection (ICSI)	This option is used for men who have no sperm in their semen; it is possible to fertilize an ovum from a single sperm; the sperm is micro surgically aspirated from the epididymis or testes. Assisted fertilization occurs by IVF-ET
Donor insemination	Where there are barriers such as cost, a limitation on a couple's time, frustration with timing optimal fertilization, complexity of the procedure and severe male infertility, insemination with donor sperm is a preferable option for many couples who are infertile. The donor sperm is screened for disease and genetic aberrations. The law in the UK is changing with regards to the ability of the donor to remain anonymous. The Human Fertilization and Embryology Authority provides information regarding practices associated with assisted reproduction.

(Source: Adapted from Royal College of Nursing, 2004; Hirsh, 2003; Christmas, Dinneen and Lipshultz, 1999)

- stopping smoking tobacco, as nicotine reduces plasma antioxidants;
- reassessment of current medication (prescribed or non-prescribed) as some medications impair spermatogenesis or sexual function (see Table 11.13 below);
- having more frequent intercourse – increases output of non-senile spermatozoa;
- reducing alcohol intake – alcohol has the ability to suppress spermatogenesis;
- avoiding hot baths/saunas – heat suppresses spermatogenesis;
- wearing boxer shorts as opposed to briefs – heat suppresses spermatogenesis;
- avoiding contact with pesticides, herbicides, heat and radiation at work – all impair spermatogenesis.

The patient may need support from the practice nurse; he and his partner can be told that there are many infertile men who are becoming increasingly treated with success; previously infertile couples are able to enjoy the joys of parenthood (Christmas, Dinneen and Lipshultz, 1999).

PRESERVING SEMEN

Sperm banking may be required for some men. The effects of cancer (and other conditions) and the outcome of treatment on the man's fertility can cause much distress and upset for some men and their partners. Raising the issue of sperm banking, according to Quinn and Kelly (2000), should be a part of the role of the nurse when offering help and support to the male patient with cancer. In order to offer this support effectively the nurse must ensure that s/he understands the issues and concerns surrounding sperm banking. Steele *et al.* (1995) describe sperm banking as the preservation of sperm by freezing in order that it may be used at a later date for artificial insemination.

The practice nurse should aim to understand and, if need be, question local policy and procedure associated with sperm banking. Quinn and Kelly (2000) demonstrate

Table 11.13. Some drugs that have the ability to impair male fertility

Drug	Action on spermatogenesis
Sulfasalazine, methotrexate, nitrofurantoin, chemotherapy	Impaired spermatogenesis
Testosterone injections, gonadotrophin releasing hormone analogues	Pituitary suppression
Cimetidine, spironolactone	Anti-androgenic effects
α Blockers, antidepressants, phenothiazines	Ejaculation failure
β Blockers, thiazide diuretics, metoclopramide	Erectile dysfunction
Anabolic steroids, cannabis, heroin, cocaine	Variety of effects on spermatogenesis

(Source: Hirsh, 2003; Jenkins, Corrigan and Chambers, 2003)

a lack of understanding about sperm banking by nurses working on a male oncology ward, as well as a degree of difficulty in approaching the patient regarding this important subject. The Royal College of Nursing (RCN; 2004) has provided guidance for the management of fertility of male cancer patients.

MANAGING INFERTILITY IN PRIMARY CARE

It has been estimated that one in four couples seeks advice about their infertility from the general practice at some point in their lives (Gunnel and Ewings, 1994). The National Institute for Health and Clinical Excellence (NICE; 2004) suggests that those who are concerned about delays in conception should be offered an initial assessment in general practice; a couple-centred approach is advocated with the practice nurse or GP making a detailed history, examination, routine investigations and referral to the secondary sector to the most appropriate fertility specialist.

A number of couples who seek advice and who may go for treatment can suffer from depression, stress and anxiety. The practice nurse should aim to provide those couples with ongoing support and information-giving at each stage of the fertility management process. This approach, according to Whitman-Elia (2001), places primary care service provision at the heart of all issues related to infertility.

When recommendation is to be made for secondary care, the following details should be included in the referral letter (Jenkins, Corrigan and Chambers, 2003):

- results of semen analysis
- results of all previous investigations
- the personal details of both the man and woman, that is, contact information
- reproductive histories
- duration of trying to conceive and previous contraception.

Ongoing support means that the practice nurse needs to be aware of actual or potential issues that may arise, for example, stress as a result of investigations and treatments may affect the couple's relationship, leading to a reduction in libido and frequency of sexual intercourse, aggravating the fertility problem even further (Bagshawe and Taylor, 2003). Information may need to be given to the couple regarding contact details about fertility support groups and counselling services that may help the couple cope with the possible psychological effects of fertility and infertility. NICE (2004) recommends that counselling should be provided by someone who is not directly involved in the management and care of the couple's fertility problems.

The provision of high-quality infertility care in the primary care setting requires a coordinated team approach with effective communication between all key parties

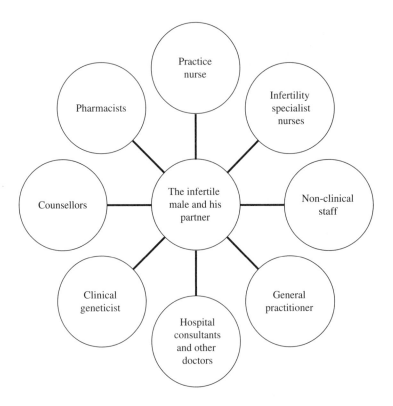

Figure 11.5. A coordinated team approach

(see Figure 11.5). Individual roles and responsibilities must be ascertained and lo-cal protocols and policies should be formulated using the best available evidence in order to provide implementation at a local level.

Coordination and a seamless transition from primary care to secondary care is vital if the care of the patient is to be effective. The risk of duplication of tests that have already been performed in the general practice must be avoided if primary care interventions are not to be undermined (Morrison *et al.*, 2001).

SMOKING CESSATION AND THE ROLE OF THE PRACTICE NURSE

The role of the practice nurse is varied. One aspect of that role is focused on health promotion. According to McEwen and West (2001), the practice nurse is at the fore-front of initiatives to combat smoking. Smokers can, without professional input, stop smoking; however, success rates improve when healthcare professionals intervene (BMA, 2004). The delivery of smoking cessation interventions delivered through the NHS is an extremely cost-effective way of preserving life and reducing ill health (West, McNeill and Raw, 2000). West, McNeill and Raw (2000) and ASH (2005) provide guidelines for healthcare professionals regarding smoking cessation:

- The practice must be aware of who their smokers are. Unless the practice know who their smoking patients are, they will be unable to provide a service concerning cessation. Practice nurses and GPs should advise smokers to stop smoking during routine consultations (at least on an annual basis), giving advice and prescribing effective medication to help the patient, as well as referral to specialist cessation services. The advice given should be documented in the patient's notes. It is important to ensure that documentation takes place, as smoking status may change after registration (United States Department of Health and Social Services, 2000).
- Provide access to specialist smokers' services that offer behavioural support. NHS specialist smokers clinics should be the first point of referral for smokers wanting help beyond the advice the practice nurse can provide.
- Offer access to specialist cessation counsellors.
- Encourage and assist smokers in the use of nicotine replacement therapies (NRT) or bupropion.

The practice nurse can use the following approach to help the patient stop smoking (British Heart Foundation, 2001):

Ask about and record smoking status, ensuring that records are kept up to date.

Advise smokers of the benefits of stopping using a personal and holistic approach, relating this to patient concerns such as issues surrounding infertility as well as any other health problems the patient may have.

Assess motivation to stop – and if possible reinforce. Smokers are much more likely to stop after experiencing significant health problems.

Assist smokers to stop: include useful tips on how best to try, the offer of support and considerations of either NRT or bupropion (with the provision of accurate information and advice about these). Bupropion is contraindicated in patients with seizure disorders as well as patients on drugs which are known to lower the threshold of seizures including antipsychotics, other antidepressants, anti-malarials, theophylline, quinolones and sedating antihistamines. There is also the possibility of potentially dangerous interactions with other drugs.

Arrange follow-up if possible – or review when next seen. Alternatively, refer the patient to a specialist smoking cessation service.

Action on Smoking and Health (2005) provides insight into the key messages associated with the licensing arrangements for NRT:

- Smokers who smoke more than 10 cigarettes per day should be offered NRT. It is safe to recommend NRT to patients with cardiovascular disease where the alternative is the patient resuming smoking. Those patients who have unstable cardiac disease must be fully assessed by the GP before the prescribing of NRT.

- It is appropriate to offer all forms of NRT to young men aged 12–17 years of age, so long as the practice nurse is sure that the patient is dependent enough to necessitate the use of NRT and he is also committed to stopping smoking.
- It is appropriate to use more than one form of NRT concurrently. Combinations of gum, patch, inhaler or other combinations in those men who have failed to quit may be required.
- NRT can be prescribed for up to nine months so long as the patient demonstrates a continued need for NRT beyond the initial 8- to 12-week treatment phase. The patient should be reviewed monthly after the prescription has been issued.

NRT comes in six different forms (see Table 11.14).

Those men who smoke have a poorer response to infertility treatments (BMA, 2004); stopping smoking improves sperm count and quality. If men stop smoking, there is a high possibility that they will prolong normal function (BMA and ASH, 1999). In recent years the Government has successfully managed to ensure the elimination of tobacco advertising and promotion. These moves will help to encourage those who wish to give up smoking. There has also been the establishment of smokers' cessation clinics providing life-saving advice and treatments for many men who wish to give up smoking, with practice nurses taking a pivotal role in devising and implementing strategies to help men stop or reduce smoking. The nurse also has an important role to play in ensuring that men recognize the impact that smoking can have on their sexual and reproductive health and the benefits smoking cessation brings.

Dorey (2001) suggests that many men may not be aware of the total adverse effects on the body and reproductive system from smoking. All men who smoke, she continues, should be offered smoking cessation treatment. Any interventions that the nurse and patient agree upon will require action that adopts an across-sector approach, taking into account the broader social, cultural, economic and physical environments that shape men's experiences of health and well-being.

Improving the nation's health will mean that a significant number of people who smoke will have to cease. Practice nurses working with other members of the primary

Table 11.14. Nicotine replacement therapy

Chewing gum (2 mg and 4 mg)
Transdermal patch (16 h and 24 h in varying dose)
Nasal spray
Inhaler
Sublingual tablet
Lozenge

(Source: Drug Therapy Bulletin, 1999)

healthcare team, and most importantly with the patient, have the ability to improve the general health of men and the rest of society. Smoking cessation should be seen by all members of the practice as high priority and clinical guidelines should be produced that assist the practice nurse in helping the patient to stop smoking. National guidance has been produced, and this should be translated into local policy addressing the specific needs of patients. Smoking cessation should be seen as integral to an NHS that is truly patient led.

CONCLUSION

The use of tobacco has a profound physical and economical effect on all of society. It is the principle avoidable cause of premature death in the UK. Smoking can have a considerable impact on male reproduction. Cardiovascular disease and cancer are also the result of cigarette smoking. The harmful effects of cigarette smoking has meant that smoking has become a public health priority.

Smoking rates increase with every marker of social disadvantage. Those from the poorer social classes are more likely to die early, owing to a variety of factors with the dominant factor in men being smoking. Other inequalities are also evident in relation to smoking; for example, some men with mental health problems and those men in prison.

A deeper understanding of the causes and possible treatments of male infertility will help to provide the patient and his partner with healthcare provision that is of a high quality. While the treatment of infertile patients is often carried out in the secondary care setting, a significant amount of care, for example, initial diagnosis and undertaking of assessment and investigation, is conducted in the primary care setting. The practice nurse must be aware that the patient will require advice and support during and after treatment.

REFERENCES

Action on Smoking and Health (2001) *Fact Sheet No 12: What's in a Cigarette*, ASH, London.

Action on Smoking and Health (2005) *Nicotine Replacement Therapy: Guidance for Health Professionals on Change in the Licensing Arrangements for Nicotine Replacement Therapy*, ASH, London.

Action on Smoking and Health and Health Development Agency (2001) *Smoking and Health Inequalities*, ASH/HAD, London.

Action on Smoking and Health and Imperial Cancer Research Fund (1999) *Tobacco Additives – Cigarette Engineering and Nicotine Addiction*, ASH/ICRF, London.

Alam, S., Niederberger, C.S. and Meacham, R.B. (2004) Evaluation and treatment of male infertility. In (eds R.S. Kirby, C.C. Carson, M.G. Kirby and R.N. Farah) *Men's Health*, 2nd edn, Taylor & Francis, London, pp. 261–266, Chapter 20.

American Council on Science and Health (2003) *Cigarettes: What the Warning Label Doesn't Tell You*, 2nd edn, ACSH, New York.

Bagshawe, A. and Taylor, A. (2003) ABC of subfertility: counselling. *British Medical Journal*, **327**, 1038–1040.

Briggs, P. (2004) Scrotal disorders (eds S. Fillingam and J. Douglas) *Urological Nursing*, 3rd edn, Bailliere Tindall, London, pp. 245–21, Chapter 13.

British Heart Foundation (2001) *Stopping Smoking Evidence Based Guidance: Factfile 8*, BHF, London.

British Medical Association (2004) *Smoking and Reproductive Life: Impact of Smoking on Sexual, Reproductive and Child Health*, BMA, Edinburgh.

British Medical Association and ASH UK (1999) Warning: smoking causes male sexual impotence, *Smoking and Threats to Men's Sexual Health*, BMA and ASH UK, London.

British Medical Association and the Board of Science and Education and Tobacco Control Resource Centre (2004) *Smoking and Reproductive Life: The Impact of Smoking on Sexual, Reproductive and Child Health*, BMA and the Board of Science and Education and Tobacco Control Resource Centre, London.

British Medical Association (2004) *The Human Cost of Tobacco: Passive Smoking: Doctors Speak Out on Behalf of Patients*, BMA, London.

Burrows, B., Schrepferman, C. and Lipshultz, L. (2002) Comprehensive office evaluation in the new millennium. *Urological Clinics of North America*, **29**, 873–894.

Christmas, T.J., Dinneen, M.D. and Lipshultz, L. (1999) *Diseases of the Testes*, Health Press, Abingdon.

Coad, J. and Dunstall, M. (2005) *Anatomy and Physiology for Midwives*, 2nd edn, Elsevier, Edinburgh.

Collishaw, S., Maughan, B., Goodman, R. and Pickles, A. (2004) *Time Trends in Adolescent Health*, Nuffield Foundation, London.

Department of Health (1998) *Smoking Kills: A White Paper on Tobacco*, The Stationery Office, London.

Department of Health (1999) *Saving Lives: Our Healthier Nation*, DH, London.

Department of Health (2000) *Permitted Additives to Tobacco Products in the United Kingdom*, DH, London.

Department of Health (2004) *Choosing Health, Making Healthier Choices Easier*, DH, London.

Department of Health (2005) *The Chief Medical Officer's Annual Report*, DH, London.

Dorey, G. (2001) Is smoking a cause of erectile dysfunction? A literature review. *British Journal of Nursing*, **10** (7), 455–465.

Drug Therapy Bulletin (1999) Nicotine replacement to aid smoking cessation. *Drug Therapy Bulletin*, **37**, 52–54.

Erens, B., Primatesta, P. and Prior, G. (2001) *Health Survey for England: The Health of Minority Ethnic Groups 1999*, The Stationery Office, London.

European Society for Human Reproduction and Embryology (1996) Guidelines to the prevalence, diagnosis, treatment and management of infertility. *Human Reproduction*, **11**, 1775–1807.

Gunnel, D.J. and Ewings, P. (1994) Infertility prevalence, needs assessment and purchasing. *Journal of Public Health Medicine*, **16**, 29–36.

Hargreave, T.B. and Mills, J. (1998) Investigating and managing infertility in general practice. *British Medical Journal*, **316**, 1438–1441.

Heffner, L.J. and Schust, D.J. (2006) *The Reproductive System at a Glance*, 2nd edn, Blackwell Publishing, *Boston*.

Hek, G., Condon, L. and Harris, F. (2005) *Primary Care Nursing in Prisons: A Systematic Overview of Policy and Research Literature*, University of West England, Bristol.

Hirsh, A. (2003) The ABC of subfertility: male subfertility. *British Medical Journal*, **237**, 669.

Information Centre Lifestyle Statistics (2006) *Statistics on Smoking: England*, Office for National Statistics, London.

Iammarrone, E., Balet, R., Lower, A.M. *et al.* (2003) Male infertility: best practice and research. *Clinical Obstetrics and Gynaecology*, **17** (2), 211–229.

Jarvis, M. and Wardle, J. (1999) Social patterning of individual health behaviours: the case of cigarette smoking. In (eds M. Marmot and R. Wilkinson) *Social Determinants of Health*, Oxford University Press, Oxford.

Jenkins, J., Corrigan, L. and Chambers, R. (2003) *Infertility Matters in Health Care*, Radcliffe Medical Press, Oxford.

Laws, T. (2006) *A Handbook of Men's Health*, Elsevier, Edinburgh.

Mackaness, R. (1985) *A Little of What You Fancy*, Fontana Paperbacks, London.

Marshall, T., Simpson, S. and Stevens, A. (2000) *Health Care in Prisons: A Health Care Needs Assessment*, University of Birmingham, Birmingham.

Meszaros, G. and Sanders, S. (2006) *Endocrine and Reproductive Systems*, Elsevier, Philadelphia.

McEwen, A. and West, R. (2001) Smoking cessation activities by general practitioners and practice nurses. *Tobacco Control*, **10**, 27–32.

McNeil, A. (2001) *Smoking and Mental Health – A Review of the Literature*, Action on Smoking and Health, London.

McQueen, A.C.H. (2006) Disorders of the reproductive system and the breast. In (eds M.F. Alexander, J.N. Fawcett and P.J. Runciman) *Nursing Practice Hospital and Home: The Adult*, 3rd edn, Churchill Livingstone, Edinburgh, pp. 253–356, Chapter 7.

Morrison, J., Carroll, L., Twaddle, S. *et al.* (2001) Pragmatic randomized controlled trial to evaluate guidelines for the management of infertility across the primary care–secondary care interface. *British Medical Journal*, **322**, 1282–1284.

National Institute for Health and Clinical Excellence (2004) *Fertility: Assessment and Treatment for People with Fertility Problems: Guideline Number 11*, NICE, London.

Quinn, B. and Kelly, D. (2000) Sperm banking and fertility concerns: enhancing practice and the support available for men with cancer. *European Journal of Oncology Nursing*, **4** (1), 55–58.

Royal College of Obstetricians (1998) *Gynaecologists: The Initial Investigation and Management of the Infertile Couple: Evidence Based Clinical Guideline, Number 2*, RCOG, London.

Royal College of Nursing (2004) *Managing the Fertility of Male Cancer Patients*, RCN, London.

Schover, L.R. and Thomas, A.J. (2000) *Overcoming Male Infertility: Understanding its Causes and Treatments*, John Wiley & Sons Inc., New York.

Steele, S.J., Bahadur, G., Shenfield, F. and Steele, J.W. (1995) Sperm banking. *Assisted Reproduction Review*, **5**, 115–119.

Tengs, T.O. and Osgood, N.D. (2001) The link between smoking and impotence: two decades of evidence. *Preventative Medicine*, **32** (6), 447–452.

United States Department of Health and Social Services (1990) *Reducing the Health Consequences of Smoking: 25 Years of Progress: A Report of the Surgeon General*, USDHSS, Rockville, MD.

United States Department of Health and Social Services (2000) *Treating Tobacco Use and Dependants*, USDHSS, Rockville, MD.

West, R., McNeill, A. and Raw, M. (2000) Smoking cessation guidelines for health professionals: an update. *Thorax*, **55** (12), 987–999.

Whitman-Elia, G.F. (2001) A primary care approach to the infertile couple. *Journal of the American Board of Family Practice*, **14** (1), 33–45.

World Health Organization (1998) *Selecting Indicators for Monitoring Reproductive Health: Number 45*, WHO, Geneva.

World Health Organization (2000) *Laboratory Manual for the Examination of Human Semen and Semen-Cervical Mucus Interaction*, Cambridge University Press, Cambridge.

12 Working with specific groups of men

INTRODUCTION

The practice nurse works with a variety of patients. When working with men s/he will also work with those who come from, or belong to, specific groups. Sometimes these groups are known as hard-to-reach groups and in certain instances may also be referred to as vulnerable groups. Burton and Kagan (2005) use the term marginalized when discussing some groups in society such as those who are poor, unemployed, discriminated against or disabled. All of these groups are at risk of being excluded by society, including being excluded from accessing healthcare.

The National Health Service (NHS) belongs to all of us, including those groups who may be classified as hard to reach. All practices, whether they are rural or urban, will have patients for whom inequalities in health exist and are also avoidable and unjust (Department of Health (DH) 2002a and 2002b). Men who fall into the groups outlined above could be classed as hard-to-reach as they may find it difficult to access and use primary care services. The provision of primary care services to men who belong to groups such as the homeless, those who work in the sex industry, travellers and asylum seekers is a recognized problem in the United Kingdom (Pfeil and Howe, 2004) and all of these groups receive unsatisfactory care.

Van Cleemput and Parry (2001) point out that for travellers access to healthcare provision is also limited and that they encounter worse health than that experienced by those in the lowest socioeconomic groups who live in deprived urban areas. Asylum-seekers, despite having the right to free access to healthcare offered by the NHS, often fail to understand how to access these services (Burnett, 2002). Lipley (1999) states that the healthcare services offered to sex workers are virtually nil due to GPs' refusal to register them. This is further compounded by sex workers' unsocial hours of employment.

The hard to reach often experience higher levels of morbidity and mortality, and have reduced access to preventative services when compared with those in the general population (DH, 2002a). Health inequalities have already been discussed in Chapter 3 from a global perspective and in relation to the health of men per se. This chapter will discuss four specific groups of men who could be deemed to be hard to reach:

- men who are homeless
- men who are a part of the prison population
- gay men (men who have sex with men)
- asylum-seekers.

The NHS Plan (DH, 2000) made reducing health inequalities a priority. The cross-cutting spending review (DH, 2002b) provides for a whole-Government focus on health inequalities, establishing priority areas for action and setting targets to be achieved. *The NHS Plan* (DH, 2000) along with the various national service frameworks (NSFs) aim to address and reduce inequalities in the general population. If a fair and comparable service is to be provided, the principles associated with attempts to eradicate inequality must be applied to those groups who are seen as hard to reach.

The introduction in 2007 of the Equality Act 2006 will place a gender duty on all businesses (including general practices) to ensure that organizations promote equality, rather than the onus being on individuals to highlight discrimination. The introduction of this Act sees the biggest change in equality law in 30 years.

The provision of high-quality care for the vulnerable and marginalized may provide a challenge for those workers in the primary care setting. Understanding the challenges that men from various groups may experience can help the practice nurse plan care interventions accordingly, as well as ensuring that they offer services that are responsive to need. Practice nurses must explore new and innovative approaches to care provision for this group who may be seen as hard to reach, in order to provide a service that is commensurate with the ethos of the *Code of Conduct* (Nursing and Midwifery Council (NMC), 2004). Primary care, according to the Department of Health (DH, 2002a), has a strong role to play in tackling and reducing inequalities, providing services that reach those in greatest need.

King *et al.* (2007) explain that the increase in mortality, morbidity and the burden of disease, along with other adverse health experiences, is the result of illness, social conditions and social policy conspiring to undermine healthcare barriers to care. Pfeil and Howe (2004) point out that those who are described as hard to reach report feeling humiliated when visiting the general practice. These feelings arise from thoughtless comments and negative non-verbal communication made by staff, as well as being stared at by other patients.

Healthcare workers such as practice nurses and other members of the general practice may be ill prepared when caring for vulnerable patients; they may feel uncomfortable. According to King *et al.* (2007), the groups that healthcare workers feel uncomfortable providing care for include:

- chronically ill
- elderly
- addicts
- mentally ill
- victims of violence
- those from disadvantaged backgrounds
- those from minority groups.

Stockwell (1984) made similar observations in her work over two decades ago. She noted that some patients (in ward settings) were seen as being difficult by some nurses and as a result received poorer standards of care. It was noted by Stockwell (1984) that certain characteristics helped determine the patient's lack of popularity among nurses, for example, being a foreigner or having a perceived defect such as a psychiatric illness. Healthcare workers become the third factor in the triple jeopardy that hard-to-reach populations have to contend with when it comes to healthcare. The three factors are:

- accessing healthcare provision;
- their illness;
- healthcare workers.

STIGMA

Stigma, according to Goffman (1963), occurs when society labels someone as tainted, less desirable or handicapped; stigmatization can apply to all groups of men in this chapter. Stigma can have far-reaching effects in so far as the individual may feel stressed as a result of their illness, which can contribute to psychological and so-cial morbidity. It also has the potential to jeopardize personal identity and social and economic opportunities; furthermore, it can seriously affect families and significant others (Ablon, 2002). Fife and Wright (2000) point out that spoilt identity, guilt and shame are dimensions that are often associated with stigma.

ACCESSING HEALTHCARE

The needs of hard-to-reach groups cannot be met by using conventional approaches and as a result specific primary care services with a more flexible approach are required (Pfeil and Howe, 2004), encouraging the vulnerable of society to use and engage with primary healthcare services. Communities most at risk of ill health (the vulnerable, hard to reach and marginalized) often experience the least satisfactory access to care. Accessing healthcare is problematic for these patients; they are ill and when they eventually do receive or gain access to care it is less than optimal. Mar-ginalization associated with the groups discussed in this chapter face discrimination in many ways and barriers to access exist in many forms, including:

- services that are intimidating or stigmatizing
- access and transport difficulties
- lack of interpreters
- inflexible service hours or appointment systems
- staff attitude
- waiting times
- fear of clinical settings

- communication and/or literacy problems
- gender differences
- insensitivity.

Patients will be discouraged from seeking help and accessing care provision unless the nurse provides services that are appropriate and welcoming. Care provision must be enhanced along with improved prevention, early intervention and targeted approaches; when these issues have been addressed, this may go some way to reducing inequalities in health.

HOMELESS MEN

Homelessness is the consequence of several complex interactions that occur between structural and individual factors. They are not always solely related to housing, and usually there is no one single occurrence that results in homelessness. Life events that are associated with several unresolved issues can accumulate and result in, or lead to, homelessness (Centre for the Analysis of Social Exclusion, 2002). The majority of homeless people in the United Kingdom are men (Bunce, 2000).

Homeless men have no address and therefore no fixed abode, and as a result may be unable to register with a general practitioner (Crane and Warnes, 2001). These men may suffer poorer health and experience more mental ill health than those who have homes (St Mungo's, 2004). Those men who sleep rough are one of the most vulnerable groups in society and many men will suffer from acute health problems (Office of the Deputy Prime Minister, 2002). Table 12.1 provides some of the characteristics that reflect the homeless population.

Table 12.1. Some features of homeless men

- 90 % of rough sleepers are male
- 75 % are aged over 25 years
- The life expectancy of a homeless person is 42 years compared with the male national average of 75 years
- This population is 35 times more likely to kill themselves than the general population
- These men are four times more likely to die from unnatural sources, for example, accidents, assaults, murder, drugs or alcohol poisoning
- Half of this population is reliant upon alcohol
- Just under three-quarters of these men are misusing drugs
- Between 30 % and 50 % have mental health problems
- 5 % of this population are from black and ethnic minority groups

(Source: Adapted from Office of the Deputy Prime Minister, 2002)

Homelessness has a broad meaning; it can be used for those men who are living in homes that are unsuitable as well as for men who sleep rough (Diaz, 2006). A person is defined as homeless in the Homelessness Act 2002 if they have:

- no accommodation that they are entitled to occupy;
- accommodation that is available, but it is unreasonable for them to continue to occupy, for example, because of the risk of violence;
- accommodation that they are entitled to occupy and it is reasonable to continue to occupy, but is not available to occupy.

The Government has improved homelessness legislation and reduced the number of men who sleep rough by two-thirds; however, there are many men who experience problems leading to long-term health and social problems (Diaz, 2005). The target set to reduce homelessness to as near to zero as possible, but at least by two-thirds, was the result of a report published by the Social Exclusion Unit (1998). The task to reduce the numbers was taken on by the Rough Sleepers Unit (Department of Environment, Transport and the Regions, 1999).

It is not possible to quantify the number of men who are considered homeless and difficulties occur when trying to estimate how many men in the UK are homeless because of the unknown nature of the problem. Many men arrive and depart large cities and towns making the approximation of statistical representation difficult; there are some men who drift in and out of hostels or other accommodation and there are other men who sleep rough. This has implications for estimating the extent of the problem outside of large cities and towns such as London, where, because of the size and mobility of the population, data is less reliable.

Being homeless can be short-lived and for some men sporadic. Any data provided pertaining to homelessness must be treated with caution as it is not a true representation of the extent of the problem; for example, Diaz (2006) explains that those who are counting the homeless may fail to count those who have hidden themselves in disused buildings or may be staying in areas that have not been included in any count. There may also be the problem of double counting some people. It has been estimated that there are approximately 459 people sleeping rough in England on any one night (Department for Communities and Local Government, 2005). Despite this, a report from Randall and Brown (2000) suggests that the number of people sleeping rough over the course of a year is estimated to be at least ten times higher than the snapshot on any given night provided by street counts.

While there are challenges associated with the ability to estimate the numbers of homeless men, data is available, such as that collected and collated by the Office of the Deputy Prime Minister. This data is provided on a quarterly basis detailing the number of households that contact local authorities and those that have been provided with support if they meet the requirements provided in legislation related to homelessness, for example, the Housing (Homeless Person) Act 1996 as well as the amended Homelessness Act 2002.

St Mungo's is London's largest homelessness agency, providing support for homeless people. This charity has undertaken the most comprehensive survey of the problems of the homeless in the United Kingdom (St Mungo's, 2004). The survey took into account the experiences and challenges endured by over 1534 homeless people.

There appears to be a correlation between those men who find themselves homeless and having had or experienced an institutional background – for example, having been in care, the armed forces or prison (approximately one-third of prisoners lose their housing on imprisonment (Office of the Deputy Prime Minister, 2002), those having experienced family breakdown, sexual and/or physical abuse as a child or in adolescence, or a previous experience of family homelessness. The most common starting point for homelessness, according to the Centre for the Analysis of Social Exclusion (2002), is family conflict. Other factors, including:

- drug and alcohol misuse
- problems at school
- poor educational attainment
- poor physical and mental health
- involvement in criminal acts from an early age

play a key role in a person's susceptibility to becoming homeless (Diaz, 2006).

Low income, unemployment and poverty, according to Anderson (2001), are universal factors linked with homelessness. A result of these factors is that the unemployed man will be unable to pay the mortgage or rent. An outcome of low income can result in an inability to rehouse. This is further complicated by having no fixed address, making the securing of employment difficult, if not impossible, causing further financial hardship – making this vicious cycle difficult to break.

Home can mean many things to many people. A home can mean a place that provides security, a sense of safety, and it can also provide networks for social and community support to occur. However, there are some homes, maybe those where abuse takes place, that are seen by some men and boys as prisons. Often homelessness is considered to apply only to those people who sleep rough; a definition of rough sleepers is given by the Government as:

> sleeping rough, or bedded down in the open air (such as on the streets, or in doorways, parks or bus shelters); people in buildings or other places not designed for habitation (such as barns, sheds, car parks, cars, derelict boats, stations, or bashes. (Department for Communities and Local Government, 2006)

A bash is a makeshift shelter often comprising cardboard boxes (Diaz, 2006).

THE HEALTH AND SOCIAL IMPLICATIONS OF HOMELESSNESS

Bunce (2000) points out that once a man becomes homeless he will automatically become susceptible to a variety of illnesses, diseases, injuries and other health complaints such as psychological trauma. Homeless men are often among those most

Table 12.2. Some specific health issues: homeless men

Physical health	• Higher rates of tuberculosis and hepatitis than the general population, poor conditions of the feet and teeth, respiratory problems, skin diseases, injuries following violence and infections
Mental health	• Serious mental illnesses such as schizophrenia and also depression and personality disorders
Drug and alcohol dependency	• High misuse of heroin, crack cocaine and alcohol

(Source: Adapted from Office of the Deputy Prime Minister, 2002)

in need of treatment and healthcare as a result of their life circumstances; however, they often face obstacles in accessing primary healthcare services. The homeless man may ignore or leave issues concerning his health untreated until this becomes critical. The result is that he will need to rely on treatment and care at accident and emergency departments or walk-in centres presenting with multiple and well-established health and social care problems. If health inequalities and homelessness are to be tackled then local authorities and primary healthcare services must work together to provide accessible and appropriate services to men (Office of the Deputy Prime Minister, 2002).

Pleace and Quilgars (1996) suggest that those who are homeless experience health problems that are related to an increased risk of contracting infectious diseases as they often live in overcrowded places that are damp and cold. They may also experience unsanitary environments as well as sleeping and living in close proximity to others. Often the homeless man will have a combination of illnesses, both physical and psychological, as well as drug addiction. Table 12.2 identifies some specific health issues that have been associated with men who sleep rough.

Homeless men, just as men in the general population, bring to the practice nurse myriad challenges; they also experience health problems such as prostate cancer, osteoporosis and erectile dysfunction, and the practice nurse must be cognizant of this, providing high-quality care that is flexible and responsive. Pfeil and Howe (2004) provide details about the provision of daily clinics for homeless people with a nurse who is available to see and advise patients in the morning and a general practitioner undertaking consultation in the afternoon. The clinics are provided by the Salvation Army in specially designed rooms.

CARING FOR PRISONERS

Healthcare provided by prison services in the United Kingdom (Scotland, England and Wales and Northern Ireland) now reflects what is provided in the wider community (Royal College of Nursing (RCN), 2001). Concerns about healthcare have been discussed many times in the past. It was over a decade ago that long-standing concerns about health standards in prisons were raised (HM Inspectorate of Prisons for England and Wales, 1996) and the establishment of formal partnership between the prison service and the NHS emerged (Joint Prison Service and the National Health Service Executive Working Group, 1999). The provision of healthcare in prisons is undergoing transformation.

There have been a number of primary healthcare developments within the prison service in recent years. Good primary care is the essential foundation on which any good healthcare system is built and this, according to the Department of Health and Her Majesty's Prison Service (DH and HMP; 2002), is especially the case in prison settings. There are many challenges facing those nurses who provide primary care services to the prison population. One of them is the ability to apply mainstream NHS standards in primary care nursing to the prison setting.

The NHS Plan (DH, 2000) has primary care at its heart, providing a modern health service with new opportunities for nurses to take on. There are several opportunities that primary care nurses can take on in an attempt to improve the health of the nation (DH, 2002c). These can include for those at the first point of contact for patients:

- ordering diagnostic investigations
- prescribing
- clinic management
- protocol management of certain patient groups.

Primary care nurses are described as 'gatekeepers' of the NHS, providing treatment and care and making appropriate referrals to other healthcare professionals (DH and HMP, 2002). The service itself – primary care – has been described as having four principles of practice, see Table 12.3.

The principles alluded to in Table 12.3 should also be applied and be seen to be applied to the care of those men who are prisoners. Good, effective primary care should happen wherever the patient is. It has been noted (DH and HMP, 2002)

Table 12.3. The four principles underpinning the provision of good primary care

Fairness	Accessibility	Responsiveness	Efficiency
Services provided across the country should not vary in range or quality	Services should be reasonably accessible to people who need them, irrespective of age, sex, ethnicity or health status	The service should reflect the user's needs and their preferences as well as the health and social needs of the population	Services provided should be based on research evidence of clinical effectiveness and resources should be used efficiently

(Source: Adapted from DH, 2000)

that most healthcare provided to prisoners is of a primary care type with the nurse providing key elements of care. The nurse, providing care to prisoners, is ideally placed to offer care that utilizes his/her full range of skills and attributes, in line with the views espoused in *Making a Difference* (DH, 1999), *The NHS Plan* (DH, 2000) and *Liberating the Talents* (DH, 2002c). Prisoners are just like any other NHS patient, and as such they are allowed to and should receive the same primary care services that any other NHS patient would be entitled to receive. It is just that they are temporarily residing at another address for the time being. The same quality and range of services offered to patients in the general community setting, such as access to a primary healthcare professional within 24 hours and a primary care doctor within 48 hours, is a baseline standard that applies to all (DH, 2004).

Prisoners are a vulnerable population, many men who are incarcerated may have experienced high levels of social exclusion prior to coming into the prison system and may have experienced, according to Hek, Condon and Harris (2005), the following:

- being in care as a child
- being excluded from school
- being homeless
- being unemployed.

The combination of these past life experiences with the effect prison can have on the person's physical and psychological health means that these men will have specific healthcare needs that will need addressing while they are in prison. Parrish (2003) notes how satisfaction surveys have demonstrated that patients are highly satisfied with nurse alternatives to GP care; this coupled with the opportunistic nature of primary care nursing means that the prison population may also benefit from primary care nurses taking on additional roles within prisons in respect to the health of the prison population.

MALE PRISON POPULATION

In England and Wales it has been estimated that at any one time there are approximately 74 000 people detained in 140 prisons. In 2004 (House of Lords/House of Commons Joint Committee on Human Rights, 2004), the Scottish prison service population stood at 6779, while the Northern Ireland prison population is approximately 1313 (Prison Reform Trust, 2006). One-quarter of the prison population at the end of June 2005 was reported to be from a minority ethnic group compared to 1 in 11 of the general population (Home Office, 2005). In England and Wales 35 % of minority ethnic prisoners were foreign nationals; of the British national prison population 10 % were black and 4 % were Asian (Hollis, Cross and Olowe, 2003).

Foreign national prisoners come from over 168 countries but over half are from just six countries:

- Jamaica
- Republic of Ireland
- Turkey
- India
- Pakistan
- Nigeria.

The single largest group (a quarter) are Jamaicans (Prison Reform Trust, 2006).

In some prisons there is overcrowding and this, in some cases, may mean that some prisoners spend 23 hours of the day in a cell that is shared with another man with an unscreened toilet (HM Inspectorate of Prisons for England and Wales, 2004). The overcrowding of prisons can lead to both poor physical and psychological health.

THE HEALTH OF THE PRISON POPULATION

Prisons are not healthy places; Hek, Condon and Harris (2005) suggest that generally prisoners are not healthy people. Seventy-two per cent of men in prisons suffer some form of mental illness; this is much higher than the general population, with 95 % of the younger prison population, those aged between 15–21 years, experiencing some form of mental distress (Social Exclusion Unit, 2002), and 20 % of men having previously been admitted to a mental hospital.

According to Hek, Condon and Harris (2005), there are three major health concerns within prisons: mental health (including self-harm), substance abuse and alcohol-related problems. While these are important health concerns, there are other issues such as:

- communicable diseases (i.e. HIV, sexually transmitted infections, hepatitis B and C and tuberculosis)
- diet (obesity and overweight)
- ischaemic heart disease and cardiovascular problems
- diabetes mellitus
- exercise (musculoskeletal problems)
- smoking (respiratory problems, i.e. asthma)
- epilepsy
- accidents (accidental and non-accidental).

There is a growing evidence base that will provide the nurse with information and insight into the specific healthcare needs of the male prisoner (Hek, Condon and Harris, 2005). Understanding the issues that impinge on the physical and psychological health of the male prisoner can help the nurse plan appropriate approaches to care provision.

GAY MEN (MEN WHO HAVE SEX WITH MEN)

The healthcare needs of gay men are similar to heterosexual men: their needs do not differ significantly. There are, however, certain issues that are specifically related to gay men. For the practice nurse to provide high-quality care to this group of patients, s/he will need to think about gay men from a social, physical and emotional perspective. The older gay man, suggests Kitchen (2003), wants acceptance and equality. They have stated that they want the right to be themselves. These requests should be reflected in the care that the practice nurse provides. The nurse is better placed to be able to shape services to meet individual needs by understanding the inequalities in care provision that are actual, perceived or potential. The provision of healthcare for gay men is not about providing special treatment; it is concerned with respecting the individual and their diversity.

If the practice nurse wishes to consider a gay man as part of a social network, then this will mean that s/he will have to engage with the social and cultural factors that shape his experience. Gay men are a highly heterogeneous population; they are autonomous people and come from socially mobile populations deriving from a range of social, ethnic and geographical backgrounds (Keogh *et al.*, 2004a). As a result of this diverse heterogeneity the practice nurse will need to devise and develop a diverse portfolio of interventions in order to address the diverse healthcare needs this population may present with.

Keogh *et al.*'s (2004a) study focused on the care gay men received in general practice. The study confirmed that nearly a third of gay and bisexual men registered with a GP reported that the staff in the practice did not know they had sex with men and, furthermore, that they would be unhappy if the practice did know. These findings demonstrate some of the challenges that gay men may need to deal with when accessing and using healthcare provision.

Chapter 1 provided an overview of masculinity and discussed hegemonic masculinities as well as how it is possible to stereotype and prejudge certain types of masculinities. Those men who have sex with men can also suffer stigma, prejudice and discrimination; gay men may be blamed for the spread of HIV and AIDS. Much research evidence has centred on the healthcare needs of gay men in relation to their sexual health. While the work in this area has been influential in service provision, it may also be detrimental to the health of gay men, who have healthcare needs other than those associated with sexual health and the prevention of HIV. Some gay men are celibate or live in a monogamous relationship and so if the practice nurse focuses solely on giving the man information related to safer sex, because s/he assumes that this is the man's only health need s/he will be providing inadequate healthcare. The assumption brings with it an emphasis on what the man might do as opposed to who he is. Younger gay men or men who are unsure about their sexuality may pick up on this preoccupation with sex and also assume that this (sex) is what it is to be a gay man.

TERMINOLOGY AND EXPRESSIONS

The term gay has been adopted in this chapter for the sake of ease. Many men use many terms to describe themselves and their sexuality and from the beginning of the nurse–patient relationship the nurse must respect the term or expression that the patient wishes to use when identifying his individual sexuality. In certain circumstances, gay men are men who have sex with men; however, it must be noted that not all men who have sex with men are gay men (Jones, 2004). The nurse must remember this when working with men as well as the language that s/he decides to use.

It is estimated that 5–7 % of the population belong to a gay, bisexual or transgendered group (Keogh *et al.*, 2004). This data, however, must be treated with caution, as reliable data concerning sexual orientation is unavailable.

There are some men who will not, or may even refuse to, identify with being referred to as gay or bisexual. Several reasons for this may be apparent; for example, there may be political reasons why some men prefer one term as opposed to another. On the other hand there are men who are proud to be identified as gay as this can provide them with a sense of a shared identity. The term gay can also be seen as a cultural or community term as opposed to a label attached or imposed on this group by others. Some men may engage in sex with other men but they may not identify with gay men; they may have sex often or occasionally with men or/and women and may prefer to be identified/defined as a man who has sex with men. Bisexual men are often identified as men who are attracted to both men and women and in this case he may wish to identify or define himself as gay or bisexual.

There are also men from minority ethnic groups who also have sex with men and they too might choose not to identify with gay men. Some reasons for this may be associated with issues concerning race and exclusion. Patel, Orhan and Maharaj (1999) state that in some cultures terms or concepts that are associated with being gay may not exist. Sexual identity is complex and for some this is not so easy to compartmentalize. Often it is a fluid and dynamic entity and therefore to label an individual as gay, bisexual or heterosexual can be misleading and, hence, have the potential to misrepresent those involved.

Society's homophobic treatment of gay men (in general) may be the reason why some men do not wish to be identified as gay. There are men who are 'situationally' homosexual, according to Jones (2004). The examples he provides include those men who are not or do not identify as gay, such as those men in prison, those who may have female partners and who identify as a man who has sex with another man, for example, sex workers. It should be noted incidentally that not all male prostitutes are gay.

The diversity associated with identity as discussed above means that the nurse should be sensitive and, as far as possible, aware of the personal situation and circumstances of the individual s/he is caring for. Opportunities for the provision of health promotion activities may be missed and may fail if the needs of all parties described above are not addressed; it is imperative, therefore, that any attempts at reducing risk-taking behaviours include the preferences of the man.

Health education material that has been produced for men who have sex with men may be met with resistance from those men who identify themselves as gay, and vice versa.

Confidentiality and the disclosure of information by men who identify as men who have sex with other men, whether gay or bisexual, are issues that must be given due consideration as these men may be cautious about disclosing the type of sexual activity they engage in. They may be anxious as to how the nurse may respond to these disclosures, fearing they will be judged or patronized.

HETEROSEXISM AND HOMOPHOBIA

Gay men may face barriers to accessing healthcare at all levels; barriers that prevent them from being themselves, often because healthcare providers are discriminatory. The Royal College of Nursing (2003) notes that discrimination, stigma and prejudice occur towards lesbian, gay, bisexual and transgender people. The Nursing and Midwifery Council (2004) clearly demonstrates in their code of professional conduct that every registered nurse, midwife or specialist community public health nurse must respect the patient or client as an individual. Failure to respect this could be deemed to be professional misconduct.

Homophobia can make access to healthcare provision inaccessible. It has been established that there is widespread homophobia among healthcare professionals (Douglas-Scott, Pringle and Lumsdaine, 2004). Homophobia impacts negatively on a gay man's health outcomes.

Douglas-Scott, Pringle and Lumsdaine (2004) define heterosexism as the belief that heterosexuality is inherently superior to homosexuality or bisexuality. They state that homophobic behaviours are irrational fears that can lead to hatred, resulting in verbal and physical attacks and abuse. Those who subscribe to these beliefs justify domination and the imposition of their values and beliefs, believing that everyone is heterosexual. Cosis-Brown (1998) makes the point that in general sexual orientation is not usually visually obvious and assumptions are made that people are all heterosexual. There are several nurses who do not hold the views expressed above, and errors in care provision may be related to a lack of awareness as opposed to the prejudices described.

While heterosexual patients do not have a need to reveal their heterosexuality and may not have any problems or concerns regarding who is aware of their sexuality, this may not be the same for some gay men (Keogh et al., 2004). Gay men may feel exposed and vulnerable; in some smaller, close-knit communities they may encounter spiteful or accidental exposure and as such face the resulting prejudice by others, for example, insurance companies. There are some gay men who have voiced concerns about being seen as deviant if they disclose their sexuality (Keogh et al., 2004).

There is a shortage of evidence available that demonstrates insight and understanding of the needs of gay men in the general practice setting. This lack of knowledge can impact on the practice nurse's ability to develop policies and inform their practice, that is, care that is based on the best available evidence. It has been established that there are health inequalities between the healthcare needs of gay men and the needs of men in general (D'Augelli, 2004; Green, 2003; King *et al.*, 2003).

Many gay men do not have the confidence to be open and honest about their sexuality, even if this is pertinent to their healthcare. Some gay men are concerned that the nurse might react in a hostile and judgemental manner towards them and some have experienced intimidating and judgemental care. If the nurse does intimidate and judge the man, there is a danger that isolation will occur. Guidance has been produced by the RCN and UNISON (2004) focusing on healthcare for lesbian, gay and bisexual service users and their families.

INEQUALITIES EXPERIENCED BY GAY MEN

Health inequalities and social exclusion are experienced by some gay men, Douglas-Scott, Pringle and Lumsdaine (2004) discusses these in detail. Many of the factors that influence the health of the individual are within their control. Very often, social exclusion – a reality expressed by gay men – includes not only social but also economic and psychological isolation. Those people who are socially integrated, it has been demonstrated (Kawachi and Kennedy, 1997), will live longer compared with those who are socially isolated. They are also at risk of an earlier death. Table 12.4 outlines some of the social indicators that affect gay men differently from the general population.

The experiences of being socially excluded and discriminated against have been correlated with poor mental health (Douglas-Scott, Pringle and Lumsdaine, 2004). Links have also been demonstrated between self-harm and poor social support as well as internalized homophobia. Poor mental health may also be the outcome of the long-term effects of bullying.

Table 12.4. Social indicators that affect gay men differently from the general population

- Higher levels of depression, suicide and self-harm are correlated with being gay (King and McKeown, 2003)
- There is also a high prevalence and a high incidence of sexually transmitted infections, such as syphilis, among gay men
- There appears to be a higher incidence of eating disorders among gay men (Bloomfield, 2005)
- Higher levels of substance misuse, for example, use and abuse of alcohol (Alcohol Concern, 2004; Dyter and Lockley, 2003)
- The effects of bullying, for example, harassment relating to sexual orientation, such as homophobic remarks or jokes, offensive comments relating to a person's sexual orientation, threats to disclose a person's sexual orientation to others (King and McKeown, 2003)

Suicide among young men has been identified as a public health priority (Health Development Agency, 2004). It has been estimated that between 20 and 40 % of gay and bisexual men have attempted suicide (Remefedi, 1999). The evidence Remefedi (1999) provides is statistically significant in relation to the association between suicide and male homosexuality. Rivers (2001) states that there are higher levels of attempted suicide or self-harm among young lesbian, gay and bisexual people.

Sex between men continues to be the group at greatest risk of acquiring and transmitting HIV in the United Kingdom; of those infections diagnosed in 2002, 80 % were associated with gay men. There are disproportionate numbers of gay men affected by STIs such as syphilis and hepatitis B (Health Protection Agency, 2004).

A considerable number of gay men experience bulimia nervosa (Douglas-Scott, Pringle and Lumsdaine, 2004). This health concern may be related to body image and the apparent association with eating disorders. Higher levels of body image disturbance are reported by gay men compared with their heterosexual counterparts. Douglas-Scott, Pringle and Lumsdaine (2004) do not provide the number of cases of bulimia nervosa, but they estimate that the levels of binge eating between gay and heterosexual males is 25 % and 10 % respectively with purging occurring in 11.7 % and 4.4 % respectively. Schneider, O'Leary and Jenkins (1995) report similar disordered eating patterns associated with bulimia nervosa in gay men and heterosexual women when comparing them with lesbians and heterosexual men.

Problem drinking and the use of other substances, for example, illegal drugs, is a concern within the gay community (Hughes and Eliason, 2002). Young gay men are said to be more likely than heterosexual men to take illegal drugs (Mullen, 1999; Thiede *et al.*, 2003), for example:

- ecstasy
- cocaine
- marijuana.

Many reasons are provided as to why this might be. For example, the venues in which some gay men tend to gather together, that is, pubs and clubs, may result in an increased use of alcohol, tobacco and drugs.

Homophobic behaviour often begins in the early school years and young people at school can suffer the adverse effects of homophobic bullying resulting in poor health (Douglas-Scott, Pringle and Lumsdaine, 2004; Department for Education and Skills (DfES) and DH, 2004). Those boys who identify as gay or have trouble in expressing their sexuality face the danger of family disruption and rejection, isolation from friends and peers and higher levels of emotional and physical bullying (Corsaro, 2005). It has also been identified that these boys experience difficulties in gaining access to support from teachers and healthcare professionals including those in primary healthcare (DfES and DH, 2004). Wells (1999) states that for those gay youths adolescence can be traumatic, and in some cases life threatening.

There is little opportunity for gay youths, a marginalized group, to voice their exclusive needs – often they are voiceless (Dootson, 2000). This can be further compounded by the fact that there may be a lack of recognition or acceptance by healthcare providers. Some healthcare providers have homophobic attitudes and are unaware of the healthcare needs of the vulnerable gay male adolescent (Wells, 1999).

Practice nurses should aim to offer a service that does not discriminate on the basis of sexuality; they should be prepared to provide tangible evidence that the care they offer does not ignore the patient's sexuality if need be. Assessment of needs should not ignore an individual's sexuality; it should take it into account as appropriate (Kitchen, 2003). Keogh *et al.* (2004) suggest that a key aspect of making people feel at ease (gay friendly) in the practice is to let them know that they will be treated equally and with respect. The practice should endeavour to let all patients know this, including gay men.

MIGRANT POPULATIONS

The increase in asylum-seekers to the United Kingdom has generated much media interest and debate in recent years (Keogh *et al.*, 2004). Despite being seen by some as a 'burden on society', refugees contribute considerably to the economic well-being, knowledge base and cultural life of host countries. The British Medical Association (2006) reports that in 2005 1087 refugee doctors were recorded on the British Medical Association refugee doctor database.

An asylum-seeker or refugee is defined by the 1951 United Nations Convention on the Status of Refugees as an individual who has a well-found fear of being persecuted for reason of religion, nationality, membership of a particular social group or political opinion; is outside the country of his nationality; and is unable, or owing to such fear, is unwilling to avail himself of the protection of that country. In the United Kingdom a person becomes a refugee only when the Home Office has accepted their asylum claim. The person remains an asylum-seeker while they wait for a decision in respect of their claim

Irrespective of status, that is, asylum-seeker or refugee, the person has full and equal entitlement to NHS services. These entitlements also include the right to permanent registration with a general practitioner. Unlike other overseas visitors, asylum-seekers do not pay for general practice or other NHS services.

Most asylum-seekers/refugees in the UK are men (Heath and Jefferies, 2005). German (2004) states that many of these men have been subjected to experiences such as:

- public beatings
- abuse
- persecution

- forced labour
- involuntary conscription
- detention
- torture
- witnessing killings
- separation from families.

These experiences can, according to Tribe (2005), be exacerbated by having to negotiate an asylum system in a foreign language. Feldman (2006) points out that some refugees and asylum-seekers have difficulties in registering with general practitioners and specific issues with needs not being met in relation to mental health and chronic illnesses. Many men, on arrival in the United Kingdom, can feel isolated. They may find it difficult adapting to a new life; they may have to come to terms with their loss of role; some may have lost control of their daily lives and many of them find themselves living in extreme poverty (Burnett, 2002). It is well recognized that the health of men is problematic and this is compounded even further if the man happens to be an asylum-seeker or refugee.

Blackwell (2005) suggests that detention (the holding of asylum-seekers, usually in detention centres while claims for asylum are being assessed) can add to the sense of isolation and may exacerbate fear and aggravate psychological distress, such as, stress, anxiety, distress and post-traumatic stress disorder (PTSD), all as a result of the trauma that the individual has already experienced. Some men may find access to skilled health professionals, such as nurses in detention centres, limited or restricted, inflicting further harm on an already traumatized person's mental and physical health. According to Tribe (2005), PTSD may be the consequence of exposure to:

- war
- loss of family members
- persecution
- imprisonment
- organized violence
- torture.

The effects of PTSD can be further compounded with the loss of access to family members as well as social support systems, coupled with a future that is uncertain. There are a number of asylum-seekers and refugees who live in poor conditions which can be damaging to their physical and psychological well-being (London Assembly and Mayor of London, 2003).

Asylum-seekers and refugees present a high suicide risk (Medical Foundation for the Care of Victims of Torture, 2003). The psychological and physical well-being of all asylum-seekers and refugees, and in particular men, given the fact that men account for the majority of asylum seekers/refugees, as well as the fact that men have particular issues surrounding access to healthcare systems and coupled with the fact that men are at a higher risk of suicide in the population generally, means that the health of these men must be given serious consideration by all nurses, no matter what their political associations may be.

The harmful effects of detention can hinder men's ability to recover from mental distress/disorders such as PTSD and severe depression. This is made even worse for asylum-seekers/refugees (just as it is for men in the general population who may be incarcerated), referral to a mental healthcare professional can be stigmatizing (Razban, 2005) and as a result men may wait and fail to ask for help until problems become overwhelming. The implications for men in the general population when they fail to seek help concerning their health is discussed by White and Banks (2004).

The nurse working in general practice may come into contact with male asylum-seekers or refugees; if s/he is aware of the specific mental health and physical needs of these men, they may have the potential to enhance the quality of care provided as well as reducing the considerable amount of stress experienced. Providing care for the male asylum-seeker/refugee can encourage the nurse to widen their field of focus as well as appreciating other expressions of distress, contextual meanings, cultural constructions of behaviour and explanatory health beliefs.

CONCLUSION

Caring for diverse populations in the general practice setting brings with it many challenges and opportunities. The practice nurse needs to develop insight and understanding of the diverse needs of the whole population, and often this is complex. This chapter has only begun to highlight some of the specific healthcare needs of four groups of men who may be classified as hard to reach, that the practice nurse may come into contact with and need to provide care for.

Inequalities in access to care for some of these groups of men discussed are problematic. New and innovative ways of providing services that address the needs of these men must be developed if the central premise of primary care is to be respected, namely:

- fairness
- accessibility
- responsiveness
- efficiency.

The nature of primary care nursing means that the practice nurse is ideally placed to begin to address the health concerns of the more vulnerable members of our society. The NHS belongs to all of us including the men discussed in this chapter.

REFERENCES

Ablon, J. (2002) The nature of stigma and medical conditions. *Epilepsy and Behavior,* **3** (6), S2–S9.

Alcohol Concern (2004) *Gay and Lesbian People's Fact Sheet,* Alcohol Concern, London.

Anderson, I. (2001) *Pathways through Homelessness: Towards a Dynamic Analysis,* University of Stirling, Scotland.

Blackwell, R.D. (2005) *Counselling and Psychotherapy with Refugees,* Jessica Kingsley, London.

Bloomfield, S. (2005) *Eating Disorders and Men: The Facts,* Eating Disorders Association, Norwich

British Medical Association (2006) http://www.bma.org.uk/ap.nsf/Content/RefugeeDocsB riefingPaper?OpenDocument&Highlight=2,refugee,doctors#RefugeeDoctorsDatabase, accessed 10 June 2006.

Bunce, D. (2000) Problems faced by homeless men in obtaining health care. *Nursing Standard,* **14** (34), 43–45.

Burnett, A. (2002) *Guide to Health Workers Providing Care for Asylum Seekers and Refugees,* Medical Foundation Series, London.

Burton, M. and Kagan, C. (2005) Marginalization. In (eds G. Nelson and I. Prilleltensky) *Community Psychology: In Pursuit of Liberation and Well Being,* Palgrave, Basingstoke, 291–308.

Corsaro, W.A. (2005) *The Sociology of Childhood,* 2nd edn, Pine Forge Press, Thousand Oaks, CA.

Centre for the Analysis of Social Exclusion (2002) *Routes into Homelessness,* Centre for the Analysis of Social Exclusion, London.

Cosis-Brown, H. (1998) *Social Work and Sexuality: Working with Lesbians and Gay Men,* Macmillan, London.

Crane, M. and Warnes, A. (2001) Primary health care services for single homeless people: defects and opportunities. *Family Practice,* **18** (3), 272–276.

D'Augelli, A.R. (2004) High tobacco use amongst lesbian, gay and bisexual youth: mounting evidence about a hidden population's health risk behaviour. *Archives of Pediatric and Adolescent Medicine,* **158** (4), 309–310.

Department for Communities and Local Government (2005) *National Rough Sleeping Estimated in England,* DCLG, London.

Department for Communities and Local Government (2006) Notes and definitions for homelessness data, http://www.communities.gov.uk/index.asp?id=1156301, accessed September 2006.

Department of Environment, Transport and the Regions (1999) *Coming in from the Cold,* DETR, London.

Department for Education and Skills and Department of Health (2004) *Stand Up for Us: Challenging Homophobia in Schools,* DfES, London.

Department of Health (1999) *Making a Difference,* DH, London.

Department of Health (2000) *The NHS Plan: A Plan for Investment, A Plan for Reform,* DH, London.

Department of Health (2002a) *Addressing Inequalities: Reaching the Hard-to-Reach Groups: National Service Frameworks: A Practical Aid to Implementation in Primary Care,* DH, London.

Department of Health (2002b) *Tackling Health Inequalities: Summary of the 2002 Cross-Cutting Review*, DH, London.

Department of Health (2002c) *Liberating the Talents*, DH, London.

Department of Health (2004) *Standards for Better Health*, DH, London.

Department of Health and Her Majesty's Prison Service (2002) *Developing and Modernising Primary Care in Prisons*, DH and HMP, London.

Diaz, R. (2005) *Young People and Homelessness*, Shelter, London.

Diaz, R. (2006) *Street Homelessness*, Shelter, London.

Dootson, L.G. (2000) Adolescent homosexuality and culturally component nursing. *Nursing Forum*, **35** (3), 13–21.

Douglas-Scott, S., Pringle, A. and Lumsdaine, C. (2004) *Sexual Exclusion: Homophobia and Inequalities: A Review*, UK Gay Men's Health Network, London.

Dyter, R. and Lockley, P. (2003) *Drug Misuse Amongst People from the Lesbian, Gay and Bisexual Community: A Scoping Study*, Home Office, London.

Feldman, R. (2006) Primary health care for refugees and asylum seekers: a review of the literature and a framework for services. *Public Health*, **120** (9), 809–816.

Fife, B. and Wright, E. (2000) The dimensionality of stigma: a comparison of its impact on the self of persons with HIV/AIDS and cancer. *Journal of Health and Social Behavior*, **41** (1), 51–67.

German (2004) Enabling re-connection: educational psychologists supporting unaccompanied, separated, asylum seeker/refuge children. *Educational and Child Psychology*, **21** (3), 6–29.

Goffman, E. (1963) *Stigma*, Prentice Hall, Upper Saddle River, NJ.

Green, A.L. (2003) Chem friendly: the institutional basis of 'Club-Drug' use in a sample of urban gay men. *Deviant Behavior*, **24** (5), 427–447.

Heath, T. and Jefferies, R. (2005) *Asylum Statistics: United Kingdom 2004*, Research Development Statistics Directorate, Home Office, London.

Health Development Agency (2004) *Youth Suicide Prevention: Evidence Briefing*, HDA, London.

Health Protection Agency (2004) *Focus on Prevention: HIV and Other Sexually Transmitted Infection in the United Kingdom in 2003: An Update: November 2003*, HPA, London.

Hek, G., Condon, L. and Harris, F. (2005) *Primary Care Nursing in Prisons: A Systematic Overview of Policy and Research Literature*, University of the West of England, Bristol.

Hollis, V., Cross, I. and Olowe, T. (2003) *Prison Population Brief: England and Wales*, Home Office, London.

Home Office (2005) *Population Custody, Quarterly Brief April to June 2005*, Home Office, London.

HM Inspectorate of Prisons for England and Wales (1996) *Patient or Prisoner? A New Strategy for Health Care in Prisons*, Home Office, London.

HM Inspectorate of Prisons for England and Wales (2004) *Annual Report of HM Chief Inspector of Prisons for England and Wales 2002–2003*, The Stationery Office, London.

House of Lords/House of Commons Joint Committee on Human Rights (2004) *Deaths in Custody: Third Report of Session 2004–5, vol. 1*, The Stationery Office, London.

Hughes, T.L. and Eliason, M. (2002) Substance use and abuse in lesbian, gay, bisexual and transgendered communities. *Journal of Primary Prevention*, **22** (3), 263–298.

Joint Prison Service and National Health Service Executive Working Group (1999) *The Future of Prison Health Care*, DH, London.

Jones, M. (2004) Working with gay men in society of sexual health advisors. In (eds Society of Sexual Health Advisors) *The Manual for Sexual Advisors*, SSHA, London, 326–338.

Kawachi, I. and Kennedy, B.P. (1997) The relationship of income inequality to mortality: does the choice of indicator matter? *Social Science Medicine*, **45** (7), 1121–1127.

Keogh, P., Weatherburn, P., Henderson, L. *et al.* (2004) *Doctoring Gay Men: Exploring the Contribution of General Practice*, Sigma Research, London.

King, M. and McKeown, E. (2003) *Mental Health and Social Wellbeing of Gay Men, Lesbians and Bisexuals in England and Wales*, MIND, London.

King, M., McKeown, E., Warner, J. *et al.* (2003) Mental health and quality of life of gay men and lesbians in England and Wales: controlled, cross-sectional study. *British Journal of Psychiatry*, **183**, 552–558.

King, T.E., Wheeler, M.B., Bindman, A.B. *et al.* (2007) *Medical Management of Vulnerable and Underserved People*, McGraw Lange, New York.

Kitchen, G. (2003) *Social Care Needs of Older Gay Men and Lesbians on Merseyside*, Get Heard, Southport.

Keogh, P., Henderson, L., Dodds, C. and Hammond, G. (2004) *Morality, Responsibility and Risk: Gay Men and Proximity to Risk*, Sigma Research, London.

Lipley, N. (1999) Street life. *Nursing Standard*, **13** (48), 13.

London Assembly and Mayor of London (2003) *Access to Primary Care: A Joint London Assembly and Mayor of London Scrutiny Report*, Greater London Authority, London.

Medical Foundation for the Care of Victims of Torture (2003) *Suicide in Asylum Seekers and Refugees*, The Medical Foundation for the Care of Victims of Torture, London.

Mullen, A. (1999) *Social Inclusion: Reaching Out to Bisexual, Gay and Lesbian Youth*, Reach Out, Reading.

Nursing and Midwifery Council (2004) *Code of Professional Conduct: Standards for Conduct, Performance and Ethics*, NMC, London.

Office of the Deputy Prime Minister (2002) *Addressing the Health Needs of Rough Sleepers*, ODPM, London.

Parrish, C. (2003) The future of primary care. *Nursing Standard*, **17** (26), 12–13.

Patel, G., Orhan, A. and Maharaj, K. (1999) *Hard to Reach, Hard to Teach: Research into the Sexual Health Needs of South Asian Men Who Have Sex with Men*, Naz Project, London.

Pfeil, M. and Howe, A. (2004) Ensuring Primary Care Reaches the 'Hard to Reach'. *Quality in Primary Care*, **12** (3), 185–190.

Pleace, N. and Quilgars, D. (1996) *Health and Homelessness in London*, King's Fund, London.

Prison Reform Trust (2006) *Bromley Briefings Prison Fact File*, PRT, London.

Randall, G. and Brown, S. (2000) *Helping Rough Sleepers off the Streets: A Report to the Homelessness Directorate*, Office of the Deputy Prime Minister, London.

Remefedi, G. (1999) Suicide and sexual orientation: nearing the end of controversy?. *Archives of General Psychiatry, American Medical Association*, **56**, 876–885.

Razban, M. (2005) An interpreter's perspective. In (eds R. Tribe and H. Raval) *Working with Interpreters in Mental Health*, Brunner-Routledge, London.

Rivers, I. (2001) The bullying of sexual minorities at school: its nature and long term correlates. *Educational and Child Psychology*, **18** (1), 33–46.

Royal College of Nursing (2001) *Caring for Prisoners: Guidance for Nurses*, RCN, London.

Royal College of Nursing (2003) *The Nursing Care of Lesbian and Gay Male Patients or Clients: Guidance for Nursing Staff*, RCN, London.

Royal College of Nursing and UNISON (2004) *Not 'Just' a Friend*, RCN/UNISON, London.

Schneider, J., O'Leary, A. and Jenkins, S. (1995) Gender, sexual orientation and disordered eating. *Psychology and Health*, **10**, 113–128.

Social Exclusion Unit (1998) *Rough Sleeping*, Her Majesty's Stationery Office, London.

Social Exclusion Unit (2002) *Reducing Re-offending by Ex-Prisoners. Social Exclusion Unit*, Her Majesty's Stationery Office, London.

St Mungo's (2004) *St Mungo's Big Survey into the Problems and Lives of Homeless People*, St Mungo's, London.

Stockwell, F. (1984) *The Unpopular Patient*, RCN, London.

Thiede, H., Valleroy, L., MacKellar, D. *et al.* (2003) Regional patterns and correlates of substance use among young men who have sex with men in 7 US urban areas. *American Journal of Public Health*, **93**, 1915–1921.

Tribe, R. (2005) The mental health needs of refugees and asylum seekers. *Mental Health Review*, **10** (4), 8–15.

Van Cleemput, P. and Parry, G. (2001) Health status of gypsy travellers. *Journal of Public Health Medicine*, **23** (2), 129–134.

White, A.R. and Banks, I. (2004) Help seeking in men and the problems of late diagnosis. In (eds R.S. Kirby, C.C. Carson, M.G. Kirby and R.N. Farah) *Men's Health*, 2nd edn, Taylor & Francis, London.

Wells, S.A. (1999) The health beliefs values, and practices of gay adolescents. *Clinical Nurse Specialist*, **13** (2), 69–73.

13 Psychological issues and the male

INTRODUCTION

It has already been stated that men are prone to risk (physical risk) as a result of their gender. The mental health of men is poorly understood and as a result is often undervalued (Men's Health Forum, 2006); little is known about how to devise effective ways to help men aspire to good mental health. Men are prone to specific psychological risks that may require intervention by the practice nurse in order to alleviate their suffering. These conditions may be managed in the practice setting or the practice nurse may need to refer the patient to the most appropriate healthcare professional. The following three issues are discussed here:

- suicide
- rape
- domestic violence.

The numbers of men who have been formally admitted to NHS hospitals in England and Wales under the Mental Health Act 1983 (Sections 2, 3 and 4) has risen significantly. In England in 1990, 8673 men were admitted formally; this rose to 13 400 between 2003 and 2004 (Depatment of Health (DH), 2004). During the same period in Wales this rose from 547 to 759 (Health Statistics Analysis Unit, 2004).

Black men have higher admission rates than white men under Sections 2, 3 and 4 of the Mental Health Act; these men are also over-represented in secure units. Many men who have no formal diagnosis of a mental health illness may, nonetheless, be attempting to cope with their problems alone. There are a number of men who are far more likely to become alcohol dependent, commit suicide and misuse drugs (Men's Health Forum, 2006). The key to achieving good mental health means that people need to have the maximum chances in life in order to experience positive mental health.

There is evidence that points to the fact that some common mental health problems, such as depression and anxiety, have increased as well as the markers that point to a society that is discontent, for example, violence in public places, substance misuse and family breakdown (James, 1998).

The issues of mental well-being and mental health are important to the public. The Government's publication *Our Health, Our Care, Our Say* (DH, 2006) demonstrates its commitment to reducing suicide, after extensive consultation with the general public these issues emerged as issues of importance. The Government has recognized and responded to the need to take mental health seriously by the publication of a number of documents, for example, the *National Service Framework*

(NSF) for Mental Health (DH, 1999a). The NSF (DH, 1999a) calls upon the NHS to promote mental health for all.

The benefits to the nation in striving to achieve, enhance and improve mental well-being are outlined by the National Institute for Mental Health in England (NIMHE; 2005) which states that positive mental health has the potential to improve the physical health of the person, improve quality of life, reduce crime, enhance educational attainment and lead to an increase in personal dignity.

Trying to define or characterize mental well-being or positive mental health is difficult. These states, according to the Men's Health Forum (2006), are slippery objects to grasp. Most people know what it is like for them to feel happy and content, to love and feel loved; these add up to and contribute to what it is to have positive mental health or a good sense of mental health and well-being; they are, however, subjective and very personal entities.

Layard (2005) makes an analysis of seven identifiable factors that influence an individual's chances of achieving a sense of well-being:

- family relationships
- financial situation
- work
- community and friends
- health
- personal freedom
- personal values.

Five of those key aspects above are discussed by the Men's Health Forum (2006); they also include a sixth factor – school, in so far as mental health and the road to achieving well-being are often instigated in childhood. The six factors outlined by the Men's Health Forum (2006) are considered in Table 13.1(below).

The aspects outlined in Table 13.1 can be seen as complex factors that interact with each other and have the potential to impinge significantly on a person's well-being. These factors will affect men and women differently.

Schizophrenia is one of the most disabling mental health disorders. While it is equally distributed among the sexes, men, however, have a worse prognosis and the illness in men runs a more severe course (Walters and Tylee, 2003).

SUICIDE

Suicide is a major public health issue with approximately 5000 people in England taking their own lives (DH, 2002). Every suicide is both an individual loss as well as a loss to society. Over 75 % of suicides in the UK are committed by men, with the majority of suicides occurring in men under 40 years. Women attempt suicide three or four times more often than men; however, four times as many men than women die from suicide each year (Lloyd, 2001). The gender difference associated with deaths as a result of

Table 13.1. Six factors that are recognized to have a significant impact on the mental well-being of the man

Aspect	Component
Family	The family has the ability to socialize boys, creating traditional male attitudes; boys and girls in families are often brought up to exhibit different attitudes and to have different expectations. Some of these attitudes associated with the traditional male role may be detrimental to men's well-being. Men tend to demonstrate a number of damaging tendencies, such as a relative lack of emotional expressiveness, and these predispositions may have their roots in the ways in which boys are raised; boys are often encouraged to minimize the expression of hurt; for example, 'big boys don't cry', 'soldier on'. When boys do express vulnerability or do indeed cry they may suffer at the hands of others and be called 'poof', 'faggot', 'gay' or 'sissy'. The way boys are socialized or raised at home or at school have the potential to impinge on their ability to enjoy positive mental health when they grow older. Stable, long-term adult relationships are protective of men's mental health; there is evidence to suggest that when fathers are more actively involved with the upbringing of their son(s) then they will have a better chance of enjoying a more satisfying adult life. A strong father/son relationship increases the likelihood of a boy growing up to enjoy positive mental health.
Financial circumstances	An important precursor of positive mental well-being is being able to afford (financially) the daily necessities of life. The greater the gap between the rich and poor in society, then the greater the chances of poorer mental and physical health. Increased wealth may not correlate with increased happiness.
Work	Enjoying satisfaction at work can be a very important predisposing factor for positive mental health. However, not having a job and being unemployed can lead to distress, anxiety and depression; psychological and psychiatric morbidity increases as a result of unemployment and when the man finds employment these effects are reversed. One reason may be associated with the importance of being a breadwinner and a cultural indicator of the male role; men remain the breadwinner in most traditional families despite major social changes having occurred over the years. The burden of having to work and produce results can also be detrimental to a person's mental health and can result in work-related stress. Men more than women are likely to suffer from work-related stress. Work-related stress can also predispose a man to diabetes and heart disease. Men in the UK work the longest hours in Europe. The outcome of working long hours can have a detrimental effect on a man's ability to engender family relationships.

(continued)

Table 13.1. (*Continued*)

Aspect	Component
School	The issue of school does not usually impact on the mental health of the adult male; however, the effects of a positive experience at school or a traumatic experience can have a lifelong effect on a person and potentially hinder the achievement of positive mental health. The evidence demonstrates that boys, particularly from black and minority ethnic (with the exception of those of Indian and Chinese origin) communities, are performing less well at school. The effects of this are that these boys may grow up to experience a less positive mental health. Some of the discrepancies associated with academic under-achievement may be explained by higher levels of deprivation experienced by these pupils. Black Caribbean boys are twice more likely as white boys to be classified as having behavioural, social and emotional problems. Most pupils excluded from schools are boys. There is a clear correlation between achieving at school and mental well-being, albeit a modest correlation; higher educational achievement is correlated with increased chances of obtaining a more satisfying job. Young gay men are particularly susceptible to bullying and the outcome of this can be detrimental to mental health. Nearly 50 % of all gay men stated that they have experienced homophobic attitudes at school from both teachers and pupils.
Community and friends	The concept social capital is associated with a feeling of being connected to others as well as the wider society – broadly it is related to the engagement between citizens and civil processes. A correlation between low social connectedness and poor mental health has been established. Men are known to score low social capital: they do not appear to have as much contact with friends, trust in others or participation in social activity as women have. Men tend to shy away from physical and social engagement with men stating they feel unsupported from a social and emotional perspective; the result is a higher risk for poorer mental health; lack of social support clearly correlates with poor mental health. Men may find it difficult to belong to or find membership to communities and in an attempt to fit in may use other means to ease a sense of belonging, for example, the use of alcohol. The reasons men tend to have lower levels of social capital have not been fully explored; the reasons are complex and multifactorial; there is a need for further research in this area.

(*continued*)

Table 13.1. (*Continued*)

Aspect	Component
Health	Being seriously ill or having a disability does not necessarily mean the men will be unable to enjoy positive mental health; good health is not a prerequisite of mental well-being. Some men have the ability to adapt to their illness and the physical limitations that may be the result of poor health or disease. However, chronic pain and mental illness in particular can impinge on mental well-being.

(Source: Adapted from Men's Health Forum, 2006)

suicide is pan-European. For example, the ratio of deaths in men compared to women in Portugal is 2 : 1 and in the Republic of Ireland is 11 : 1 (Men's Health Forum, 2000).

It is acknowledged that more women than men are diagnosed with depressive illnesses. What must be considered, however, is if male-specific symptoms are being taken into account when making a diagnosis of depression. Depression, according to the Men's Health Forum (2006), is less easily recognized in men, as opposed to depression being less common in men. This may mean that there are potentially large numbers of men who are not receiving the treatment and support they need in order to enjoy good mental health. Figure 13.1 provides data concerning the death rate of intentional self-harm and injury of undetermined intent in England.

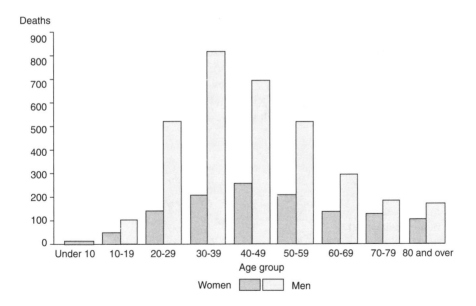

Figure 13.1. Death rate of intentional self-harm and injury of undetermined intent in England 2004. (Source: CSIP and NIMHE, 2006)

In the last 30 years the rate of suicide in older men has fallen but in younger men it has risen. There has been, and continues to be, a sustained fall in the numbers of younger men who commit suicide but the numbers still remain high in comparison with the general population (CSIP and NIMHE, 2006).

There are several indicators of unhappiness that men may experience and these may not be recognized by healthcare professionals as potential indicators of emotional distress, for example, heavy drinking and drug misuse, the outcome of which can be death by suicide. The prison population (as discussed earlier in Chapter 12) suffer with poor mental health. Being male and black means that you are more likely to be diagnosed with a psychiatric mental health problem than a white man is. Gay men as opposed to the male population in general experience more depression and anxiety. It may be that these men are at risk of depression and anxiety because they belong to a minority community group and, as is the case with most minority groups, they can experience discrimination.

The practice nurse must give more consideration to the male patient who presents with the issues described above and offer him support. Consideration is also required for those who care for people with mental health problems. Adaptation of care provision is required in order to meet the man's needs in a more effective manner. This may help to improve their mental well-being and also to save lives.

SUICIDE AND RISK FACTORS

In order to reduce the rates of suicide the practice nurse must develop the skills required to assess suicidal risk. Appleby (1996) notes that a number of men who commit suicide are known to have visited their general practice three months prior to death. Approximately 25 % of people who commit suicide have been in contact with mental health services in the year prior to their death (Appleby *et al.*, 1999). Biddle *et al.* (2004) note, however, that only 1 in 5 young men aged between 16 and 24 years with suicidal thoughts would seek help from the general practice. There are many risk factors for suicide (Men's Health Forum, 2000) and they include:

- being male
- living alone
- being unemployed
- misusing alcohol
- misusing drugs
- being mentally ill
- being a member of the lower social classes (4 and 5)
- living in an area of economic and social deprivation
- living in rural areas.

The most common form of suicide for men (accounting for half of deaths) is hanging and suffocation. Death by drug overdose and carbon monoxide poisoning (car exhaust fumes) has decreased.

Table 13.2. Suicide attempters versus completers

Characteristic	Attempters	Completers
Gender	Female	Male
Age	Predominantly young	Risk increase with age
Method	Low lethality (pills, cutting)	More violent (gun, jumping)
Circumstances	Intervention likely	Precautions against discovery
Common diagnosis	Borderline personality disorder	Major mood disorder, alcoholism, schizophrenia
Motivation	Change in situation, cry for help	Death
Dominant affect	Depression with anger	Depression with hopelessness

(Source: Adapted from Fremouw, Perczel and Ellis, 1990)

The definition of suicide varies; the World Health Organization (WHO; 1992) defines it as: 'suicide and deaths from injury and poisoning undetermined whether accidentally or purposely inflicted'. As there are differences in the way in which suicide is defined, this can mean that a reporting bias may exist and as such any data that is presented may be significantly underestimating the extent of the problem. It may be helpful when caring for men who have suicidal ideation to consider suicide, as Hawton (1992) suggests, as a spectrum, extending from vague thoughts about suicide to more significant thoughts, a preparation towards the completed suicidal act.

It is possible to make comparisons between those individuals who attempt suicide as opposed to those who successfully commit the act. The distinctions between the two groups are highlighted in Table 13.2.

In most of the Western world, according to Wheat (2000), suicide is not unlawful. Section 1 of the Suicide Act 1961 abolished the crime of suicide. Under Section 2 of the Act, however, it is unlawful to aid and abet a suicide.

DELIBERATE SELF-HARM

Self-harm is more prevalent in females than males; it is four times more common and also occurs more frequently in younger adults. In the past self-harm may have been referred to as self-mutilation or self-injury. Walsh (2006) defines self-harm as:

Intentional, self-effected, low lethality bodily harm of a socially unacceptable nature, performed to reduce psychological distress.

Many cases of self-harm are associated with drug overdoses. A definition of self-harm in relation to overdose is defined by Pratt *et al.* (2005) as:

A non-fatal act in which a person causes self-injury or ingests a substance in excess of any prescribed or generally recognized therapeutic dosage.

According to Bhugra (2004), suicide may be preceded by attempted suicide, parasuicide or deliberate self-harm; these terms are often used interchangeably. It is also noted that not all cases of attempted suicide, parasuicide or deliberate self-harm lead to suicide.

Data indicating the numbers of people who self-harm are very unreliable. The information and data provided in association with self-harm may only indicate the minimum number of people who self-injure; many cases of self-injury – for example, scalding, cuts and burns – are often managed at home and as a result do not become statistically apparent.

METHODS USED TO COMMIT SUICIDE

A good knowledge of the methods used for committing suicide is essential if the practice nurse is to devise, develop and take part in effective suicide prevention programmes (Bertolote, 2001). Males and females tend to use different methods in order to commit suicide; when comparing males with females, it would appear that the key feature is associated with the lethal intention with which the act is committed. This accounts for the rates of actual suicide in males and the rates of attempted suicide in females. Hanging is a relatively quicker process than, for example, the taking of drugs. When hanging does occur, there is far less chance that a life-saving intervention will be attempted as opposed to drug-taking, where gastric lavage may be the life-saving intervention.

A selection of techniques are used in order to commit suicide. The Men's Health Forum (2000) suggests that there has been an increase in hanging and suffocation since 1983. This rise is noticeable in the 15–44 age group. Other methods include suicide by the use of firearms and explosives, jumping from high places and lying in front of trains or buses. Table 13.3 outlines some of the methods men use to commit suicide.

POSSIBLE CAUSES OF MALE SUICIDE

It may never be possible to understand why people commit suicide and what the likely underlying causes are; however, there are notable relationships between suicide and

Table 13.3. Methods used to commit suicide

Hanging and suffocation	34 %
Poisoning by gasses and vapours	23 %
Poisoning by substance	20 %
Drowning	5 %
Other methods	18 %

(Source: Men's Health Forum, 2000)

Table 13.4. Some of the multifaceted issues contributing to suicide

---

- Individual characteristics such as mental illness, drug use, gender identity issues and a genetic or biological component
- Family problems such as child abuse, a suicide in the family and family breakdown
- Social isolation
- Psychosocial (the effects that issues such as ill health, stress and inequality have on an individual's health status)

(Source: Adapted from Durkheim, 1952, Wilkinson, 1996)

some particular factors. In men they are psychiatric illness, in particular depression and schizophrenia, alcoholism, drug addiction, cerebral disorders such as epilepsy, and brain injury, personality disorder and neuroses (Men's Health Forum, 2000). Hart and Flowers (2001) state that gay men are particularly vulnerable to mental health problems, and as such they are at a higher risk of attempting suicide. Table 13.4 provides a list of some of the multifaceted causes of suicide.

Often depression, which may lead a man to take his own life, according to Wasserman (2001), centres on a man's occupation and workplace. When a man becomes unemployed he may not only lose his job but also suffer the loss of his social support networks, his friends and colleagues, structure to his daily life and loss of status. Those men who are unemployed, have schizophrenia and a previous history of attempted suicide are in the high-risk category as schizophrenia appears to be one of the most significant factors. A large number of men who commit suicide have had a depressive illness (Wasserman, 2001).

Young people who have a past history of suicide attempts are at a greater risk of engaging in further suicide attempts (Lewinsohn, Rhode and Seeley, 1994). Adolescents who engage in self-harm and have suicidal thoughts often experience more problems and life events than those adolescents who do not deliberately self-harm or have suicidal thoughts (Samaritans, 2003). The adolescents identified by the Samaritans (2003) were also noted to be more anxious and depressed and also had lower self-esteem than those who did not engage in self-harm. Mental illness in youth suicide is the strongest risk factor, as is a family history of mental illness and/or suicide (Agerbo, Nordentoft and Bo-Mortensen, 2002).

PREVENTING SUICIDE

As far back as 1998, the Acheson Report (Department of Health, 1998) recommended that policies be formulated to prevent suicide among young people. The report singled out in particular young men and those with psychiatric illness. When considering inequalities in health, the report stated that social issues such as unemployment, alcohol and substance misuse and social isolation were major contributing factors (Gunnell *et al.*, 1999). Several recommendations were made in that report to reduce social isolation:

- offering social support for parents
- developing of 'lifelong skills'
- preventing substance and alcohol misuse
- provision of adequate housing
- relieving poverty
- increasing the numbers of those in employment and the promotion of health in the workplace.

These approaches, it could be suggested, will go some way to promote social cohesion. The number, duration, strength and quality of social relations are all inversely related to suicide risk. Those who enjoy kinship, occupation, friendship and other social ties are generally at a much lower risk of suicide as opposed to those who do not experience social cohesion (Mäkinen and Wasserman, 2001).

Our Healthier Nation (DH, 1999b) calls for a reduction in the numbers of suicides by at least a fifth by 2010. Standard 7 of the mental health NSF (DH, 1999b) (preventing suicide) sets out how that target is to be achieved; the NSF highlights nine interventions to prevent suicide at a local level. The framework also includes how those working in prisons can instigate measures to reduce the rates of suicide through assessing the risk of suicide among prisoners. The *National Suicide Prevention Strategy for England* (DH, 2002) states that there is no single route to achieving the Government's targets to reduce suicide by a fifth by 2010; a multidisciplinary approach is advocated. A call is made for a coherent approach to address the multifaceted influences such as:

- social circumstances
- biological vulnerability
- mental ill health
- life events
- access to means.

There are several initiatives that are designed to be implemented at a local level by and with the general practice. Suicides can be prevented by:

- the promotion of mental health for everybody, working with individuals and communities;
- the provision of high-quality primary mental healthcare;
- ensuring that those with mental health problems can access local services;
- guaranteeing that those with severe or enduring mental health problems have an individualized care plan that allows access to services around the clock;
- the provision of safe hospital accommodation for those who need it;
- providing support to those who care for people with severe mental illness in order that they can continue to do this;
- supporting prison staff in preventing suicide;
- ensuring staff are equipped to assess the risk of suicide competently among those at greater risk;

- targeting young men in schools to ensure that they are provided with clear opportunities to talk about their personal concerns;
- developing audit to appraise suicide activities and to learn lessons from this.

There are some specific factors that may predispose a man to consider taking his own life. One of the key factors appears to be associated with poor mental health. If the practice nurse is aware of the predisposing factors and undertakes a full and holistic assessment of the patient, this may help to stem the numbers of unnecessary deaths that occur as a result of suicide.

Practice nurses who demonstrate an awareness of the population most at risk – for example, those young men from lower social classes, those who are socially isolated, men with mental health problems and those with gender identity issues – will in the process help to single out those men who may be at risk of attempting suicide. Care must also be taken by the nurse not to stereotype men; remember that each man is an individual and may not conform to the stereotypical 'macho' male image.

RAPE AND SEXUAL ASSAULT

The numbers of male sexual assault remain underreported; this is also the case with female sexual assault. It is difficult to find accurate data related to male rape. Underreporting means that research into the issues that men face following sexual assault are limited and it is, therefore, a poorly understood phenomenon. Male rape is cloaked in myth and taboo. The statutory offence of male rape was introduced in 1996 and data has been collected since this date. Before this date no data had been collected on male sexual assault.

DeVisser *et al.* (2003), in an Australian study, focused on men and several aspects of their sexual health and relationships. The report demonstrated that 4.8 % of men had experienced sexual coercion, 2.8 % disclosed to the researchers that this had occurred when they were aged less than 16 years.

Year on year there has been an increase in reporting of the offence. This may demonstrate that there is an increasing awareness of the problem. Sexual assault has the potential to impact on a man from medical, social and psychological perspectives.

LEGAL DEFINITION OF RAPE

The age of consent of any sexual activity is 16 years for men and women in England, Scotland and Wales; in Northern Ireland it is 17 years of age (Family Planning Association, 2004). Prior to the Sexual Offences Act 2003 the definition of rape only included penile penetration of the vagina and anus. In Scotland rape is defined as vaginal penetration and anything else is classed as indecent assault (Sexual Offences Act, Scotland) 1976. Male rape in Scotland is not a recognized offence and the perpetrator would be convicted under aggravated assault. In Northern Ireland a man would commit rape if he had anal or vaginal intercourse with a male or female without their

Table 13.5. Numbers of male rape 1996–2001

Year	Reported numbers of male rape
1996	227
April 1997–March 1998	375
April 1998–March 1999	504
April 1999–March 2000	600
April 2000–March 2001	664

(Source: Her Majesty's Crown Prosecution Service Inspectorate, 2002)

consent (Criminal Justice (Northern Ireland) Order 2003). Other serious offences such as forced oral sex were treated only as indecent assault. Penetration of the mouth by the penis is now classed as serious and can be construed as rape. This is the only sexual offence that can be committed by a man. In England and Wales a woman may be charged with sexual assault by penetration. This new offence was introduced by the Sexual Offences Act 2003. A crime has been committed if a person intentionally touches another person in a sexual manner without reasonable belief that that person has consented, and the purpose must be sexual. The Sexual Offences Act 2003 is the most sweeping overhaul of legislation in relation to sex crimes in England and Wales for 50 years; it advocates equality with regards to issues such as consent and rape for both men and women. Those practitioners who conduct intimate examinations or intimate searches are exempt from this offence.

The offence of male rape is relatively new, and as a result of this reporting and the way in which male victims are managed and cared for and encouraged to report the crime needs to be developed and improved. The number of male sexual assaults reported and recorded is outlined in Table 13.5.

There are several reasons why a man may not report rape or sexual assault; most reasons centre on shame and guilt (see Table 13.6).

Table 13.6. Some reasons why men do not report rape or sexual abuse

- Thinking that the person is the only one this has happened to
- Guilt, shame
- Fear of ridicule
- Fear of not being believed
- Fear of reprisal from the rapist
- Concern about what family and friends might think
- Dislike of talking about feelings and emotions
- Men are supposed to be able to better protect themselves
- Men cannot be victims of rape
- The man experienced an erection and/or ejaculated during the attack
- Fear of being accused of being gay – only gay people get raped
- Unable to come to terms with the feelings of fear and the threat to your life
- Self-blame

There are many myths and taboos surrounding the issue of male rape. Low reporting rates, according to Armitage (2004), perpetuate these myths and taboos. Many people are of the opinion that men are assertive sexually and socially, that they have the wherewithal to defend themselves and that they enjoy all sexual encounters. More often than not men are seen as perpetrators when it comes to crime and not the victims (see Table 13.7.)

Table 13.7. Myths and facts associated with rape

Myth	Fact
Men cannot be sexually assaulted	Men can and are sexually assaulted every day. Any man, regardless of his age or size, strength, occupation, race or sexual orientation, can be sexually assaulted. Male rape can occur at home, at work, outdoors, any place the rapist wants to commit the act
Only gay men are raped	More gay men are raped than their heterosexual counterparts; gay men can be the target of anti-gay violence
It is only gay men that sexually abuse other men	Many men who sexually assault other men describe themselves as exclusively heterosexual. Sexual assault is often about violence, domination and control as opposed to sexual attraction
Men cannot be sexually assaulted by women	The majority of male rape perpetrators are male; nevertheless women can and do sexually assault men
Male rape victims do not suffer as much as female victims	All rape victims regardless of gender suffer the effects of sexual assault. Often male rape involves a higher use of violence and weapons and is more likely to involve multiple assailants. Male rape victims are more prone to commit suicide than their female counterparts
Most rape victims are strangers	The majority of rapists are known to the victim, just as is the case with women victims; it is, however, acknowledged that gang rape can and does occur
Erection and ejaculation during rape means the victim consented	Erection and ejaculation is the result of both physical stimulation and neural activity. The rapist may use lubrication with the sole aim of causing an erection and subsequent emission
Rape in gay couples does not exist	Rape in any relationship can and does exist – heterosexual or homosexual

(Source: Adapted from Coxell *et al.*, 1999; Armitage, 2004)

There are certain factors that identify both men and women as being at risk of sexual assault. Armitage (2004) suggests that the following factors make a man more vulnerable to sexual violence:

- youth
- poor educational attainment
- past history of sexual assault
- works in the sex industry
- is in prison.

HEALTH IMPLICATIONS

The impact of rape can impinge on the man's health from a physical and psychological perspective as well as having a detrimental effect on the individual's social life. Survivors of sexual assault report a range of psychological and emotional disorders, including shock, anxiety, depression, post-traumatic stress disorder and other trauma-related mental health issues. They can also experience disturbed sleep, loss of self-esteem, sexual dysfunctions and behavioural and eating disorders. Psychological and emotional trauma can also manifest itself as psychosomatic illnesses; for example, stomach aches, headaches and back problems. The World Health Organization (2002) notes that sexual assault victims are more likely to attempt or to commit suicide.

The survivor may come to the practice nurse, accident and emergency nurse or nurses working in genitourinary medicine clinics for help and advice. Some of the injuries (physical and psychological) sustained during an attack may require admission to hospital.

The primary aim of care should be to provide the patient with an all-inclusive sexual health service, that is, one that is sensitive, compassionate, discreet and respectful. Protocols and policies advocate that a multidisciplinary approach be taken to devise policy and protocol; the team must also take into account local and national policy; these policies and protocols should be made available to nurses in the general practice setting. Guidelines have been produced by the Association for Genitourinary Medicine and the Medical Society for the Study of Venereal Diseases (AGUM and MSSVD; 2001) with respect to the management of adult survivors of sexual assault.

EXAMINATION AND ASSESSMENT

It is important to understand that care for the victim should only be limited to the diagnosis, treatment and psychological support. An examination required for the collection of specimens for forensic purposes must not be undertaken by the nurse. It should be noted that not all attacks will result in physical injury. If the patient wishes to consent to a forensic examination, it is vital that no other examination is performed as this may invalidate any evidence collected during the forensic examination. The nurse needs to approach the situation with compassion; the nurse, as the patient's advocate, has to judge the need of taking specimens against the patient's suffering.

Any investigations that are necessary will be done in accordance with need – for example, Sexually transmitted infection screening; investigations will vary depending on local policy. Reynolds, Peipert and Collins (2000) note that survivors of sexual assault have higher rates of STIs compared with the general population, and opportunist screening may be beneficial. The following issues will need to be addressed if a patient requests an examination (Reynolds, Peipert and Collins, 2000; Wakely, Cunnion and Chambers, 2003):

- screening for STIs (i.e. gonorrhoea, chlamydia with swabs being taken from all sites exposed during the attack, for example, anus, pharynx and urethra);
- hepatitis B and C, HIV testing (if indicated);
- provision of antibiotic therapy;
- provision of post-exposure prophylaxis (HIV) therapy (if indicated);
- provision of hepatitis B vaccination (if appropriate);
- provision of emotional and psychosexual support if needed (consider referral for counselling);
- analgesia may be required;
- tetanus toxoid (if appropriate).

There is a risk of HIV transmission from one act of unprotected penetrative intercourse; however, despite this the risk is very low. It is recommended that the patient uses a condom until a diagnosis of HIV has been ruled out – usually within three months (Mein *et al.*, 2000).

THE FORENSIC EXAMINATION

A physician trained in forensic medicine is required to undertake the forensic examination (Rogers, 1996). A forensic examination may have already been undertaken if the patient has reported the incident to the police; however, it should be noted that the forensic examination may not have included screening for, and treatment of, STIs. The treatment of any injuries sustained during the assault take priority over the examination. Immediate medical care may be needed if the assault has occurred recently. The aim of this examination is to collect evidence for any legal proceedings that may ensue.

It may be that the patient may decline a forensic examination and if so this should be respected. Some patients prefer a same-sex healthcare practitioner to undertake the examination; this needs to be determined. The patient's best interests are what the nurse must be guided by, which means respecting the person's wishes in all instances.

Any DNA evidence on or in the body of the survivor, in moist areas, degrades rapidly; usually over 2–10 days. Forensic examination needs to be undertaken as soon as possible but within ten days of an assault (Hampton 1995). If the patient has agreed to have a forensic examination, he should be advised as follows:

● do not shower or bathe
● do not clean the teeth or rinse the mouth out
● ensure all clothes worn remain unwashed.

Note: the patient should be asked to retain underclothes worn during the assault in paper bags as opposed to plastic bags, this reduces the speed at which the DNA degrades.

RISK OF HIV AND STIs

An increased risk of HIV and or other STIs can occur to those survivors of sexual assault or rape because:

● the use of force may have been traumatic, resulting in a tearing injury to the genital tract, increasing the risk of contracting STIs/HIV;
● perpetrators tend to belong to a category of individuals who have higher rates of STIs/HIV;
● co-infection with an STI can also increase the risk of HIV transmission.

Forced anal penetration, according to Armitage (2004), has a greater risk than penile–vaginal rape with an HIV-positive assailant. Each case should be assessed individually with regards to risk, explaining issues carefully to the patient in order for them to make an informed decision. What must be borne in mind is that risk assessment is difficult when the HIV status of the attacker may be unknown.

Legal support may also be needed if the patient wishes to bring about legal charges; the nurse can support the patient, acting as coordinator if referral is required. The practice nurse can help the survivor from a physical and psychological perspective; if the patient wishes to go through with a forensic examination only an appropriately trained person can conduct this examination; no other examination should be conducted. However, if the patient decides not to proceed with a forensic examination (and this is his choice), then an examination to screen and treat any possible STIs should be offered.

It may be appropriate to offer hepatitis B vaccination as well as post-exposure prophylaxis after an unprotected assault. The survivor should be offered counselling and a follow-up appointment must be made to determine the effects of treatment as well as assessing how the person is coping. It is vital that the care offered and provided be non-judgemental, sympathetic as well as discreet. Table 13.8 (below) outlines options for healthcare after an assault has occurred.

The male survivor may experience similar feelings to his female counterpart who has been sexually abused; often these feelings are centred on feeling guilty, self-blaming and shame. For a man, however, these feelings may be amplified further as they may have to contend with the common myth that men should be self-sufficient

Table 13.8. Options for healthcare after an assault has occurred

Injuries	Genital or bodily injuries should be managed in the accident and emergency department. In general practice it may be appropriate to manage more minor injuries. If the injuries (physical or psychological) are so severe, this may necessitate hospital admission
Screening for STIs	Many opportunities are available in general practice to offer the man STI screening in the surgery; if this is not the case, then referral may need to be made to a local genitourinary medicine clinic
Psychological support	Ongoing support may be needed and can be arranged by the practice nurse or the genitourinary medicine clinic
Forensic examination	This examination is undertaken by a specialist physician through the police or sexual assault referral centres. Consent must be gained from the patient prior to forensic examination taking place. It must be remembered that any acute injury or medical need has to take precedence over forensic examination
Personal safety	If the assault has occurred in the man's home, he may not wish to return there. Contact details of local support agencies and refuges should be made available

(Source: Adapted from Armitage, 2004)

and that they should be able to protect themselves, the 'macho image'. This can lead to depression, social alienation, isolation and a suppression of emotions that may later manifest in other harmful ways, such as violence and domestic violence (Armitage, 2004). King, Coxell and Mezey (2002) suggest that all forms of sexual molestation may result in self-harming behaviour, such as drug and alcohol misuse.

The practice nurse may be required to arrange support and counselling for the man after the attack has occurred; providing support may encourage the man to talk through the issues, allowing him the opportunity to express his feelings. The nurse should have contact details available for any patient, male or female, who may need to be referred to sexual assault referral agencies in the locale. Figure 13.2 (below) encapsulates the agencies who may be involved with the provision of support.

DOMESTIC VIOLENCE

In many health and social care publications domestic violence is generally confined to abuse and violence associated with the female population. Very little is known

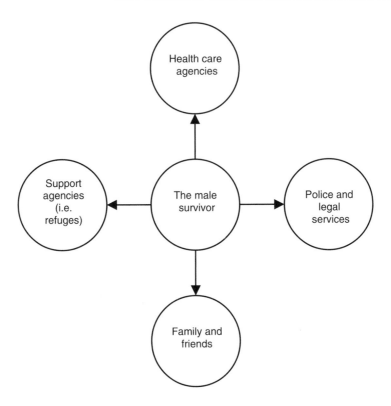

Figure 13.2. The various agencies who may become involved in the provision of support for the male survivor

about family violence that occurs to men. Just as the data associated with rape (male and female) is unreliable, as the instances of rape may go unreported and therefore unrecorded, so too is the case with male cases of domestic violence where the male is the victim; often the needs of men who are victims of domestic abuse go unmet. It is estimated that 90 % of cases of domestic violence cases are committed by men against women; the practice nurse must recognize and be prepared to assist men who also experience abuse. Figure 13.3 (below) provides data concerning the estimated incidents of male and female victims of domestic violence.

Some women do abuse men and those men who live in same-sex relationships may be abused (DH, 2005). Violence at the hands of a current or past partner with whom they share or have shared an intimate relationship does occur. Domestic violence accounts for approximately 15 % of all violent crime and will involve one in four women and one in six men at some point in their lives (Home Office and Association of Chief Police Officers, 2006). The Home Office is currently considering the needs of men who may experience domestic violence.

Similar myths are associated with men who find themselves victims of domestic violence as do men who are survivors of rape and sexual assault, making it difficult

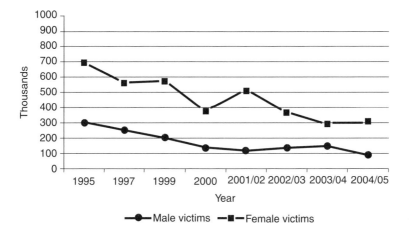

Figure 13.3. Estimated numbers of incidents of male and female victims of domestic violence. England and Wales 1995–2004/2005. (Source: Dewar Research, 2005)

for the man to confide in anyone, leading to isolation, low self-esteem, depression and despair. Men who are victims of domestic violence should be encouraged to:

- keep a diary of all incidents of abuse with dates, times and details of abuse;
- if injuries have been inflicted, seek care and treatment as soon as possible from the practice nurse/general practitioner, telling them that they are injured as a result of domestic violence;
- photograph the injuries if possible;
- stay resident in the home unless it is unsafe to stay (physically and psychologically unsafe);
- try to tell family and friends what is happening and try not to make excuses for the perpetrator;
- avoid provocation, making every effort not to retaliate;
- seek legal advice as soon as possible;
- seek emotional and psychological support (i.e. counselling) as soon as possible.

CONCLUSION

Mental well-being and the impact this has on men is currently poorly understood. Further evidence is required in order to improve a man's ability to experience happiness, contentment and peace of mind. The consequences of poor mental health for the man, his partner and carers are seriously undervalued.

The aim of public policy should be to improve the health of the nation; it must also address the important issues associated with the mental health of men. There are several mechanisms that prevent men from achieving an optimal level of mental well-being, for example, current policies, statutory services and legislative systems;

these are complex and multifactorial. The practice nurse must question and act upon policy and procedure to determine if they address, in a satisfactory and adequate manner, the complex mental health needs of men.

The practice nurse is ideally placed to promote positive mental health among male patients; for example, the practice may be informed of a patient's admission to hospital for care after a drug overdose. Such awareness will alert the nurse to consult with the patient after discharge to determine if he is adequately supported from a social and healthcare perspective. The practice nurse can, if needed, make referrals to appropriate agencies. In the primary healthcare setting a strategy should be devised that would lead healthcare providers to early detection and prompt treatment of men with depression.

Health promotion activities that attempt to tackle mental health must take into account the needs of men and boys, considering the complex issue of masculinity. The effective approaches that the practice nurse uses with women in respect of mental health well-being may not be as effective with the male patient; for example, encouraging a man to 'open up' during consultations or to recognize and admit their vulnerability may fail to encourage them to seek and take up any help that may be available.

REFERENCES

Agerbo, E., Nordentoft, M. and Bo-Mortensen, P. (2002) Familial, psychiatric and socioeconomic risk factors for suicide in young people: nested case-control study. *British Medical Journal*, **325**, 74.

Appleby, L., Shaw, J., Amos, T. *et al.* (1999) Suicide within 12 months of contact with mental health services: national clinical survey. *British Medical Journal*, **318**, 1235–1239.

Appleby, L. (1996) General practitioners and young suicides. *British Journal of Psychiatry*, **168**, 330–333.

Armitage, C. (2004) In a lonely place. *Student British Medical Journal*, **12**, 200–201.

Association for Genitourinary Medicine and the Medical Society for the Study of Venereal Diseases (2001) *National Guidelines on the Management of Adult Victims of Sexual Assault*, MSSVD, London.

Bertolote, J.M. (2001) Suicide in the world: an epidemiological overview 1959–2000. In (ed. D. Wasserman) *Suicide: An Unnecessary Death*, Martin Dunitz, London, pp. 3–10, Chapter 1.

Biddle, L., Gunnell, D., Sharp, D., and Donovan, J.L. (2004) Factors influencing help seeking in mentally distressed young adults: a cross sectional survey. *British Journal of General Practice*, **54**, 248–253.

Bhugra, D. (2004) *Culture and Self-Harm: Attempted Suicide in South Asians in London*, Psychology Press, London.

Care Services Improvement Partnership and (National Institute of Mental Health in England) (2006) *National Suicide Prevention Strategy for England: Annual Report on Progress 2005*, CSIPNIMHI, London.

Coxell, A., King, M., Mezey, G. and Gordon, D. (1999) Lifetime prevalence, characteristics and associated problems of non-consensual sex in men. *British Medical Journal*, **318**, 846–850.

Department of Health (1998) *Independent Enquiry into Inequalities in Health Report*, Department of Health, London.

Department of Health (1999a) *National Service Framework for Mental Health*, The Stationery Office, London.

Department of Health (1999b) *Saving Lives: Our Healthier Nation*, Department of Health, London.

Department of Health (2002) *National Suicide Prevention Strategy*, DH, London.

Department of Health (2004) *Statistics on Formal Admissions under the Mental Health Act*, DH, London.

Department of Health (2005) *Responding to Domestic Abuse: A Handbook for Health Professionals*, DH, London.

Department of Health (2006) *Our Health, Our Care, Our Say*, The Stationery Office, London.

DeVisser, R.O., Smith, A.M., Rissel, C.E. *et al.* (2003) Sex in Australia: experiences of sexual coercion among representative samples of adults. *Australia and New Zealand Public Health*, **27** (2), 198–203.

Dewar Research (2005) *Government Statistics on Domestic Violence: Estimated Numbers of England and Wales: 1995–2004/2005*. Dewar Research, Ascot.

Durkheim, E. (1952) *Suicide: A Study in Sociology*, Routledge & Kegan Paul, London.

Family Planning Association (2004) *Fact Sheet: The Law on Sex*, FPA, London.

Fremouw, W.J., Perczel, W.J. and Ellis, T.E. (1990) *Suicide Risk: Assessment and Response Guidelines*, Pergamont, New York.

Gunnell, D., Lopatatzidis, A., Dorling, D. et al. (1999) Suicide and unemployment in young people: analysis of trends in England and Wales: 1921–1995. *British Journal of Psychiatry*, **175**, 263–270.

Hampton, H. (1995) Care of the woman who has been raped. *New England Journal of Medicine*, **332**, 234–237.

Hart, G. and Flowers, P. (2001) Gay and bisexual men's general health. In (eds N. Davidson and T. Lloyd) *Promoting Men's Health: A Guide for Practitioners*, Bailliere Tindall, London, pp. 225–34, Chapter 2.

Hawton, K. (1992) By their own young hand. *British Medical Journal*, **304**, 1000.

Health Statistics Analysis Unit (2004) *Report SB/2004 Admission of Patient to Mental Health Facilities in Wales 2003/2004 (Including Patients Admitted Under the Mental Health Act 1983*, National Assembly for Wales, Cardiff.

Her Majesty's Crown Prosecution Service Inspectorate (2002) *A Report on the Joint Inspection into the Investigation and Prosecution of Cases Involving Allegations of Rape*, HMCPSI, London.

Home Office and Association of Chief Police Officers (2006) *Lessons Learnt from the Domestic Violence Enforcement Campaigns 2006: Police and Crime Standards Directorate*, Home Office, London.

James, O. (1998) *Britain on the Couch*, Random House, London.

King, M., Coxell, A. and Mezey, G. (2002) Sexual molestation of males: association with psychological disturbance. *British Journal of Psychiatry*, **181**, 153–157.

Layard, R. (2005) *Happiness from a New Science*, Penguin, London.

Lewinsohn, P.M., Rhode, P. and Seeley, J.R. (1994) Psychosocial risk factors for future adolescent suicide attempts. *Journal of Consulting and Clinical Psychology*, **62** (2), 297–305.

Lloyd, T. (2001) Men and health: the context for practice. In (eds N. Davidson and T. Lloyd), *Promoting Men's Health: A Guide for Practitioners*, Bailliere Tindall, London, pp. 3–34, Chapter 1.

Mäkinen, I.H. and Wasserman, D. (2001) Some social dimensions of suicide. In (ed D. Wasserman), *Affective Disorders and Suicide*, Martin Dunitz, London, pp. 101–108, Chapter 12.

Mein, J.K., Palmer, C.M., Shand, M.C. et al. (2000) Management of acute adult sexual assault. *Medical Journal of Australia*, **178**, 226–230.

Men's Health Forum (2000) *Young Men and Suicide: Strategy Guidelines for Health Authorities*, Men's Health Forum, London.

Men's Health Forum (2006) *Mind Your Head*, Men's Health Forum, London.

National Institute for Mental Health in England (2005) *Making it Possible: Improving Mental Health and Well- Being in England*, DH, London.

Pratt, S., Davis, S., Sharpe, M. and O'May, F. (2005) Contextual effects in suicidal behaviour: evidence, explanation, and implications. In (ed. K. Hawton), *Prevention and Treatment of Suicidal Behaviour*, Oxford University Press, Oxford, pp. 53–70, Chapter 4.

Reynolds, M.W., Peipert, J.F. and Collins, B. (2000) Epidemiologic issues of STDs in victims of sexual assault. *Obstetrics and Gynecological Surveillance*, **1**, 51–57.

Rogers, D. (1996) Physical aspects of alleged sexual assault. *Medicine Science and the Law*, **36** (2), 117–122.

Samaritans (2003) *Youth and Self Harm: Perspectives – A Report*, University of Oxford and Samaritans, Oxford.

Wakely, G., Cunnion, M. and Chambers, R. (2003) *Improving Sexual Health Advice*, Radcliffe Medical Press, Oxford.

Walsh, B.W. (2006) *Treating Self-Injury: A Practical Guide*, Guilford Press, New York.

Walters, P. and Tylee, A. (2003) Understanding depression in men. *The Practitioner*, **247** (1648), 598–602.

Wasserman, D. (2001) Suicide – an unnecessary death. In (ed. D. Wasserman) *Affective Disorders and Suicide*, Martin Dunitz, London, pp. 40–510, Chapter 4.

Wheat, K. (2000) The law's treatment of the suicidal. *Medical Law Review*, **8**, 182–209.

Wilkinson, R. (1996) *Unhealthy Societies*, Routledge, London.

World Health Organization (1992) *The ICD-10 Classification of Mental and Behavioural Disorders: Clinical Descriptions and Diagnostic Guidelines*, WHO, Geneva.

World Health Organization (2002) *World Report on Violence and Health*, WHO, Geneva.

14 Male cancers

INTRODUCTION

It is estimated that one in three people will develop cancer at some stage in their lives and one in four will die as a result of the disease (Quinn *et al.*, 2001). Gender appears to play an important role in some adolescent male cancers with a particular impact on testicular cancer. This may be due to the reality that early recognition is impeded by some young men's lack of knowledge and their probable reluctance to seek help. The incidence of bone and brain tumours and of leukaemias is twice as high in male adolescents as in females, and the reason for this is unknown (Health Development Agency, 2001).

While testicular cancer appears to favour men and boys at the lower end of the age spectrum, the opposite is true for prostate cancer. Prostate cancer is said to be a disease of the older man.

Early diagnosis in testicular cancer is crucial; it is vital that nurses working in primary care settings such as general practice are comfortable talking about what can be embarrassing issues, particularly for young men. Improved knowledge of symptoms and risk factors can lead to an early diagnosis (Beckford-Ball, 2006).

Cancer of the penis is very rare and is predominantly diagnosed in men aged over 60 years. It is estimated that in the UK there are around 360 cases per year. The exact cause of penile cancer is unknown; however, it has been noted that the disease is much less common in those men who are circumcised, and as such an inference regarding personal hygiene is made. A build up of smegma may increase risk; however, there is no data to confirm or refute this. Risk is also increased with the viral infection human papilloma virus (HPV). As with most cancers, smoking is also a risk factor associated with cancer of the penis. Symptoms of penile cancer can include:

- any unusual discharge from the penis
- bleeding
- lumps, sores or growths.

Biopsy is taken of the lesion(s) in order to provide a diagnosis. Surgery, chemotherapy and/or radiotherapy may be used in the treatment of penile cancer. Early detection may mean that the cancer is easier to control and possibly cure.

This chapter addresses two male-specific cancers – prostate and testicular cancer.

MEN AND CANCER

Each year in the UK there are more than 134 000 men who are diagnosed with cancer; one in three men during their lifetime will be diagnosed with cancer (Cancer

Table 14.1. Numbers and incidence rates per 100 000 for prostate, lung, bowel and testicular cancer in men (2000)

Cancer	England	Wales	Scotland	Northern Ireland	UK
Prostate	23 109	1607	1892	541	27 149
Lung	19 035	1267	2446	497	23 245
Bowel	15 538	1114	1842	462	18 956
Testicular	1648	76	213	68	2005

(Source: Cancer Research UK, 2004)

Research UK, 2004). The most commonly diagnosed cancer in men is cancer of the prostate gland with lung and colorectal cancer following. These three cancers are responsible for more than half of the cancers in men in the UK. Table 14.1 provides insight into four cancers – prostate, lung, bowel and testicular.

It is estimated that 85 000 men die from cancer and approximately 1 in 4 of all men in the UK will die from cancer. The number of deaths and mortality rates for prostate, lung, bowel and testicular are shown in Table 14.2.

While the number of deaths associated with lung cancer have fallen, this type of cancer is responsible for over 25 % of all cancer deaths in men. Since the 1970s male mortality rates have fallen by 46 % in response to the fall in incidence in lung cancer, which is the biggest cause of cancer deaths in men (Wood *et al.*, 2005).

Prostate cancer follows lung cancer as the second biggest cause of death from cancer in men in the UK. Eighty-five per cent of deaths from prostate cancer occur in men aged 70 years or over (Cancer Research UK, 2004).

Eleven per cent of all male deaths from cancer are attributed to bowel cancer. There are almost 34 900 cases of bowel cancer in the UK. The rates of male bowel cancers have been falling since the early 1990s. The exact cause of bowel cancer is often unknown. A male to female ratio of 1.5:1 exists for colorectal cancers (Rowan and Brewster, 2005).

Table 14.2. Numbers of deaths and mortality rates per 100 000 for prostate, lung, bowel and testicular cancer in men (2002) UK

Cancer	England	Wales	Scotland	Northern Ireland	UK
Lung	16 361	1059	2317	487	20 224
Prostate	8	529	775	193	9937
Bowel	7057	470	851	205	8583
Testicular	56	3	11	4	74

(Source: Cancer Research UK, 2004)

Table 14.3. One-, five- and ten-year survival rates for men diagnosed in England and Wales, prostate, lung, colon, rectum and testicular cancer

Cancer	1971–75 One-year (%)	1996–99 One-year (%)	1971–75 Five-year (%)	1996–99 Five-year (%)	1971–75 Ten-year (%)	1996–99 Ten-year (%)
Prostate	65	87	31	65	21	n/a
Lung	15	23	4	6	4	n/a
Colon	39	67	22	47	23	n/a
Rectum	50	73	25	47	23	n/a
Testicular	82	98	69	95	67	n/a

(Source: Cancer Research UK, 2004)

Survival rates for men with prostate, lung, bowel and testicular cancer have improved since the 1970s. Table 14.3 demonstrates the survival rates at one, five and ten years for men diagnosed with prostate, lung, bowel and testicular cancer. Bowel cancers have been shown separately – colon and rectum.

INEQUALITY AND CANCER CARE

Cancer is an important cause of poor health and illness globally; there are large geographical differences in the incidence, mortality and survival rates of cancer. In the UK there are inequalities associated with who gets cancer: those who live in less affluent and more deprived areas are more likely to get certain types of cancer and overall are more likely to die from cancer after being diagnosed with it (DH, 2000). There may be many reasons why these inequalities exist. Genetic variation may account for some of the reasons associated with ethnic-specific cancers. Exposure to certain risk factors such as diet and smoking are important factors that need careful consideration. Lack of or lower awareness of the signs of cancer in some social groups may lead to late presentation to general practice. This may also be combined with failure to attend for follow-up, low uptake of screening and unequal access to service provision. These are important factors that may lead to inequality. If all men of working age, regardless of socioeconomic group, had the same mortality rates from lung cancer as those in professional groups, then there would be 2300 fewer deaths from lung cancer per year (DH, 2000).

Cancer screening programmes in the UK have achieved some excellent results in attempting to access all communities in our society. There are, however, some indications that some communities are prevented from accessing services, for example, those from minority ethnic groups, those with a learning disability and people who live in deprived areas (Chui, 2003).

If those disadvantaged groups (the socially excluded) have difficulties in engaging with mainstream services such as healthcare provision, then it could be suggested that they will also fail to engage fully with services associated with cancer care, for example, screening programmes. Problems may occur for this section of our society in getting into the system and then once in the system successfully navigating it. The practice nurse needs to take those factors into account when referrals are being made or agencies are requesting information as to why a patient may have failed to attend an appointment. It is acknowledged that attention must be paid to providing fair and equal access to services as well as ensuring that the patient once in the system is supported through it.

Primary care has an important role to play in the care of patients with chronic conditions and in particular cancer care. The general practice is central in ensuring that there is access for all patients in receiving high-quality cancer care. If access is prevented, for whatever reason, this can impact on the patient's survival as well as their quality of life. Improvements must be made in ensuring that access to cancer services is the same for all members of the practice population, including those who may be seen as socially excluded (Campbell, Macleod and Weller, 2003; Pascoe *et al.*, 2004).

THE NATIONAL CANCER PLAN

Cancer is a major public health issue and diagnosis of cancer for both men and women is a feared diagnosis. The *NHS Cancer Plan* (DH, 2000a) is not just about providing extra money for cancer services; it is also concerned with reforming the way cancer services are delivered. The *NHS Cancer Plan* was published soon after the publication of the *NHS Plan* (DH, 2000b); the aim of the *NHS Plan* was to give the people of Britain a first-class health service by investing in the service and the people who work in the service.

The National Cancer plan has four key aims:

1. to save more lives;
2. to ensure that those who have cancer get the right professional support, care and treatment;
3. to end the inequalities associated with cancer care;
4. to expand and improve cancer care by investigating in more nurses, doctors and other key staff as well as investing in equipment and screening services.

Death rates related to cancer are falling steadily and survival rates from all major cancers are improving. Ninety-nine per cent of patients suspected with cancer are seen by a specialist within two weeks of being referred urgently by their general practitioner; more staff and equipment are now in place as a result of the cancer plan (DH, 2004).

BENIGN AND MALIGNANT PROSTATE CANCER

Often prostate cancer is referred to as a disease of old age. Prostate cancer is the most common cancer in men in the UK accounting for nearly 25% of all new male cancer diagnoses. Surgery for benign prostatic hyperplasia (BPH) and the use of prostate-specific antigen (PSA) testing accounts for much of the increase in the detection of prostate cancer (Cancer Research UK, 2006). As the population ages it seems likely, according to Kirby and Brawer (2004), that the incidence of prostate cancer worldwide will continue to rise.

Despite the fact that BPH is one of the most common diseases to affect men of middle age and above (Kirby and McConnell, 2005), this chapter will focus primarily on prostate cancer. BPH is rarely life-threatening; however, the patient may experience problems associated with urinary outflow with the risk of acute urinary retention a reality (Kirby, 2000); approximately half of men with BPH have a reduced quality of life (Girman *et al.*, 1999). There are many treatment options for those patients with BPH to choose from, according to Girman *et al.* (1999) and Kirby, (2000); the choice of treatment will depend on a balance between several factors, for example:

- clinical need and considerations related to the prevention of disease progression;
- patient preference and, if appropriate, his family;
- cost/benefit ratio and long-term effectiveness of therapy.

The practice nurse must provide the patient with as much information as possible for him to make an informed decision. Treatment options must be based on individual need, underpinned by the best possible evidence.

THE PROSTATE GLAND

This gland is approximately 2.5 cm in length and lies at the base of the urinary bladder surrounded by the upper part of the urethra. The function of the prostate gland is not well understood (Laws, 2006).

Marieb (2004) describes the gland as chestnut-shaped and, that it is made up of 20–30 compound tubular alveolar glands that are embedded in a mass of smooth muscle and dense connective tissue. A thin milky fluid is secreted by this gland adding bulk to semen on ejaculation. Prostatic fluid accounts for approximately one-third of semen volume. The prostate consists of three distinct zones (see Figure 14.1 below):

- the central zone
- the peripheral zone
- the transition zone.

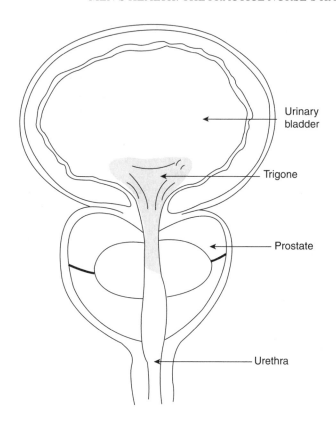

Figure 14.1. The prostate gland

RISK FACTORS

There are no easily modifiable risk factors for prostate cancer (Cancer Research UK, 2006); this means that there is insufficient evidence on which to build prevention strategies. However, age, ethnicity and family history are known to increase risk.

AGE

Prostate cancer in men aged less than 50 years is rare, and risk below this age is very low (Kirby and Brawer, 2004); the disease is more prevalent in those men who are aged over 60 years; 60% of cases occur in men aged over 70 years of age. Selley *et al.* (1997) note that 15–30% of men over 50 years have histological evidence of cancer of the prostate, rising to 60–70% by the time the man reaches 80 years of age; as a result of this it should be noted that most men are likely to die *with* prostate cancer, not *from* it.

FAMILY HISTORY

The risk of developing prostate cancer increases two to three times if a family member, a brother or father, developed the disease at a young age. Monroe *et al.* (1995) suggest that prostate disease may be recessive or linked to the X chromosome. There is also evidence that those men who have a family history of breast cancer may also have an increased risk of contracting the disease (Cancer Research UK, 2006).

RACE

Variation in incidence, as well as racial difference, is noted around the world; therefore, ethnicity should be seen as a risk. Prostate cancer is more prevalent in men of African decent. The highest rates in the world are recorded in African American men, lowest rates are recorded in Asian men and in England the rates in men of South Asian origin are considerably lower than other ethnic groups (Winter *et al.*, 1999). Southern and Eastern Europe have the lowest rates; highest rates are found in Scandinavian countries and countries in northern Europe (Ferlay *et al.*, 2002).

GEOGRAPHICAL VARIATION

Globally, it is estimated that 670 000 men are diagnosed with prostate cancer per year. Worldwide after lung cancer, prostate cancer is the second most common cancer in men (Ferlay *et al.*, 2002). The incidence and mortality rates for the United States are twice as much as the reported rate in the United Kingdom. Gann (1997) suggests this may be due to the high rates of PSA testing in the USA.

DIET

Western diet may be implicated in the high rates of prostate cancer found in developed countries and in particular the high rates of animal fat consumed; however, evidence is inconclusive. Hypercholesterolaemia and hyperlipidaemia have been associated with an increased risk of prostate cancer (Bravi *et al.*, 2006). A small but significant increased risk for men drinking more than 50 g/day of alcohol with a slightly higher risk for those men who consume more than 100 g/day has been reported in a meta-analysis published by Bagnardi *et al.* (2001).

OCCUPATIONAL AND ENVIRONMENTAL FACTORS

Evidence suggests that there are some environmental and occupational factors that may be potential promoters of prostate cancer (Kirby and Brawer, 2004). Those men who are exposed to cadmium and men who work in the nuclear power industry are said to be at increased risk of prostate cancer. This is also the case in those men who are or have been exposed to environmental factors such as industrial chemicals.

Table 14.4. Presenting symptoms of localized prostate cancer

Local disease	Locally invasive disease
• Asymptomatic	• Haematuria
• Elevated PSA	• Dysuria
• Weak urinary stream	• Perineal and suprapubic pain
• Hesitancy	• Erectile dysfunction
• Sensation of incomplete emptying of the urinary bladder	• Incontinence
• Frequency	• Loin pain or anuria resulting from obstruction of the ureters
• Urgency	• Symptoms of renal failure
• Urge incontinence	• Haemospermia
• Urinary tract infection	• Rectal symptoms including tenesmus

(Source: Kirby and Brawer, 2004)

SIGNS AND SYMPTOMS

Prostatic hypertrophy can cause urinary tract obstruction. Localized prostate cancer may present in a similar way that BPH presents; the patient may complain of dysuria, bladder outflow obstruction, frequency of micturition, hesitancy and on occasion haematuria. It must be noted that some men with localized prostate cancer may be asymptomatic and those men with metastatic spread can experience skeletal pain and in particular back pain (Cancer Research UK, 2006). Table 14.4 outlines some presenting symptoms.

STAGING AND GRADING

The majority of prostate cancers are adenocarcinomas and 70 % arise in the peripheral zone of the gland; 5–15 % occur in the central zone and the remainder from the transition zone. BPH predominantly develops within the transition zone (Kirby and Brawer, 2004). Tumours are usually staged using the tumour, node and metastasis (TNM) system.

The Gleason System is most often used to grade prostate cancers and is based on an histological picture assessing the extent to which the tumour cells are arranged into recognizably glandular structures (Gleason, 1966) (see Table 14.5).

Table 14.5. The Gleason System – prostate cancer grading

Grade 1	Tumours consist of small, uniform glands with minimal nuclear changes
Grade 2	Tumours have medium-sized acini, still separated by stromal tissue but more closely arranged
Grade 3	Tumours show marked variation in glandular size and organization and generally infiltration of stromal and neighbouring tissues
Grade 4	Tumours demonstrate marked cytological atypia with extensive infiltration
Grade 5	Tumours are characterized by sheets of undifferentiated cancer cells

(Source: Adapted from Gleason, 1966)

Table 14.6. TNM classification of prostate cancer

Primary tumour		
Tx		Primary tumour cannot be assessed
T0		No evidence of primary tumour
T1		Clinically inapparent tumour, not palpable or visible by imaging
	T1a	Tumour incidental: histological finding in 5 % or less of tissue resected
	T1b	Tumour incidental: histological finding in more than 5 % of tissue resected
	T1c	Tumour identified by needle biopsy (e.g. because of elevated PSA)
T2		Tumour confined within the prostate[a]
	T2a	Tumour involves one lobe
	T2b	Tumour involves both lobes
T3		Tumour extends through the prostate capsule[b]
	T3a	Extracapsular extension (unilateral or bilateral)
	T3b	Tumour invades seminal vesicle(s)
T4		Tumour is fixed or invades adjacent structures other than seminal vesicles: bladder neck, external sphincter, rectum, levator muscles and/or pelvic wall
Regional lymph nodes		
Nx		Regional lymph nodes cannot be assessed
N0		No regional lymph node metastasis
N1		Regional lymph node metastasis
Distant metastasis[c]		
Mx		Distant metastasis cannot be assessed
M0		No distant metastasis
M1		Distant metastasis
	M1a	Non-regional lymph node(s)
	M1b	Bone(s)
	M1c	Other site(s)

(Source: Adapted from Cancer Research UK, 2006; Parkinson and Feneley, 2004)

[a]Tumour found in one or both lobes by needle biopsy, but not palpable or visible by imaging is classified as T1c.

[b]Invasion into the prostatic apex or into (but not beyond) the prostatic capsule is not classified as T3, but as T2.

[c]When more than one site of metastasis is present, the most advanced category should be used.

Schroder *et al.* (1992) describe the TNM classification system, which demonstrates pattern of disease and spread (see Table 14.6).

Those tumours that are confined within the prostatic capsule are often referred to as 'early disease' (T1 and T2). T3/T4 tumours are known as 'locally advanced' disease; in these instances the tumour has spread beyond the prostate gland and into the surrounding tissue but not to other parts of the body. Metastatic disease (M1) may occur despite an increased trend towards early detection.

TREATMENT OPTIONS

There is currently no consensus regarding the best treatment for men who have early prostate cancer; current knowledge prevents a definitive answer to the options that are available that will result in the most favourable outcome for the patient. Table 14.7 outlines some of the treatment options (with intent and drawbacks) for men with localized prostate cancer.

Watchful waiting is not advised for those patients who are aged less than 60 years; however, in men aged 60 and 70 years best practice is unclear. The management of early prostate cancer is controversial and it cannot be over-emphasized that the patient be fully informed of the options available to him.

Selection of men to be offered the watchful waiting approach is based on the premise that many of the men are elderly with a relatively short life expectancy; their prostate cancer is likely to progress very slowly, may not cause symptoms and will not be their cause of death (Cancer Research UK, 2006). The role of the practice nurse in this instance is to act as the man's advocate and to ensure that he is given sufficient information to understand the rationale for the approach that has been selected for him. The nurse must also encourage the man to engage in the process that is undertaken with regard to treatment options. Most men under 70 years of age are offered radical prostatectomy (Emberton, 1999).

The aim of treatment with respect to 'early disease' (sometimes called localized disease (Kirby and Brawer, 2004)) is to aim to cure. Two curative options are available and each approach is based on individual assessment of the person:

- radical prostatectomy
- radical radiotherapy.

Table 14.7. Some treatment options available for localized prostate cancer

Watchful waiting	Radical prostatectomy (retropubic, perineal or laproscopic)	External radical radiotherapy (external beam, conformal) Bracytherapy
Surveillance	Aim to cure	Aim to cure
Non-invasive	Impotence up to 80 %[a]	Impotence up to 60 %[a]
	Incontinence up to 20 %[a]	Incontinence up to 5 %[a]
Metastatic cancer may develop	Mortality – range between 0.2–1.2 %. 40 % have residual tumour after surgery	Long-term diarrhoea/bowel problems in up to 10 %[a]
Uncertainty		
Unacceptable		

(Source: Adapted from Cancer UK, 2006; Kirby and Brawer, 2004)

[a]These percentages will vary according to case selection, surgical expertise and the length of follow-up.

Table 14.8. Ten-year survival rates for three approaches to the management of early prostate cancer

Approach	Estimated ten-year survival
Radical prostatectomy	80–90%
Radical radiotherapy	65–90%
Watchful waiting	70–90%

(Source: Adapted from Donovan *et al.*, 1999; Cancer Research UK, 2006)

In all three approaches the use of hormone therapy may also be considered. Survival rates for the three approaches are high; ten-year survival rates are outlined in Table 14.8.

Active surveillance, according to Cancer UK (2006), is a fourth option that is also available; this involves careful monitoring of localized prostate cancer in efforts to determine its biological aggressiveness with the option of offering curative treatment if the disease significantly progresses.

The practice nurse should offer the patient the reason why (if appropriate) watchful waiting is the mode of treatment being suggested. Review should also include measurement of PSA levels at regular intervals. If there is a sequential rise in PSA levels, or the patient becomes concerned, he may be offered re-biopsy and the option of initiation of therapy considered. The patient needs as much information as possible to enable him to make an informed decision; the possibility and probability of side effects of treatment must be explored. Some of the prognostic indicators are outlined in Table 14.9.

Table 14.9. Some prognostic indicators associated with progression of disease

- Grade
- Clinical stage
- Pathological stage
- Tumour volume (digital rectal examination)
- PSA testing
- Neovascularity (generation of new blood vessels)
- Oncogenes

(Source: Adapted from Cancer UK, 2006; Kirby and Brawer, 2004)

RADICAL PROSTATECTOMY

Surgical and radiological improvements in relation to treatment of prostate cancer continue to improve. Radical prostatectomy involves the removal of the entire prostate and seminal vesicles with anastomosis of the urethra to the bladder; the procedure can be performed under general or local anaesthetic (Resnick, 2003). There are a number of approaches that may be used:

- retropubic
- perineal
- laparoscopic (robotic-assisted laparoscopic prostatectomy).

Radical prostatectomy is performed when the man has been fully assessed and it is deemed possible to remove the tumour completely. The advantage of a radical prostatectomy is that the surgeon is able to remove all prostatic tissue and thus the entire tumour, providing the patient with a definitive cure but only when the tumour is contained within the prostate gland (Kirby and Brawer, 2004). There are, however, adverse side effects associated with the procedure, including incontinence and erectile dysfunction.

RADICAL RADIOTHERAPY

Conformal radiotherapy provides high doses of radiation to the tumour in an effective manner at the same time minimizing damage to the healthy tissue surrounding the cancer. This approach, according to Kirby and Brawer (2004), is offered to men who may be unsuitable candidates for radical prostatectomy; the treatment lasts for approximately six weeks. Despite the new technology associated with conformal radiotherapy, there are also side effects related to this approach; they can include urinary frequency, bladder damage, proctitis, rectal bleeding and erectile dysfunction. Modulated radiotherapy is a relatively new approach currently under development and is a more sophisticated version of conformal radiotherapy.

BRACHYTHERAPY

The word brachytherapy means slow therapy. This technique uses radioactive implants as an alternative to external beam radiation; these may be seeds or wires. The implants may be placed in the tumours (interstitial implants) or near tumours (intracavitary therapy and mould therapy) (Watson et al., 2006), but not all centres in the United Kingdom are able to offer this approach. Iodine-125 or palladium-103 seeds are placed into the prostate using the trans-perineal route along with transrectal ultrasound (TRUS) as guidance (Kramer and Siroky, 2004). Careful assessment of the patient is needed to determine suitability. Jani and Hellman (2003) report that this approach may result in a lower incidence of rectal and neurovascular side effects, for example, erectile dysfunction, although it should be acknowledged that urinary side effects may be higher. Kirby and Brawer (2004) suggest that brachytherapy should be avoided in those men with severe bladder outflow obstruction; after seed implantation the gland may become swollen and this can further exacerbate the problems the man is already experiencing.

Currently there are other technologies, such as high-intensity focused ultrasound (HIFU) and cryoablation being developed (Donnelly *et al.*, 2002); however, in both approaches there are no long-term randomized controlled trials available that will allow these two newer technologies to be compared with the more established treatment options available. Kirby and Kirby (2004) recommend that both of these newer technologies, for the time being, should be regarded as experimental.

Table 14.10 provides an outline of the advantages and disadvantages of radiotherapy, brachytherapy and radical prostatectomy in the treatment of localized prostate cancer.

Table 14.10. Advantages and disadvantages of radiotherapy, brachytherapy and radical prostatectomy as treatments for localized prostate cancer

Radiotherapy

Advantages	Disadvantages
Potential cure	The gland is left *in situ*
Avoids surgical interventions	Difficult to asses cure
Can be undertaken as an outpatient	No definitive staging process possible
May be enhanced by hormone ablation therapy	Patient anxious during follow-up period
	Has associated morbidities:
	• Rectal injury
	• Urinary incontinence
	• Erectile dysfunction
	• Damage to urinary bladder
	• Haematuria
	• Cystitis
	Surgery after radiotherapy not possible

Brachytherapy

Advantages	Disadvantages
This is a one-off treatment	Not able to use this procedure after prostate surgery
Can be performed as a day case or as an overnight stay	Relatively new technology – limited experience of long-term effects
Limited period of catheterization	Difficulty assessing cure
Low risk of incontinence	Subsequent surgery will be made more dangerous
Lower risk of erectile dysfunction	

Radical prostatectomy

Advantages	Disadvantages
Cure if the tumour is pathologically confined	This is a major operative procedure
Definitive staging possible	Potential mortality associated with the procedure
Decreased patient anxiety during follow-up	Has associated morbidities:
Easy monitoring for recurrent disease	• Erectile dysfunction
Possible to provide radiotherapy post surgery	• Persistent incontinence
	• Pulmonary embolism
	• Rectal injury
	• Blood transfusion
	• Bladder neck stricture

(Source: Adapted from Kirby and Brawer, 2004; Cancer Research UK, 2006; Kramer and Siroky, 2004)

LOCALLY ADVANCED DISEASE

Patients who have evidence of locally advanced disease, defined by Kirby and Brawer (2004) as those men who have stage tumour stage 3 (T3), no regional lymph node metastasis (N0) and no evidence of distant metastasis (M0), may receive radiotherapy and hormone therapy (Cancer Research UK, 2006). This combines the use of external beam radiation and endocrine therapy with a luteinizing hormone releasing hormone analogue and antiandrogen as an adjuvant treatment prior to radiotherapy, with the aim of reducing the tumour. Advanced disease means that the tumour is no longer confined to the gland itself, but there is no evidence of spread to local lymph nodes or other more distant sites.

Active surveillance is advocated by Kirby and Brawer (2004) in those patients who are elderly and as such may have a relatively short life expectancy; most of these men, they suggest, will succumb to other co-morbid conditions.

Hormonal therapy along with radiotherapy may play an important role in increasing survival (Bolla *et al.*, 2002). Bilateral orchidectomy with adjuvant antiandrogen treatment and hormones may offer a survival advantage for those men who have had a tumour upstage following radical prostatectomy.

Locally advanced disease may also bring with it a number of urologic emergencies, for example, acute or chronic retention of urine necessitating transurethral resection of the prostate gland. Kirby and Brawer (2004) discuss these issues further.

METASTATIC DISEASE

Those men who present with metastatic disease face the future knowing that there is no curative option available. Short-term control of the cancer can be achieved by the administration of hormone treatment in an attempt to lower the levels of androgens; bilateral orchidectomy has been used in the past as the chosen method of causing androgen deprivation. In nearly all cases of advanced prostate cancers treated with hormone therapy the cancer will eventually begin to grow back again. Kirby and Brawer (2004) note that 75% of post-bilateral orchidectomy patients report a decrease in bone pain and a reduction in PSA levels. Dearnaley (1994) states that androgen deprivation has the ability to achieve a median survival time of approximately 2.5 years. Orchidectomy, however, for some men may be an unacceptable option.

The biggest challenge faced by those patients with metastatic disease when hormone therapy is no longer effective is bone pain. Spinal cord compression and pathological fracture are cited by Kirby and Brawer (2004) as concerns. They suggest that sudden low back pain and weakness in the lower limbs with or without difficulty in voiding in those men with metastatic prostate cancer should be considered a urologic/neurosurgical emergency (see Figure 14.2 below). Pathologic fractures can also occur in the femur or humerus. Pain relief becomes a priority using a progressive approach from paracetamol to non-steroidal anti-inflammatories to opioids,

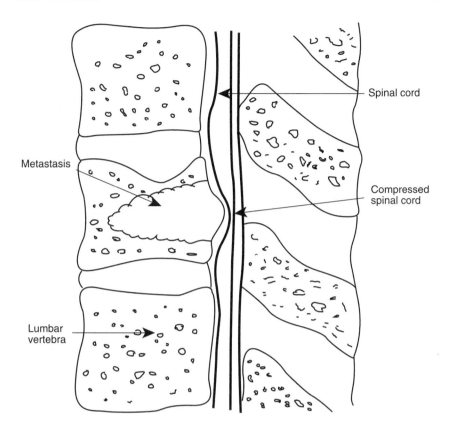

Figure 14.2. Spinal cord compression. (Source: Adapted from Kirby and Brawer, 2004)

in response to the patient's condition (British Association of Urological Surgeons, 2005). A multidisciplinary approach is advocated in caring for those men who may have metastatic disease.

SCREENING

There is controversy surrounding the screening of asymptomatic men for prostate cancer. Many cases of prostate cancer are diagnosed when the disease is advanced and incurable (Cancer Research UK, 2006). Despite there being a number of methods of screening the population, some of these methods are problematic. Three key screening approaches are available. All three approaches have drawbacks:

- digital rectal examination (DRE)
- prostate-specific antigen (PSA)
- trans-rectal ultrasound (TRUS).

Table 14.11. Clinical data identifiable on DRE

Size	The normal prostate gland is said to be slightly smaller than a golf ball, approximately $20\,cm^3$
Consistency	A normal prostate should feel smooth to touch, symmetrical and elastic.
Anatomical landmarks	The examiner should be able to identify through palpation and touch the median sulcus, lateral and cranial borders of the gland. There should be no other structure in the anatomical region.

(Source: Adapted from Watson *et al.*, 2006; Kirby and McConnell, 2005; Kirby and Brawer, 2004)

DIGITAL RECTAL EXAMINATION

It has been estimated that the accuracy of DRE in diagnosing and staging prostate cancer is in the region of 30–50%; underestimation, suggest Watson *et al.* (2006), is a result of subjective interpretation by the examiner. The examiner may be able to identify the size of the gland, its texture and changes in its architecture. DRE provides some important clinical data about several aspects of the prostate gland (see Table 14.11).

Kirby and McConnell (2005) in the context of BPH suggest that DRE is the cornerstone of the physical examination; the same could be suggested when assessing the patient in relation to cancer of the prostate gland.

THE EXAMINATION

When conducting the examination the nurse must gain the patient's consent for this intimate examination. Privacy and dignity must be provided and a full explanation of the proposed procedure given to the patient. Many men find this aspect of the consultation the most embarrassing, and a number of men dread DRE. The examination should be over with quickly; the patient may experience some discomfort. The finger is inserted into the rectum and past the anal sphincters, and the nurse may encourage the man to take deep breaths during the assessment. The nurse will be feeling the posterior aspect of the prostate gland during the examination. If possible, the patient should be placed in the left lateral position (see Figure 14.3 below); the nurse can request help or assistance from another colleague in order to provide patient safety and comfort.

Gloves must be worn for the procedure and a suitable water-soluble lubricant used. The Royal College of Nursing (RCN; 2006) provides guidance for nurses to adhere to when performing DRE and the manual removal of faeces. Nurses who undertake this type of examination for the purpose of prostate assessment must have the necessary knowledge and skills required to carry out the examination in a competent and confident manner. The nurse must at all times

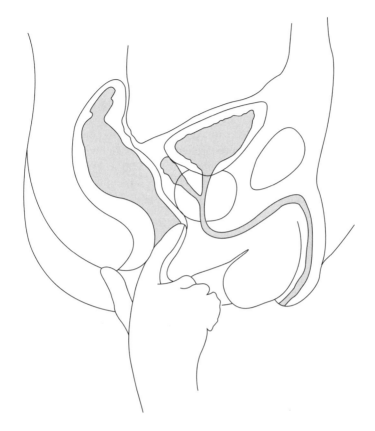

Figure 14.3. Digital rectal examination

remember that s/he is accountable for his/her actions or omissions (Nursing and Midwifery Council, 2004). Local policies and procedures must be adhered to. The findings of the examination or the outcome must be documented in the patient's notes and if necessary shared with other appropriate healthcare professionals.

PROSTATE-SPECIFIC ANTIGEN

PSA is a biological marker that can be used as an adjunct to the staging and histological classification of prostate cancer; this is a glycoprotein that is secreted by prostatic cells (Watson *et al.*, 2006). In those men with prostate cancer there is a reasonable correlation between PSA levels and the pathological stage of the disease. PSA levels, according to Kirby and Brawer (2004), that are above 10–20 ng/ml are indicative of tumour extension beyond the prostate capsule; those who have levels above 40 ng/ml are suggestive of the presence of bony or soft tissue metastasis. Watson *et al.* (2006) suggest:

PSA above 4 ng/ml: clinical suspicion
PSA of 11 to 20 ng/ml: 66 % of patients have cancer
PSA over 50 ng/ml: often the patient has distant metastasis

Leakage of PSA into the bloodstream can occur as a result of malignant epithelium and distortion of prostatic glandular architecture and, but not exclusively, the presence of prostate cancer (Parkinson and Feneley, 2004). However, there are some issues that need to be taken into account with this screening test. The value of using PSA as a tool to screen men is very difficult to assess. There are several reasons why PSA may be elevated and they include:

- urinary tract infection or prostatitis
- BPH or enlarged prostate
- recent ejaculation (within the last 48 hours)
- trauma as a result of recent instrumentation, biopsy for example

Some patients may approach the practice nurse requesting an assessment of their PSA. The practice nurse will need to be prepared to provide advice to those men in order for them to fully understand the potential and limitations of PSA as a screening tool. Table 14.12 (below) provides some advice that the practice nurse may consider offering to the man who requests a PSA test.

SENSITIVITY AND SPECIFICITY

Lack of specificity brings with it problems related to the test. Klotz (1997) reports that only 25 % of asymptomatic men with abnormally high PSA levels will have prostate cancer, with nearly two-thirds of men with elevated PSA levels not having prostate cancer but who will have endured the anxiety, discomfort and risk of follow-up investigations.

The test also lacks sensitivity. Up to 20 % of all men with prostate cancer have normal PSA levels.

Inter-laboratory reliability also confounds the problem further. There are other variables that must be taken into account and adjusted when using PSA levels, for example, age and gland size. The use of PSA alone to detect prostate cancer is unacceptable. The diagnosis must be confirmed with other tools such as DRE and TRUS, as PSA alone is not diagnostic.

Indiscriminate use of PSA testing should be avoided. A false positive result can cause the patient and his family much discomfort and anxiety. The UK Prostate Cancer Risk Management Programme is to introduce guidance on standardization of tests. It aims to produce a protocol that practitioners should adhere to if standard results are to be obtained.

Table 14.12. Some advice that the practice nurse may wish to offer the patient when he requests a PSA test

---

- The PSA test is not very accurate; it cannot predict that having the test even if it is positive will help the man live longer. In most men with prostate cancer death is the result of other causes
- There are no side effects to having the test; you must provide a blood sample. If the test is positive, there is always a risk that this may be a false positive result and you may, as result of the test, have to needlessly undergo other tests such as the taking of a biopsy of the prostate gland via the rectum. There is always a risk that this may cause bleeding and in some men (1–5%) infection may occur
- Only one in three men who have a high PSA test result will have prostate cancer
- You may experience anxiety and worry if later tests are all negative
- In general even if cancer is detected there is nothing than can be done until it begins to impinge on your health and well-being. Treatment can be recommended but, again, these treatments are not without risk
- Often there is controversy concerning the most appropriate way of treating men with prostate cancer
- Screening for prostate cancer does not appear to be associated with lower-prostate-specific mortality
- Ultimately you must decide for yourself what you want; please take some time to think about it and get back to me

---

(Source: Longmore, Wilkinson and Rajagopalan, 2005)

TRANS-RECTAL ULTRASOUND (AND GUIDED BIOPSY)

If DRE and PSA are suggestive of prostate cancer, TRUS is indicated. TRUS can also facilitate the passage of a biopsy needle to take a biopsy from the gland as well as helping to determine prostate size. Kirby and Brawer (2004) point out that TRUS provides accurate images of the prostate gland by inserting an ultrasound probe into the rectum adjacent to the prostate gland (see Figure 14.4 below). Spring-loaded biopsy needles are used. When the trigger is pressed a number of biopsies (sometimes up to 12) are taken for histology.

There are potential complications associated with TRUS, for example, bleeding and infection. Infection is estimated at approximately 2% (Longmore, Wilkinson and Rajagopalan, 2005); in order to counteract the risk, the patient is prescribed prophylactic antibiotic therapy pre and post procedure. These may be given in suppository format or orally, usually for three days. There is little consensus on the best regimen (Taylor and Bingham, 1997).

PREPARATION FOR THE EXAMINATION

Preparation of the patient will include the giving of information in an accessible manner in order for the patient to provide signed informed consent; the whole examination should take approximately 30 minutes. It is advisable that the patient

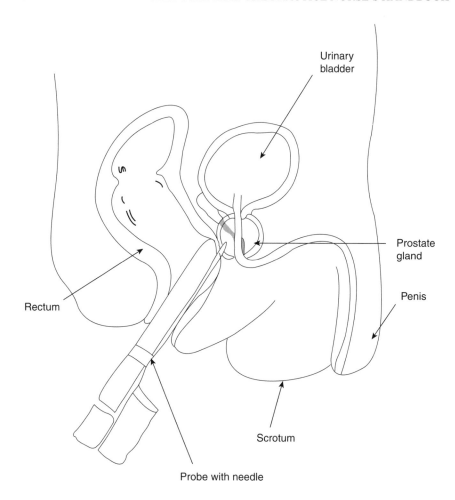

Urinary
bladder

Prostate
gland

Penis

Rectum

Scrotum

Probe with needle

Figure 14.4. TRUS with biopsy needle *in situ*. Multiple biopsies can be taken with an automatic biopsy gun. (Source: Kirby and McConnell, 2005)

bring somebody with them to the appointment as they may not feel like driving home or travelling home alone after the examination has been performed.

There is no particular physical preparation for the examination; however, those men who are on anticoagulant therapies will need specific consideration. If possible, the patient should try to evacuate the bowels prior to the procedure. The patient is placed in the left lateral position and an anaesthetic gel will be squeezed into the rectum, and in some centres local anaesthetic is injected into the prostate gland itself. The procedure is not normally painful; however, when taking the biopsy this may cause a stinging feeling; the patient should be

Table 14.13. Information that may be provided to the patient, with respect to TRUS

Suggested advice:
- Rest for the remainder of the day; work may be resumed the following day
- To drink plenty of fluids (at least two to three pints) – avoiding alcohol
- You may take a bath or shower
- After 24 h sex may be resumed (this includes masturbation)
- You may notice blood in your semen for 2–3 days
- There may be pain and discomfort after the examination and this can usually be treated by taking paracetamol

Possible complications:
- There may be blood from the rectum, in the stool and in the urine for 1–2 days, this is expected; however, if this is prolonged and becomes heavy, contact the general practice
- There may be a possibility (rarely) that during the procedure heavy bleeding can occur; this may necessitate admission to hospital
- Infection can occur and this can be treated with antibiotics at home; however, if the infection is severe, this can require admission to hospital. The nurse should explain to the patient the possible signs and symptoms of infection

---

told that he may hear several loud clicks as the biopsies are taken. During the preparation stage it may be advisable to show and let the patient hear the noise the gun makes when the biopsies are taken. The role of the nurse at this stage is to provide comfort as well as ensuring that privacy and dignity are maintained. The patient is asked to stay in the department where the procedure was carried out until he has passed urine.

Advice to be given to the patient after the procedure may include that cited in Table 14.13. Written information to promote retention should be provided. This will include the information/advice that is outlined in Table 14.13, and it may also be wise to provide contact telephone numbers.

It is important that the patient is informed of when the results will be available to him and what the next steps are. A follow-up appointment will be required.

TESTICULAR CANCER

Cancer of the testes is the most common form of cancer in men aged between 15 and 45 years (Everyman, 2006) and accounts for 1–2% of all male cancers. It is rare in the UK for men to die from testicular cancer; however, cure is dependent upon an early diagnosis, prompt treatment of the primary lesion, careful staging and correct initial treatment (Hendry and Christmas, 2004). Over 90% of cases of testicular cancer are curable (Cancer Research UK, 2002).

Testicular cancer is a relatively rare cancer with approximately 1900 new cases registered each year in the UK. It is important that patients attend for follow-up, as vigilance is essential in allowing early detection of relapses to be dealt with. Early detection and treatment increase survival prospects (Peate, 1997). The practice nurse can play a pivotal role in supporting and encouraging men to engage with treatment regimens.

INCIDENCE

The rates of testicular cancer worldwide are increasing; there has been a fourfold increase in the last 50 years and the reasons are unknown (Everyman, 2006). Latest available data (from 1998) demonstrates that there were 1900 new cases of testicular cancer. See Table 14.14 for the number and rates of new cases of testicular cancer in the UK.

Approximately 50% of all cases occur in men who are aged less than 35 years; in men under 55 years this is 93%. It is rare for the disease to occur before puberty with peak incidence rates of about 16–17 per 100000 population in those men aged between 30 and 39 years of age (Cancer Research UK, 2002).

There is no clear association between incidence and socioeconomic status; however, in Scotland, Harris et al. (1998) suggest that the highest rates were registered for least deprived men. Davies (1981) notes that in England and Wales death rates are highest among professional, administrative and clerical workers, with lowest rates among manual workers. Despite both sources being dated there is no other information available to contest the data cited.

THE TESTES

The testes develop near the kidneys and travel through the external inguinal ring at approximately eight months' gestation and at nine months they migrate into the

Table 14.14. The number and rates of new cases of testicular cancer (1998)

Country	Rates
England	1541
Wales	89
Scotland	210
Northern Ireland	47
UK as a whole	1887

(Source: Cancer Research UK, 2002)

scrotum when the boy is born. The testes are paired oval organs approximately 4–5 cm in length, suspended below the penis in the scrotal sac by the spermatic cords. Three layers encase the testis:

- tunica vaginalis
- tunica albuginea
- tunica vasculosa.

Both testes contain between 200 and 300 lobes containing the tightly coiled seminiferous tubules (see Figure 14.5). The process of spermatogenesis begins in the testes (see Chapter 10). Lymphatics from the penis and scrotum drain into the regional nodes through the spermatic cord (Anderson *et al.*, 2005).

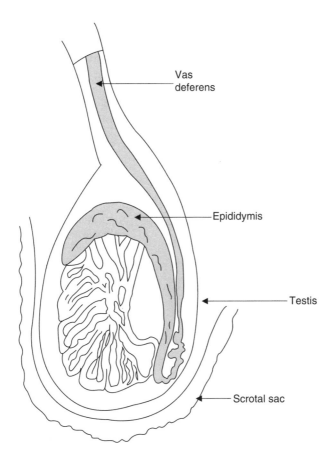

Figure 14.5. The testis

RISK FACTORS

The aetiology of testicular cancer is poorly understood; however, several risk factors have been identified. It is well established that testicular cancer has an unusual age distribution, occurring most commonly in young and middle-aged men. Other risk factors will be discussed below. Table 14.15 provides reference to some of the risk factors associated with testicular cancer.

RACE AND GEOGRAPHICAL VARIATION

There is an appreciable difference in the incidence of testicular cancer throughout the world. The incidence of testicular cancer is rising particularly in white Caucasian populations but has remained only one-third as common among black racial groups, and the reason for this is unknown. Scandinavian countries (with the exception of Finland) have the highest incidence, with lowest rates in African and Asian countries (Cancer Research UK, 2002). Men with testicular cancer in Denmark account for 6.7 % of all cancers, with men from Japan, in comparison, accounting for 0.8 % of all cancers (McQueen, 2006). In Europe Spain has the lowest rate of testicular cancer followed by Finland, Greece and Portugal (Ferlay *et al.*, 1997).

Table 14.15. Risk factors for testicular cancer

Demographic factors	• Age 20–49 years • High social class[a] • Caucasian
Medical characteristics	• First born • Low birth weight[a] • Cryptorchidism • Carcinoma *in situ* • Previous testicular tumour • Inguinal hernia • Testicular torsion[a] • Mumps orchitis[a] • Early puberty[a]
Prenatal factors	• Oestrogen exposure[a]
Genetic factors	• Close family relative with testicular cancer • Certain rare familial syndromes
Other factors	• Lack of physical exercise[a] • Sedentary lifestyle[a] • Maternal smoking[a]

(Source: Adapted from Cancer Research UK, 2002)
[a]These factors are still under evaluation.

Harland (2000) suggests that environmental factors both parentally and after the onset of puberty are important risk factors. The man's genetic makeup is said to be significant in determining the outcome of environmental exposure.

GENETIC FACTORS

The consistently lower rates reported for black American men in comparison with their white counterparts suggest, according to Cancer Research UK (2002), that there may be an inherited genetic component to the disease. There are certain rare familial syndromes as well as a close family history that are known to carry a higher risk of the disease. Brothers of a patient with testicular cancer and sons of fathers with the disease carry a higher risk of developing testicular cancer. Dieckmann and Pichlmeier (1997) note that about 2% of patients have an affected relative. An area on the chromosome Xq27 may be responsible for 25% of familial testicular cancer (Rapley *et al.*, 2002).

MEDICAL CONDITIONS

Cryptorchidism is a common congenital abnormality in males particularly among low-birth-weight babies. At birth approximately 6% of all male babies have undescended testes with most of these descending spontaneously by the time the child is three months old. Cryptorchidism is an established risk factor; however, only 10% of those men with testicular cancer have a history of the condition; cryptorchidism cannot therefore be responsible for all the increases of testicular cancer. Men with cryptorchidism have approximately 5–10 times the relative risk of the general population of developing testicular cancer, the risk increases in those men with bilateral undescended testes. Orchidopexy under the age of 4 years and at the latest by the age of 10 years reduces risk but it still remains higher than that for the general population (Cancer Research UK, 2002).

The United Kingdom Testicular Cancer Study Group (1994) notes that a decrease in risk occurs when there is an increase in exercise; risk increases when the man leads a sedentary lifestyle. There are certain medical conditions that increase risk two- to threefold and are positively associated with testicular cancer, for example, infantile inguinal hernia, testicular torsion and mumps orchitis after puberty.

PARENTAL FACTORS

A number of male reproductive disorders have been associated with exposure to high levels of maternal oestrogen during early foetal development; these disorders, it is noted, are increasing in frequency. Sharpe and Dkakkebaek (1993) cite the following male reproductive abnormalities as a result of exposure to high levels of maternal oestrogens:

- testicular cancer
- cryptorchidism
- urethral abnormalities
- poor semen quality (volume and count).

In a study conducted by Hsieh *et al.* (2002) it was determined that there is no correlation between oestrogen levels and testicular cancer incidence rates when comparing oestrogen levels in two different populations of pregnant women.

OTHER FACTORS

The United Kingdom Testicular Cancer Study Group (1994) and Møller, Jørgensen and Forman (1995) postulate that, as most cases of testicular cancer occur after the age of puberty, it may be that this tumour is driven by male sex hormones. A Swedish study (Clemmesen, 1997) noted that low birth weight was an indicator of an elevated risk of non-seminomas. The United Kingdom Testicular Cancer Study Group (1994) has found that there is no association between patient cigarette smoking and increased risk, just as there is no clear occupational exposure linked with the disease.

SIGNS AND SYMPTOMS

Often the patient may present with a painless lump or swelling on one testicle. Discovery may be an accident, examination by the patient or his partner. Other important symptoms that may also be present are outlined in Table 14.16.

In those men who present with the disease in the late stage (and this is rare) they may complain of breast tenderness, back pain, abdominal pain, supraclavicular tenderness (as a result of lymph node masses), shortness of breath and haemoptysis.

It may be difficult to diagnose testicular cancer for a number of reasons. Painless and painful lumps in the scrotum may be due to infection and may be mistaken for epididymitis (Hendry and Christmas, 2004). An attempt must be made to distinguish between lumps arising from the body of the testis and other intra-scrotal swellings.

Table 14.16. Presenting symptoms

- Enlargement of the testicle
- An increase in testicular firmness
- Pain in the testicle
- An unusual difference between one testicle and the other (it is normal for one testicle to hang lower than the other and for one to be slightly larger than the other)
- An ache in the lower stomach or groin
- A feeling of heaviness in the scrotum

(Source: Adapted from Cancer Research UK, 2002; McQueen, 2006)

A full history is required and the practice nurse needs to ask questions about recent trauma, paediatric events such as crypto-orchidism, orchidopexy, current or recent antibiotic therapy, recent surgery and sexual activity. In the latter case swelling may be related to sexually transmitted infection. It cannot be over-emphasized that a full and detailed history is required in order to arrive at a definitive diagnosis.

Careful physical examination is required as clinical examination of the testes is the best method of detecting a tumour (Hendry and Christmas, 2004). Ultrasound may help to confirm diagnosis. Surgical exploration is an option that can be used when ultrasound is inconclusive. Biopsy may demonstrate the presence of a carcinoma *in situ*.

Investigation of serum helps to identify tumour markers and can help to confirm diagnosis as well as being a helpful tool in monitoring treatment progression. The following investigations, depending on patient presentation, may also be considered:

- chest X-ray
- CT scan
- lymphangiography
- abdominal X-ray
- abdominal ultrasound
- intravenous pyelography.

STAGING AND GRADING

The terms associated with embryonic tissue as opposed to adult testes tissue are used to classify cell types of testicular cancer. Ninety-five per cent of testicular tumours are germ-cell tumours (GCT), 4 % are lymphomas and 1 % are made up of various rare histologies. In those men aged over 40 years most are lymphomas and are treated differently than GCT. The Testicular Tumour Panel of Great Britain has provided details concerning the histological classification of testicular tumours (see Table 14.17).

GCT are divided into two main groups:

- seminomas (accounting for nearly 40–45 %)
- non-seminomas (responsible for approximately 40–45 %).

Table 14.17. Histological classification of testicular tumours

Seminoma

Teratoma
- TD: teratoma differentiated
- MTI: malignant teratoma intermediated
- MTU: malignant teratoma undifferentiated
- MTT: malignant teratoma trophoblastic

Combined tumour: a malignant tumour that is a combination of seminoma and teratoma

(Source: Read *et al.*, 1992)

Table 14.18. The Royal Marsden Hospital staging system for testicular cancer

Stage definition		
I		No evidence of metastasis
	M	Rising serum markers with no other evidence of metastasis
II		Abdominal node metastasis
	A	2 cm diameter
	B	2–5 cm diameter
	C	>5 cm diameter
III		Supra diaphragmatic nodal metastasis
	M	Mediastinal
	N	Supraclavicular, cervical or axillary
	O	No abdominal disease
IV		Extra lymphatic metastasis
	L1	<3 lung metastasis
	L2	>3 lung metastasis all <2 cm in diameter
	L3	>3 lung metastasis, one or more >2 cm in diameter
	H+	Liver metastasis
	Br+	Brain metastasis
	Bo+	Bone metastasis

(Source: Huddart *et al.*, 2006)

Men aged between 20–30 years experience more teratomas and those aged 35–45 years seminomas; 10–15 % of tumours are a mix of seminoma and non-seminoma (Cancer Research UK, 2002; Simon, Everitt and Kendrick, 2005).

Staging allows the practitioner to determine how far the cancer has spread, and just as prostate cancer has distinct stages, so too does testicular cancer. The Royal Marsden Hospital staging system can be used with testicular cancer. The results of investigations, such as scans and biopsies, are considered and treatment options will be decided upon in relation to the stage of cancer. Testicular cancer has four main number stages (see Table 14.18).

TREATMENT OPTIONS

McQueen (2006) suggests that treatment is by surgery with adjuvant radiotherapy and chemotherapy. Treatment options will depend on several factors, for example, the type of tumour and serum markers, along with tumour volume. These are key variables that must be given careful consideration (Hendry and Christmas, 2004), with the key aim of maximizing benefit with minimum toxicity.

Men with seminoma often present earlier than those men with teratoma. Survival rates for seminoma are high as these tumours, as opposed to non-seminomas, are more radiosensitive and more chemosensitive. In the United Kingdom standard treatment for those men with seminoma is inguinal orchidectomy, followed by adjuvant radiotherapy (Horwich, 1991). Those men receiving radiotherapy can experience fatigue, bone marrow depression and diarrhoea (Dearnaley, Huddart and Horwich, 2001).

Teratoma patients who have early disease are also treated by inguinal orchidectomy. Huddart *et al.* (2006) suggest that radical inguinal orchidectomy is used for those men who have a primary non-seminoma. Radical inguinal orchidectomy involves removal of the testes, epididymis, a portion of the vas deferens and parts of the gonadal lymphatics and blood vessels (McQueen, 2006). Adjuvant chemotherapy is used for those men with high-risk teratoma and surveillance is provided for those patients who are classified as low risk (Cancer Research UK, 2002).

Metastatic disease (generally) is treated with chemotherapy; for example, the standard treatment is 3–4 cycles of bleomycin, etoposide and cisplatin (BEP), depending on risk status (Huddart *et al.*, 2006). Those patients (approximately 25%) with advanced disease, that is, those who have completed chemotherapy, will have residual masses in the para-arotic region or in the chest or in both sites; para-arotic lymphadenectomy may be required (Hendry and Christmas, 2004).

Post para-arotic lymphadenectomy may result in an inability of the patient to ejaculate as a result of sympathetic nerve division. Techniques are being perfected that will allow for sparing of the sympathetic nerves. See Figure 14.6 of the lymphatic system.

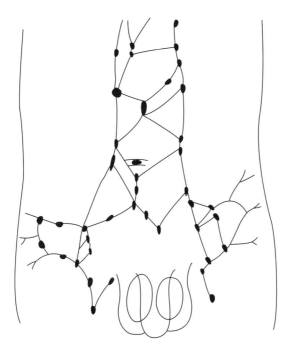

Figure 14.6. The lymphatic system

Chemotherapy can have side effects (Chaudhary and Haldas, 2003):

- secondary leukaemia
- azoospermia
- nephrotoxicity
- bone marrow suppression
- neurotoxicity
- vascular toxicities.

INFERTILITY

Infertility is a possible side effect following treatment for testicular cancer. Infertility caused by chemotherapy can be temporary and this depends on the type of drug and dose. The use of radiotherapy can lead to permanent infertility; risk is increased in relation to the dose of radiotherapy given. It may take many years for some men to return to their pre-treatment fertility level.

Reproductive function and future fertility must be discussed with the patient and his partner (if appropriate) before, during and after treatment. Seminal analysis and cryopreservation of semen are options that may be appropriate for some men if the issue of artificial insemination using cryopreserved semen is to be used. Testicular sperm aspiration (TESA) involves surgical removal of a small piece of testicular tissue or the drawing of sperm from the testicle using a syringe to identify viable sperm; this procedure is used if the sperm collected for cryopreservation is inadequate (Schover, 1997; Souhami et al., 2001).

SCREENING AND TESTICULAR SELF-EXAMINATION

Screening for testicular cancer is not effective; however, encouraging men to testicular self-examine (TSE) their testes for lumps on a regular basis is preferable (Simon, Everitt and Kendrick, 2005; Royal College of Physicians, 1991). If a reduction in the number of cases of testicular cancer is to be reduced, it is imperative that men self-examine. As survival is dependent on early detection, the practice nurse should encourage men to practise TSE at least every six months; ideally, Taylor, Lillis and LeMone (2005) suggest that TSE should be performed on a monthly basis. However, if this activity is to be effective the nurse must take into account complexities such as cultural diversity if patients are to heed vital and, in some cases, life-sustaining advice. Table 14.19 (below) outlines a proposed plan that may be used by the practice nurse when encouraging men to TSE.

Instil in the man that any abnormality must be investigated by the practice nurse or doctor, regardless of how trivial he may think it is.

The nurse must also be aware of the language s/he uses when teaching the patient to TSE. A professional approach is required at all times, but the approach used

Table 14.19. Testicular self-examination

Ensure that you provide the patient with the reason for TSE and the importance of this activity, when it is best to undertake the activity and who the patient may report any abnormalities to. Reassure the man that the abnormalities may not be the result of cancer; there are many reasons why abnormalities may occur within the scrotum.

- TSE should be performed once per month
- Take time to perform the examination
- Avoid any disruptions
- It is best to perform TSE whilst having a shower or after a warm bath
- If any abnormalities are detected, encourage the man to make an appointment with the general practice

Assess the patient's understanding prior to teaching him the correct method

- Has he been taught TSE before, what did that consist of, does he need an update?
- Why does he think it is important to perform TSE? The opportunity may arise here for the practice nurse to correct any uncertainties or to build on the patient's knowledge base
- Provide the patient with time to ask questions and if necessary seek clarification

Enhance teaching by using teaching aids/resources noting that the patient and the nurse are the most important teaching resources. The teaching aids used must take into account and acknowledge complexities such as cultural diversity and intellectual development.

- Commercially produced teaching testicular prosthesis (normal and abnormal)
- The normal testicle feels smooth, uniform and consistent
- It is normal for one testicle to be larger than the other and for one to hang lower than the other
- Diagrams and photographs may be used

Prior to the examination the patient should look at the genitalia noting redness, rashes, ulceration or swelling.

- Explain to the man that it is necessary to hold the scrotum in the palm of the hand and both hands are used during palpation

Systematically palpate the testes and the epididymis

- With the index finger and middle finger underneath the testicle and the thumb on top roll the testicle gently feeling for any evidence of a lump or abnormality
- Locate the epididymis, palpating it; this feels like a spongy cord-like structure on the top and back of the testicle. The epididymis feels soft but not as smooth as the testicle
- Repeat the process for the other testicle

(Source: Peate, 1997; Anderson *et al.*, 2005; Taylor, Lillis and LeMone, 2005; McQueen, 2006)

must be a considered approach; avoid using jargon and at the same time avoid using language that may offend the patient. Communication (verbal and written) with the patient must be:

- clear – in order for it to be understood
- straightforward – using fewer words keeping to the necessary information

- modern – using everyday language and current images (when appropriate)
- accessible – available to as many men as possible, avoiding jargon, up to date
- based on current evidence – honest
- respectful – sensitive to cultural needs and avoiding stereotypes.

CONCLUSION

The role of the practice nurse is varied; s/he may be consulted by the patient to provide advice concerning screening issues, for example, the assessment of PSA. The patient may also confer with the practice nurse on issues regarding treatment options. In order for this to be done effectively with the confidence and the patient's best interests in mind, the nurse must have the necessary knowledge, skills and attitudes.

Kirk, Kirk and Kristjanson (2004) point out that patients and relatives prefer the doctor to:

- play it straight
- stay the course
- give time
- show they care
- make it clear
- pace the information.

While the points above refer to those patients diagnosed with cancer in general, the practice nurse can also adapt the points outlined to those men who have prostate or testicular cancer.

While much cancer treatment takes place in the acute care sector, the general practice has a vital role to play. This may be in the form of referral and also follow-up review of a patient. The patient may turn to the general practice for support (physical and psychological) once a diagnosis has been made, helping them to come to terms with the diagnosis and prognosis, acting as advisor and supporter (Booker, 2004). Some men may require palliative care and this involves the management of symptoms: symptom control, caring for the dying patient and his family.

REFERENCES

Anderson, E., Gebbie, A., Smith, N. and Berrey, P. (2005) The reproductive system. In (eds F.G. Douglas, F.F. Nicol and F. C. Robertson). *Macleod's Clinical Examination*, 11th edn, Elsevier, Edinburgh, pp. 197–226, Chapter 7.

Bagnardi, V., Blangiardo, M., La Vecchia, C. and Corrao, G. (2001) A meta-analysis of alcohol drinking and cancer risk. *British Journal of Cancer*, **85** (11), 1700–1705.

Beckford-Ball, J. (2006) New initiatives to address the healthcare needs of men. *Nursing Times*, **102** (27), 23–24.

Booker, R. (2004) Chronic pulmonary disease. In (eds F. J. Martin and F. J. Lucas) *Handbook of Practice*, 3rd edn, Churchill Livingston, Edinburgh, pp. 147–159, Chapter 8.

Bolla, M., Collette, L., Blank, I. *et al.* (2002) Long-term results with immediate androgen suppression and external irradiation in patients with locally advanced prostate cancer (An EORTC Study): a phase III randomised trial. *Lancet*, **360**, 103–106.

Bravi, F., Scotti, L., Bosetti, C. *et al.* (2006) Self reported history of hypercholesterolaemia and gall stones and the risk of prostate cancer. *Annals of Oncology*, **17** (6), 1014–1017.

British Association of Urological Surgeons (2005) *Guidelines on the Management and Treatment of Metastatic Prostate Cancer*, BAUS, London.

Campbell, N.C., Macleod, U. and Weller, D. (2003) Primary care oncology: essential if high quality cancer care is to be achieved for all. *Family Practice*, **19** (6), 557–558.

Cancer Research UK (2002) *Testicular Cancer – UK*, Cancer Research UK, London.

Cancer Research UK (2004) *Men's Cancer Factsheet*, Cancer Research UK, London.

Cancer Research UK (2006) *CancerStats: Prostate Cancer – UK*, Cancer Research UK, London.

Chaudhary, U.B. and Haldas, J.R. (2003) Long term complications of chemotherapy for germ cell tumours. *Drugs*, **63** (15), 1565–1577.

Chui, L.F. (2003) *Inequalities of Access to Cancer Screening: A Literature Review*, NHS Cancer Screening Programmes, Sheffield.

Clemmesen, J. (1997) Is smoking during pregnancy a cause of testicular cancer?. *Ugeskr Laeger*, **159** (46), 6819–6819.

Davies, J.M. (1981) Testicular cancer in England and Wales: some epidemiological aspects. *Lancet*, **1**, 928–938.

Dearnaley, D.P. (1994) Cancer of the prostate. *British Medical Journal*, **308**, 780–784.

Dearnaley, D.P., Huddart, R.A. and Horwich, A. (2001) Managing testicular cancer. *British Medical Journal*, **332**, 1583–1588.

Department of Health (2000a) *The NHS Cancer Plan*: *A Plan for Investment, A Plan for Reform*, DH, London.

Department of Health (2000b) *The NHS Cancer Plan*: *A Plan for Investment, A Plan for Change*, DH, London.

Department of Health (2004) *The NHS Improvement Plan*: *Putting People at the Heart of Public Services*, DH, London.

Dieckmann, K.P. and Pichlmeier, U. (1997) The prevalence of familial testicular cancer: an analysis of two patient populations and a review of the literature. *Cancer*, **80** (10), 1954–1960.

Donnelly, B.J., Saliken, J.C. Ernst, D.S. *et al.* (2002) Prospective trial of cryosurgical ablation of the prostate: 5 year results. *Urology*, **60** (4), 645–649.

Donovan, J.L., Frankel, S.J., Faulkner, A. *et al.* (1999) Dilemmas in treating early prostate cancer: the evidence and a questionnaire survey of consultant urologists in the UK. *British Medical Journal*, **318**, 299–300.

Emberton, M. (1999) What urologists say they do for men with prostate cancer. *British Medical Journal*, **318**, 276

Everyman (2006) *Testicular Cancer Factsheet*, Everyman Campaign, London.

Ferlay, J., Bray, F., Sankila, R. *et al.* (1997) *Cancer Incidence, Mortality and Prevalence in the European Union*, IARC Press, Lyon. International Agency for Research on Cancer, CancerBase No. 4 Version 4.0.

Ferlay, J., Bray, F., Pisani, P. *et al.* (2002) *Cancer Incidence, Mortality and Prevalence Worldwide*, IARC Press, Lyon, 2002. International Agency for Research on Cancer CancerBase No. 5 Version 2.0.

Gann, P. (1997) Interpreting recent trends in prostate cancer incidence and mortality. *Epidemiology*, **8**, 117–120.

Girman, C.J., Jacobsen, S.J., Rhodes, T. *et al.* (1999) Association of health related quality of life and benign prostatic enlargement. *European Urology*, **35** (4), 277–284.

Gleason, D. (1966) Classification of prostatic carcinoma. *Cancer Chemotherapy Reports*, **50**, 125–128.

Harland, S.J. (2000) Conundrum of the hereditary component of testicular cancer. *Lancet*, **356**, 1455–1456.

Harris, V., Sandridge, A.L., Black, R.J. *et al.* (1998) *Cancer Registration Statistics Scotland 1986–1995*, Information Statistics Division, Scotland Publications, Edinburgh.

Health Development Agency (2001) *Boys' and Young Men's Health: Literature Review: An Interim Report*, HDA, London.

Hendry, W.F. and Christmas, T.J. (2004) Testicular cancer. In (eds R.S. Kirby, C.C. Carson, Kirby M.G. and R.N. Farah) *Men's Health*, Taylor & Francis, Oxford, 2nd edn, pp. 359–366, Chapter 28.

Horwich, A. (1991) *Testicular Cancer: Investigation and Management*, Chapman & Hall, London.

Hsieh, C.C., Lambe, M., Trichopoulos, D. *et al.* (2002) Early life exposure to oestrogen and testicular cancer risk: evidence against the aetiological hypothesis. *British Journal of Cancer*, **86** (8), 1362–1363.

Huddart, R., Mukherjee, R.K. Shah, R.N.H. *et al.* (2006) Chapter one. In (eds D. Brighton and M. Wood) *The Royal Mardsen Hospital Handbook of Cancer Chemotherapy*, Elsevier, Edinburgh, pp. 347–368, Chapter 1.

Jani, A.B. and Hellman, S. (2003) Early prostate cancer: clinical decision-making. *Lancet*, **361**, 1045–1053.

Kirby, R.S. (2000) The natural history of BPH: what have we learned in the last decade?. *Urology*, **56** (5) (Suppl. 1), 3–6.

Kirby, R.S. and Brawer, M.K. (2004) *Prostate Cancer* 4th edn, Health Press, Abingdon.

Kirby, R.S. and Kirby, M.G. (2004) Benign and malignant diseases of the prostate. In (eds R.S. Kirby, C.C. Carson, M.G. Kirby and R.N. Farah) *Men's Health*, 2nd edn, Taylor & Francis, Oxford, pp. 285–298, Chapter 23.

Kirby, R.S. and McConnell, J.D. (2005) *Benign Prostatic Hyperplasia*, 5th edn, Health Press, Abingdon.

Kirk, P., Kirk, I. and Kristjanson, J.L. (2004) What do patients receiving palliative care for cancer and their families want to be told? A Canadian and Australian qualitative study. *British Medical Journal*, **328**, 1343–1350.

Klotz, L. (1997) PSAdynisa and other PSA-related syndromes: a new epidemic – a case history and taxonomy. *Urology*, **50** (6), 831–832.

Kramer, A. and Siroky, M.B. (2004) Neoplasms of the genitourinary tract. In (eds M.B. Siroky, R.D. Oates, and R.K. Babayan) *Handbook of Urology: Diagnosis and Therapy*, 3rd edn, Lippincott, Philadelphia, pp. 249–299, Chapter 15.

Laws, T. (2006) *A Handbook of Men's Health*, Elsevier, Edinburgh.

Longmore, J.M., Wilkinson, I.B. and Rajagopalan, S.R. (2005) *Oxford Handbook of Clinical Medicine*, 6th edn, Oxford University Press, Oxford.

Marieb, E.N. (2004) *Human Anatomy and Physiology*, 6th edn, Pearson, San Francisco.

McQueen, A.C.H. (2006) Disorders of the reproductive system and breast: part 1. In (eds M.F. Alexander, J.N. Fawcett and P.J. Runciman) *Nursing Practice Hospital and Home: The Adult*, 3rd edn, Elsevier, Edinburgh, pp. 253–356, Chapter 7.

Møller, H.M., Jørgensen, N. and Forman, D. (1995) Trends in incidence of testicular cancer in boys and adolescent men. *International Journal of Cancer*, **61**, 761–764.

Monroe, K.R., Yu, M.C., Kolone, L.N. *et al.* (1995) Evidence of an X-linked or recessive genetic component to prostate cancer risk. *Nature Medicine*, **1**, 827–829.

Nursing and Midwifery Council (2004) *Code of Professional Conduct: Standards for Conduct, Performance and Ethics*, NMC, London.

Parkinson, R.J. and Feneley, M.R. (2004) The PSA debate, (eds R.S. Kirby, C.C. Carson, M.G. Kirby and R.N. Farah), *Men's Health*, 2nd edn, Taylor & Francis, Oxford, pp. 299–313, Chapter 24.

Pascoe, S.W., Neal, R.D. Allgar, V.L. *et al.* (2004) Psychological care for cancer patients in primary care? Recognition of opportunities cancer care. *Family Practice*, **21** (4), 432–442.

Peate, I. (1997) Testicular cancer: the importance of effective health education. *British Journal of Nursing*, **6** (6), 311–316.

Quinn, M., Babb, P., Brock, A. et al. (2001) *Cancer Trends in England and Wales 1950–1999*, Office for National Statistics.

Rapley, E.A., Crockford, G.P. and Teare, D. *et al.* (2002) Localization to Xq27 of a susceptibility gene for testicular germ cell tumours. *Nature Genetics*, **24** (2), 197–200.

Read, G., Stenning, S.P., Cullen, M.H. *et al.* (1992) Medical research council prospective study of surveillance for Stage I testicular teratoma. *Journal of Clinical Oncology*, **10**, 1762–1768.

Resnick, M.I. (2003) Carcinoma of the prostate, (eds M.I. Resnick, and A.C. Novick), *Urology Secrets*, 3rd edn, Hanley and Belfus, Philadelphia, pp. 95–97, Chapter 28.

Rowan, S. and Brewster, D. (2005) Colorectal. *Office of National Statistics 'Cancer Atlas of the UK and Ireland 1991–2000'*, ONS, London, pp. 79–90, Chapter 7.

Royal College of Nursing (2006) *Digital Rectal Examination and the Manual Removal of Faeces: Guidance for Nurses*, RCN, London.

Royal College of Physicians (1991) *Report on Preventative Medicine*, RCP, London.

Schover, L.R. (1997) *Sexuality and Fertility After Cancer*, John Wiley & Sons Inc., New York.

Schroder, F., Hermanek, P., Denis, L. et al. (1992) The TNM classification of prostate cancer. *Prostate*, **4** (Supplement), 129–138.

Selley, S., Donavan, J., Faulkner, A. et al. (1997) Diagnosis, management and screening of early localised prostate cancer. *Health Technology Assessment*, **1** (2).

Sharpe, R.M. and Dkakkebaek, N.E. (1993) Are oestrogens involved in falling sperm counts and disorders of the male reproductive tract? *Lancet*, **342**, 1392–1395.

Simon, C., Everitt, H. and Kendrick, T. (2005) *General Practice*, 2nd edn, Oxford University Press, Oxford.

Souhami, R.L., Tannick, I., Hohenberger, P. and Horiot, J.C. (2001) *Oxford Textbook of Oncology*, 2nd edn, Oxford University Press, Oxford.

Taylor, M.H. and Bingham, J.B. (1997) Antibiotic prophylaxis for transrectal prostate biopsy. *Journal of Antimicrobial Chemotherapy*, **39**, 115–117.

Taylor, C., Lillis, C. and LeMone, P. (2005) *Fundamentals of Nursing: the Art and Science of Nursing Care*, 5th edn, Lippincott, Philadelphia.

United Kingdom Testicular Cancer Study Group (1994) Aetiology of testicular cancer: association with congenital abnormalities, age at puberty, infertility and exercise. *British Medical Journal*, **308** 1393–1399.

Watson, M., Barratt, A., Spence, R.A.J. and Twleves, C. (2006) *Oncology*, 2nd edn, Oxford University Press, Oxford.

Winter, H., Cheng, K.K. and Cummins, C. *et al.* (1999) Cancer incidence in the South Asian population of England (1990–1992). *British Journal of Cancer*, **79**, 645–655.

Wood, H., Cooper, N., Rowan, S. and Quinn, M. (2005) Lung. *Office of National Statistics 'Cancer Atlas of the UK and Ireland 1991–2000'*, ONS, London, pp. 139–149, Chapter 13.

15 Exercise and sports injury

INTRODUCTION

As a part of their role many practice nurses when providing advice to patients emphasize the need for exercise. Often health campaigns promote and stress the benefits of exercise (Lucas, 2006); see Chapter 8 in this text, where the author advises and encourages the nurse to advocate exercise as one approach to disease prevention. Khot and Plomear (2006) include exercise in their text under the chapter that deals with health promotion; they state that there is evidence that points out that moving from a more sedentary lifestyle to a more active one will improve health.

Sarafino (2006) states that those people who do not undertake exercise often have other risk factors for developing serious illness, for example, being overweight or smoking. Those whose health would benefit most from physical activity appear to be the most resistant to starting or maintaining an exercise programme.

Taking part in sports and recreation can have a beneficial social, economic and health impact. The Government has set a target to increase the proportion of people in England who are reasonably active from 30 to 70 % by 2020; 'reasonably active' means moderate exercise that is undertaken for longer than 30 minutes five times per week (Department for Culture, Media and Sport/Strategy Unit, 2002). The consequence of encouraging more people to exercise brings with it a resultant increase in sports injuries; sport injuries are a side effect of sporting activity (Schneider *et al.*, 2006).

There are a number of general practices that now provide a range of services to the patient. Services vary from practice to practice with some offering sports injury care as a service through sports injury clinics. Some sports injury clinics are run by the general practitioner alone or with other healthcare professionals such as:

- nurses
- physiotherapists
- osteopaths
- chiropodists
- podiatrists
- dieticians.

The practice nurse needs to have an understanding of sports injuries, how they are to be treated and insight regarding rehabilitation and methods of prevention in order to care for the patient effectively. This chapter briefly outlines the role and function of the nurse in relation to exercise and sports injuries; it is advocated that the practice nurse adopt a gendered approach to health promotion activities with regards to exercise in order to encourage men to take up, and maintain, an exercise programme.

EPIDEMIOLOGY AND KEY DATA

Epidemiology is the discipline that deals with the occurrence, causes and prevention of disease. In the public health setting epidemiology is used to study outbreaks of disease and to design preventative measures. In sports medicine and exercise it is applied to injury as opposed to illness or disease (Sherry, 1998). Fuller (2005) suggests that epidemiological studies determine whether any association exists between risk factors and incidence. An understanding of the epidemiological issues associated with sport and exercise may help the practice nurse provide appropriate care as well as risk prevention activity.

Injury as a side effect of sport and exercise, however, is not easy to define; it is difficult to reach a consensus on one simple, convenient definition. Fuller (2005) considers the definition quagmire in more detail. For example, he states that it would be unacceptable to classify all sports injuries as those that are recorded as a result of insurance claims as this would only cover those who have insurance cover. Likewise, defining sports injury in relation to those who present at hospital is also inappropriate as the data generated will be biased to those injuries that are more severe.

Data generated in relation to sports injury and incidence is scarce; it should also be treated with caution as it may not be representative of the population as a whole. Nicholl, Coleman and Williams (1995) provide a comparison of level of injury in a range of popular sports; despite this data being dated (over a decade old) the information demonstrates how men are more at risk of injury associated with the type of sports they engage in (Table 15.1).

Table 15.1. Comparison of level of injury in a range of popular sports

Sport or activity	All injuries	Lost-time and substantive injuries
Rugby	96	58
Football	64	20
Hockey	63	14
Cricket	49	14
Badminton	29	7
Squash	24	6
Tennis	23	5
Horse riding	17	5
Running	15	5
Swimming or diving	6	2

These are self-reported injuries per 1000 occasions of participation. (Source: Adapted from Nicholl, Coleman and Williams, 1995)

Table 15.2. Comparison of location of injuries in rugby union and football

	Injuries (%)	
Injury location	Rugby Union	Football
Head or neck	11	4
Upper limb	17	3
Trunk	12	7
Lower limb	60	86
Total	100	100

(Source: Fuller, 2005)

Fuller (2005) compares the location of injuries in rugby union and football. These are two sports that are predominately played by men (Table 15.2 and Figure 15.1 below).

PARTICIPATION IN SPORTS AND EXERCISE

Results from the sports and leisure module of the *2002 General Household Survey* (GHS) (Fox and Rickards, 2004) are used to provide an understanding of the extent to which men (and women) engage in sports and physical activity. The GHS asked those over 16 years of age about their participation in relation to sports and exercise; approximately 14 800 people provided information. The following is a summary of the main findings.

The five most popular sports were:

- walking
- swimming
- keep fit/yoga (including aerobics and dance exercise)
- cycling
- cue sports (referring to snooker, pool and billiards).

On an annual basis it is estimated that (in the last 12 months prior to the question being asked) 46 % of the population engage in walking. Walking was seen as the most popular activity followed by:

- swimming (35 %)
- keep fit/yoga (22 %)
- cycling (19 %)
- cue sports (17 %).

Participation rates were different between the sexes. Men, it was noted, were more likely than women to have taken part in at least one sport, game or physical activity;

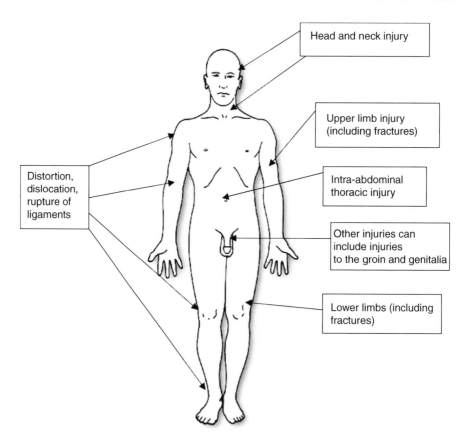

Figure 15.1. Some common sites of sports injury. (Source: Adapted from Schneider *et al.*, 2006; Fuller, 2005)

in general men were more likely to have taken part in organized competition than women; 4 in 10 men (40%) had done so in comparison with 14% of women (1 in 7). Women as opposed to their male counterparts were more likely to have engaged in tuition in order to improve their performance in a sport, game or physical activity. The largest differences between men's and women's participation rates are highlighted in Table 15.3 (below).

AGE

As individuals age it can be observed that physical activity decreases; those aged 16–19 years participated in 72% of physical activity compared to 14% of those aged 70 years or over. There is a strong association between physical activity and age (see Figure 15.2 below).

Table 15.3. Participation rates in the top ten sports, games and physical activities for men and women

Men	%	Women	%
Walking	36	Walking	34
Snooker/pool/billiards	15	Keep fit/yoga	16
Cycling	12	Swimming	15
Swimming	12	Cycling	6
Soccer	10	Snooker/pool/billiards	4
Golf	9	Weight training	3
Weight training	9	Running	3
Keep fit/yoga	7	Tenpin bowling	3
Running	7	Horse riding	2
Tenpin bowling	4	Tennis	2

(Source: Fox and Rickards, 2004)

SOCIOECONOMIC STATUS

Just as there is a clear correlation with a decrease in physical activity and age, so too is there a correlation between socioeconomic status and participation rates in sports, games and physical activities. Those who live in households that are socioeconomically more affluent take part in at least one aspect of physical activity per week when compared with those from less affluent households, where only 30 % do. Those

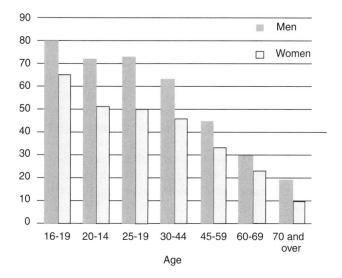

Figure 15.2. Age correlations and physical activity, age standardized ratios. (Source: Fox and Rickards, 2004)

who are unemployed (long- and short-term unemployment) demonstrated a lower participation rate than those who were employed.

EXERCISE

Regardless of age, gender or socioeconomic status, exercise plays an important part in increasing cardiovascular and musculoskeletal fitness. Taking regular exercise also has an impact on an individual's psychological well-being, reducing stress and helping with weight control: this is uncontested. Bird, Smith and James (2004) suggest that the effects of participating in physical activity can include:

- promotion of good health
- prevention of ill health
- enhancing mental health and well-being
- maintaining and/or enhancing physical activity
- improvement of health and physical capacity following illness or an accident
- reduction in the severity of particular disorders
- growth, development and health of children
- minimization of the effects of ageing
- provision of a social environment
- improvement in the capacity of an individual to cope with the physical demands of life – at whatever age.

Exercise can be defined as physical activity that is undertaken deliberately, as an individual or as a group, with the objective of enhancing health or improving physical condition (Shephard, 2004; Resnick, 2001). Physical activity, however, according to Kozier *et al.* (2004), is bodily movement produced by skeletal muscles requiring energy expenditure with production of progressive health benefits. Often the two terms, exercise and physical activity, are used synonymously.

There are a number of types of physical activity that are undertaken as part of a planned programme in a deliberate manner with the aim of enhancing health and well-being. Table 15.4 below describes some of the benefits associated with exercise.

Exercise can also play a part in certain health-related risk factors such as obesity and hypertension (Lee and Paffenbarger, 2000). Men often comment that they engage in physical exercise as part of their job and social role, for example, do-it-yourself tasks. Shephard (2004) states that for those with physically demanding occupations, do-it-yourself tasks and care of dependants can be energy-intensive activities.

Low levels of physical activity, according to Riddoch (2005), are now a major public health problem affecting adults. The impact of inactivity is as great as that of smoking or an unhealthy diet (McPherson, Britton and Causer, 2002). There may be several reasons why there has been and is a reduction in physical exercise, for example, an increase in sedentary occupation, an increase in the availability of public

Table 15.4. Some of the positive effects of exercise

Cardiovascular	Diabetes mellitus	Cancer
• Improves physiological measurements	• Decreases incidence	• Potentially has the ability to reduce the risk of cancer of the colon and prostate
• Increases cardiac output	• Improves glycaemic control	
• Decreases the risk of coronary artery disease	• Regulates blood glucose	
• Decreases symptoms associated with congestive heart failure	• Improves insulin sensitivity	• Improves quality of life and reduces fatigue
• Reduces hospitalization rates associated with congestive heart failure		
• Improves lipid profile		
Osteoarthritis	Osteoporosis	Psychological health
• Improves function	• Decreases hip and vertebral factures	• Improves the quality of sleep
• Keeps joints mobile	• Decreases the risk of falling	• Improves cognitive function
• Reduces pain		• Decreases rates of depression
		• Improves short-term memory

Economic benefits
• Money saved from reduced medical costs. Lower absenteeism and reduced disability. Physical activity is economically beneficial to the nation, communities and industry

(Source: Adapted from Nied and Franklin, 2002; Riddoch, 2005)

and private transportation, differing modes of entertainment and an increase in the use of electronic communications. Inactivity has the ability to impinge on well-being and induce much human suffering for the individual, families and society.

From a global perspective the World Health Organization (WHO; 2002) suggests that physical inactivity accounts for 1.9 million of the top ten deaths worldwide per year (see Table 15.5).

Table 15.5. Deaths related to inactivity – worldwide

12 % of strokes for men
15 % of diabetes mellitus
16 % of colon cancer
23 % of ischaemic heart disease for men

(Source: Adapted from WHO, 2002)

Table 15.6. Some reasons why men may not undertake physical activity

Lack of time
Lack of confidence/fear of injury
Embarrassment
Belief that exercise will not help them
The environment in which they exercise
Insufficient facilities available
When facilities are available they are too costly to use

(Source: Will, Demko and George, 1996; Nied and Franklin, 2002)

Inactivity also has financial implications for the nation. It is estimated that £8.2 billion is spent on the treatment and indirect effects that result in sickness absence annually (Department for Culture, Media and Sport/Strategy Unit, 2002). If inactivity was reduced by 5%, £300 million in savings per year could be realized.

There are many physical, behavioural, psychological, socioeconomical and environmental reasons why men may lack motivation to undertake exercise. The most common reason why some men do not undertake as much physical activity as they would benefit from is lack of time (see Table 15.6).

When working with the patient the skilled practice nurse has the ability to address these barriers to exercise as s/he is aware of the benefits of exercise as well as confidently being able to write an appropriate gender-specific prescription for exercise. Those practice nurses who are less familiar with the benefits of physical activity are less likely to raise and discuss the issue with the patient, potentially resulting in a missed opportunity to promote health and prevent disease. There are a number of motivators that could be cited by the practice nurse in order to try to encourage the patient (see Table 15.7).

Table 15.7. Some motivational factors that the nurse may discuss with the man to encourage the uptake/maintenance of physical activity

More energy/feeling better
Prevents some diseases/illnesses such as heart attacks
Lowers blood pressure
Look better
Lose weight
Personal accomplishments
Contact with friends
Increased strength
Sleep better

(Source: Will, Demko and George, 1996)

Government policy has now included physical activity as a priority. Most of the National Service Frameworks (NSFs) include physical activity with the aim of increasing it:

- *Mental Health* (Department of Health (DH), 1999)
- *Coronary Heart Disease* (DH, 2000)
- *Diabetes* (DH, 2001a)
- *Older People* (DH, 2001b)
- *Children, Young People and Maternity Services* (DH/DfES, 2004).

It is anticipated that the proposed NSF (expected publication autumn 2007) *Patients with Chronic Obstructive Pulmonary Disease* (COPD) will also cite physical exercise as a priority.

TYPES OF EXERCISE

Those activities such as climbing the stairs, walking to work or cycling to work can be called lifestyle activities, and are in contrast to programmed activities such as attending a fitness programme or a cycle spinning class (Riddoch, 2005). Being fit, according to Caspersen, Powell and Christenson (1985), is defined as having a set of attributes that a person has or achieves, enabling them to perform physical activity as well as the ability to perform a physical task in a specified physical, social and psychological environment (Bouchard, Shephard and Stephens, 1994). The key aspects of fitness are:

- the ability to exercise aerobically (aerobic capacity)
- power
- speed
- flexibility
- strength.

There are several types of exercise, aerobic exercise being one of them. This type of exercise (sometimes referred to as isotonic exercise) increases blood flow, heart rate and metabolic demand for oxygen; it is often sustained muscle movements that cause these phenomena to happen (Taylor *et al.*, 2005). Hand (2004) suggests that aerobic exercise (exercise in the presence of oxygen) is the most effective way of producing adenosine triphosphate (ATP) – the body's source of energy. Table 15.8 (below) provides an outline of other types of exercise with examples of each.

PRESCRIBING EXERCISE

Shephard (1994, 2004) suggests that there is a preventative value in increasing physical activity in any one of four points in the natural history of disease. He

Table 15.8. Types of exercise

Exercise type	Function	Examples
Aerobic	Improve cardiovascular fitness Assist with weight control Improve general functional ability	Rowing Skipping Walking Running Kickboxing Swimming
Strengthening	Maintain or increase muscle strength	Weight training Callisthenics Physical work T'ai chi Yoga
Isometric	Maintain muscle tone and strength	Quadriceps setting Gluteal setting Triceps setting
Isotonic	Increase and maintain muscle tone and strength Shape muscles Maintain joint mobility Improve cardiovascular fitness	Weight lifting Working with pulleys Range-of-motion exercises Performing activities of living
Isokinetic	Conditioning muscle groups	Exercise equipment Water exercises
Range-of-motion	Maintain joint movement Maintain or increase flexibility	Adduction and abduction exercises Flexion and contraction exercises

(Source: Adapted from Day, 2004)

terms the four points: primary, secondary, tertiary and quaternary prevention (see Table 15.9).

Nurses play a key role in motivating and providing patients with advice concerning their health and lifestyle; this is particularly the case when prescribing exercise to the patient. As the population of older men increases it will become even more important for the nurse to encourage the older population to begin physical activity and continue with their exercise prescription.

According to the American College of Sports Medicine (2001), there are some men who may be motivated by an individualized detailed exercise prescription. Just as the practice nurse must take a detailed medical and nursing history and a full assessment of the patient when prescribing medication, so too is the case when prescribing exercise. The principles of prescribing must be adhered to when prescribing exercise. It is vital that the nurse knows as much as possible about the patient.

Assessment will need to take into account the patient's motivation, his goals and his physical condition before any programme of exercise can be formulated in order

Table 15.9. Types of prevention

Primary prevention
  The primary preventative approach acts prior to any abnormalities of health and can
  be detected even by sophisticated laboratory testing. An example may be where a
  man who undertakes an adequate weekly amount of physical activity may be able
  to maintain his serum lipids within the recommended normal range throughout his
  life span.

Secondary prevention
  When laboratory tests have become abnormal and there is no clinical evidence of
  disease, secondary prevention can be initiated. A man, for example, who has an
  elevated serum cholesterol or other abnormal serum lipids would be recommended
  secondary prevention of ischaemic heart disease.

Tertiary prevention
  Post-coronary exercise classes are rehabilitation programmes that offer the man tertiary
  prevention. These classes are designed to maximize the recovery of cardiac function
  and reduce the possibility of a recurrence following a clinical episode of myocardial
  infarction.

Quaternary prevention
  The quaternary preventative approach aims to minimize symptoms and enhance the
  quality of life where there is little possibility of restoring full health. Moderate
  physical activity may be recommended to reduce muscle wasting in a person who has
  cancer or a wasting disease such as HIV.

(Source: Shephard, 2004, 1994)

to ensure that this is the most appropriate and most effective programme. Assessment can be carried out either formally or informally. An informal chat with the patient when he visits the surgery may have much impact. Formal assessment will include a more in-depth clinical evaluation.

Physiological assessment will provide the nurse with much data and information about the patient's physical condition. The data can be used for various purposes (Bird, Smith and James, 2004) including:

- information about the patient's current health helping the patient and the nurse to devise a prescription;
- a baseline on which to carry out further assessments – to determine effectiveness;
- assessment may detect hitherto unknown problems such as hypertension, diabetes;
- the data-collecting activity provides the nurse and the patient with an opportunity to discuss his needs.

The exact content and nature of the physiological assessment will depend on the patient's condition and the aims of the exercise prescription. The prescription needs to address the issues outlined in Table 15.10 (below).

Table 15.10. Issues to be addressed when prescribing exercise

---

Setting

There are many advantages to encouraging the man to exercise alone or in a group. The answer to this question will depend on the man's personality. There are some men who enjoy the company of others when exercising (camaraderie), just as there are others who may prefer to exercise alone.

Group events have the advantage of allowing those men who are at high risk of injury to work with others as well as having access to trained individuals who can access equipment such as cardiac resuscitation equipment.

Characteristics

The type of exercise will depend on the reason the patient wishes to undertake it or the therapeutic activity the nurse is wishing to see him achieve. Muscle groups may need to be toned; full range-of-movement exercises for the joints may be required and weight-bearing or -resisting activity to enhance bone formation can be considered depending on individual needs. Table 15.8 (above)provides information regarding various types of exercise.

Amount, intensity and frequency

It is difficult to prescribe an exact amount, degree of intensity and frequency for exercise to be effective in order to maintain health; there is confusion regarding this aspect of exercise prescribing. The necessary duration and intensity of exercise is said to be inversely related, in that the duration of effort can be reduced if the intensity is increased. A number of men of middle age (though not all men of middle age) are often only interested in the minimal amount of activity required to sustain their health.

Recommended aerobic activity is said to be at least 30 minutes of moderate intensity activity on most days of the week (see below for national guidelines). If a man's health (individual fitness) does not permit this, then the 30 minutes of activity can be accumulated as several 10- to 15-minute bouts.

To reiterate, there is little evidence available to provide consistent information regarding the best regimen concerning intensity, frequency and duration of physical activity.

(Source: Adapted from Kesaniemi *et al.*, 2001; Hardman, 2001; Shephard, 2004, 2002, 2001)

Activities that require moderate intensity exercise include:

- cycling leisurely (at below 10 miles per hour)
- walking briskly (at 3–4 miles per hour)
- swimming with moderate effort
- mowing the lawn with a power mower
- home repair activities such a painting.

GUIDELINES FOR PHYSICAL ACTIVITY

Over a decade ago recommendations for healthy levels of physical activity were devised for the nation (Department of Health and Social Security, 1996) and these

Table 15.11. Guidelines for physical activity (adults)

- Adults should achieve a total of at least 30 minutes of at least moderate intensity physical activity on five or more occasions per week
- Bouts of at least 10 minutes can be carried out in order to achieve the requisite 30 minutes
- All forms of movement will contribute to energy expenditure and are important for weight management
- Activities that produce high physical stress on the bones are recommended for bone health

---

(Source: Adapted from DH, 2004)

guidelines have been revisited again (DH, 2004). National guidance related to physical activity for adults can be found in Table 15.11.

CONTRAINDICATIONS TO EXERCISE

There may be limitations to the amount and extent of exercise prescribed based on the patient's medical condition. Excessive exercise can exacerbate physical complications and may cause injury (Lask and Bryant-Waugh, 2000). Some men who suffer with anorexia nervosa or other eating disorders may feel compelled to exercise excessively and can go to great lengths to increase activity as well as having a need to constantly maintain movement (Taylor and Cooper, 2003).

Just as there are side effects and contraindications to certain types of medication this is also the case with exercise. There may be risks associated with exercise for some patients:

- adverse cardiovascular events
- musculoskeletal problems
- metabolic disorders
- haematological disorders.

Having conducted an in-depth patient assessment (including history-taking, physical examination and physiological measurements) the nurse must be aware of the contraindications associated with some forms of exercise.

Shephard (2004) points out that the hazards associated with an episode of exercise is more than offset by a reduced risk of a cardiovascular incident during subsequent rest; men are more at risk of under-activity than over-activity. Table 15.12 (below) provides potential contraindications.

Those men who fall into the categories detailed in Table 15.12 may be able to engage safely in exercise at a low level, but only after a detailed evaluation of their physical health has been undertaken by an appropriately qualified healthcare professional and exercise is prescribed at an appropriate intensity (Bird, Smith and James, 2004).

Table 15.12. Potential contraindications

Absolute	Relative
• Recent ECG changes or myocardial infarction	• Cardiomyopathy
• Unstable angina	• Valvular heart disease
• Third-degree heart block	• Complex ventricular ectopy
• Acute congestive cardiac failure	
• Uncontrolled hypertension	
• Uncontrolled metabolic disease	

(Source: Nied and Franklin, 2002)

Another hazard that is related to exercise is associated with the use of non-prescribed anabolic steroids, used in order to increase muscle size and strength. The use of anabolic steroids among younger men is increasing. These young men often use steroids in order to boost self-confidence and improve body image. Steroid abuse is significant among men in 11 out of 20 towns surveyed in the United Kingdom (Daly, 2006). The use of steroids is commonplace among some men who are building-site workers, young professionals and students; they are used predominantly for an aesthetic effect, building muscle and leading to a toned physique.

Musculoskeletal injuries are more likely to occur as a result of exercise than a cardiac event. The extent of risk of musculoskeletal injury will depend on the type of activity the person is undertaking; for example, those who engage in skateboarding are more likely to harm themselves than those who are taking a brisk walk. Those men who have difficulties associated with sight, hearing and ataxia should be encouraged to engage in low-risk exercises. Men who do have sight and hearing problems are at risk of injury if exercising in public places, such as from road traffic accidents if running on roads; for these reasons these men should be encouraged to exercise as part of a group.

Exercise-related injuries can occur, ranging from minor aches and slight inflammations to strained muscles. These less extreme injuries may be the result of tissue being subjected to acute traumatic stress or chronic overuse. These problems can be avoided (generally) by encouraging the patient to start exercising at an easy level and progressively and gradually. Tendonitis can occur, and if this is the case, the man should be advised to stop exercising or to stop engaging in any exercise that places any stress on that particular tendon. Any pain is usually a warning sign that damage may occur or be occurring and the patient should stop what he is doing, rest and seek advice if the pain continues.

It is unwise for anyone to exercise while suffering from certain illness, for example, viral infections such as influenza. Bird, Smith and Jones (2004) suggest that exercising with a viral infection can cause a greater amount of inflammation and possibly permanent damage to body tissues. Pericarditis can occur if the virus affects the heart; furthermore, there is the possibility of cardiac arrhythmias occurring.

SPORTS INJURIES

Men differ in respect to risk. Whether it is whitewater rafting, driving fast cars or posing on a skateboard, the male engages in more risk when carrying out these activities than women do. This also includes engaging in more risky sports activities. Men and boys more than women and girls are involved in more sports injuries and fatal deaths as a result of sporting activity. Men are over-represented in dangerous leisure activities, and the social forces that encourage men to undertake these dangerous leisure activities need further investigation. Chapter 4 outlines the issues associated with men as risk takers.

Sport is a term that is often used in conjunction with physical activity; it is, according to Fox and Riddoch (2000), a subset of physical activity, involving competitive structured situations that are governed by rules. Sport is also used in the wider context and includes all exercise and leisure physical activities.

The majority of sporting activities undertaken bring risk (Fuller, 2005). Many injuries as a result of sporting activity are minor, however. Some are more serious and can leave the man with permanent injuries. Cervical spinal injuries resulting in a paraplegia/quadriplegia can be the result of diving into shallow water; knee and lower limb injuries may be the consequence of playing football or hockey and skiing. Injuries to the upper aspect of the torso, for example, may be brought about when horse riding.

Kolakowsky-Hayner *et al.* (1999) observe that the majority of spinal cord and traumatic brain injury patients are young men; they also identify that most are heavy drinkers, supporting the view that it is an interaction between traditionally male typed health behaviours and traditionally male recreational and sporting activities which place individuals at risk of traumatic spinal injury (Lee and Glynn-Owens, 2002).

Treatment for most of the injuries described above takes place within secondary care, and the majority of those sustaining injury as a result of undertaking sporting activity will go to the nearest accident and emergency unit for immediate treatment. The principles of managing sporting injuries, according to Simon, Everitt and Kendrick (2005), include:

- First Aid – **A**irway, **B**reathing and **C**irculation
- RICE:
  Rest: resting the affected part while continuing other activities to maintain overall fitness
  Ice and analgesia: apply an ice pack immediately after injury, use for a maximum of 10 minutes at a time to prevent acute cold injury
  Compression: tape or strap the injured site/limb/digit to prevent acute sprains and strains
  Elevation: decreases the risk of local swelling and dependent oedema enabling a quicker recovery
- Confirm diagnosis – clinical examination and X-ray

- Early treatment – do not delay
- Liaise with other healthcare professionals such as sports physician, sports physiotherapist
- Rehabilitation – regaining fitness, strength and flexibility. Re-examine and correct the cause of injury, for example, poor technique
- Graded return to activity
- Prevention – ensure the patient has received suitable preparation and training to undertake the activity, suitable footwear, warming-up exercises and correct equipment.

The patient should be referred to the nearest accident and emergency unit if his condition dictates this.

FITNESS TO PERFORM SPORTING ACTIVITIES

Some patients are requested by their gym or sporting facility to provide evidence that they are fit enough to undertake sporting activity. If the nurse is asked to do this, to act as a referee, s/he must ensure that this is in accordance with practice guidelines/policy.

The patient may bring a form that will need to be completed and if this is the case it should be read prior to carrying out the examination; if there is no form, then it may be advantageous to contact the sports facility requesting clarification and to check what is required of you.

It must be remembered that if you sign a form stating that the patient is fit to undertake sporting activity you may be legally liable if he is not. If possible, a caveat should be included on the form or in the letter, stating that based on the information available to you the patient appears to be fit, although you are not in a position to guarantee this. If unsure, then a professional organization such as the Royal College of Nursing should be consulted and its advice sought.

CONCLUSION

It is highly likely that readers of this chapter will agree that exercise has therapeutic health benefits; nevertheless the majority of people in the United Kingdom choose to remain inactive. There is much evidence to suggest that exercise has a positive effect on well-being and reduces the risks of developing certain diseases; despite this some men do not engage in sufficient exercise knowing the harmful effects inactivity can have on their overall health. The ability to move freely, easily and with purpose allows the man to meet his basic needs. There are many benefits associated with exercise; failure to exercise (failure to mobilize) can lead to complications for every bodily organ and bodily systems as well, causing psychosocial problems.

By adhering to the principles of this chapter the practice nurse should be able to prescribe exercise safely and effectively for the patient. It is important, however, that the nurse continues to ensure that his/her knowledge base is updated regularly in order to enhance and advance the promotion of exercise in the practice population. There is a need for the health profession population as a whole to develop a deeper understanding of the theoretical basis for exercise prescriptions. When consulting the patient the practice nurse may need to factor in more time for the consultation if s/he is to provide the patient with an exercise prescription. There may also be a need for the nurse to have an understanding of the resources that may be available to the patient to help him begin and maintain an exercise prescription; exercise prescriptions may be formulated using a multidisciplinary approach.

It is vital that the nurse understands that to be successful in encouraging the patient to appreciate the value of exercise as well as maintaining regular exercise a gender-sensitive approach should be made. The majority of chapters in this book have documented the need to encourage exercise in the prevention and reduction in incidence for several conditions, for example, obesity and depression; and most of the chapters have called for a male-specific approach in order to engage men in their health.

REFERENCES

American College of Sports Medicine (2001) *American College of Sports Medicine's Guidelines for Exercise Testing and Prescription*, 5th edn, Lippincott, Philadelphia.

Bird, S.R., Smith, A. and James, K. (2004) *Exercise Benefits and Prescription*, Nelson Thornes, Cheltenham.

Bouchard, C., Shephard, R.J. and Stephens, C. (1994) *Physical Activity, Fitness and Health: International Proceedings and Consensus Document*, Human Kinetics, Champaign, IL.

Caspersen, C.J., Powell, K.E. and Christenson, G.M. (1985) Physical activity, exercise and physical fitness: definitions and distinction of health-related research. *Public Health Reports*, **1000**, 126–131.

Daly, M. (2006) Image injection. *Druglink*, September/October, 6–8.

Day, A. (2004) Mobility and biomechanics, (ed. R. Daniel), *Nursing Fundamentals: Caring and Clinical Decision Making*, Thomson, New York, pp. 1163–1236, Chapter 38.

Department for Culture, Media and Sport/Strategy Unit (2002) *Game Plan: A Strategy for Delivering the Government's Sport and Physical Activity Objectives*, Department for Culture, Media and Sport/Strategy Unit, London.

Department of Health (1999) *National Service Framework for Mental Health*, DH, London.

Department of Health (2000) *National Service Framework for Coronary Heart Disease*, DH, London.

Department of Health (2001a) *National Service Framework for Diabetes: Standards*, DH, London.

Department of Health (2001b) *National Service Framework for Older People*, DH, London.

Department of Health (2004) *At Least Five a Week: Evidence on the Impact of Physical Activity and its Relationship to Health: A Report to the Chief Medical Officer*, DH, London.

Department of Health and Department for Education and Skills (2004) *Children, Young People and Maternity Services*, DH, London.

Department of Health and Social Security (1996) *Strategy Statement on Physical Activity*, DHSS, London.

Fox, K.R. and Rickards, L. (2004) *Sport and Leisure: Results from the Sport and Leisure Module of the 2002 General Household Survey*, The Stationery Office, London.

Fox, K.R. and Riddoch, C. (2000) Charting the physical activity patterns of contemporary children and adolescents. *Proceedings of the Nutrition Society*, **59** (4), 497–504.

Fuller, C.W. (2005) Epidemiological studies of sports injuries, (eds G.P. Whyte, M. Harries and W. Clyde), *ABC of Sports Exercise and Medicine*, 3rd edn, Blackwell, Oxford, pp. 1–3, Chapter 1.

Hand, L. (2004) Lifestyle advice, (eds J. Martin and J. Lucas), *Handbook of Practice Nursing*, 3rd edn, Churchill Livingstone, Edinburgh, pp. 63–78, Chapter 4.

Hardman, A.E. (2001) Issue of fractionalization of exercise (short vs long bouts). *Medical and Science in Sports and Exercise*, **33** (6), S421–S427.

Kesaniemi, Y.A., Danforth, E., Jensen, M.D. *et al.* (2001) Dose-response issues concerning physical activity and health: an evidence-based symposium. *Medical and Science in Sports and Exercise*, **33** (6), S351–S358.

Khot, A. and Plomear, A. (2006) *Practical General Practice: Guidelines for Effective Clinical Management*, 5th edn, Butterworth-Heinemann, Edinburgh.

Kolakowsky-Hayner, S.A., Gourley, E.V., Kreutzer, J.S. *et al.* (1999) Pre-injury substance abuse among persons with brain injury and persons with spinal cord injury. *Brain Injury*, **13** (8), 571–581.

Kozier, B., Erb, G., Berman, A. and Snyder, S. (2004) *Fundamentals of Nursing: Concepts, Process and Practice*, 7th edn, Prentice Hall, Upper Saddle River, NJ.

Lask, B. and Bryant-Waugh, R. (2000) *Anorexia Nervosa and Related Eating Disorders in Childhood and Adolescence*, 2nd edn, Psychology Press, Hove.

Lee, C. and Glynn-Owens, R. (2002) *The Psychology of Men's Health*, Open University, Buckingham.

Lee, I.M. and Paffenbarger, R.S. (2000) Associations of light, moderate and vigorous intensity physical activity with longevity: The Harvard Alumni Health Study. *American Journal of Epidemiology*, **151**, 293–299.

Lucas, B. (2006) Disorders of the musculoskeletal system. In (eds M.F. Alexander, J.N. Fawcett and P.J. Runciman) *Nursing Practice Hospital and Home: The Adult*, 3rd edn, Elsevier, Edinburgh, pp. 443–478, Chapter 10.

McPherson, K., Britton, A. and Causer, L. (2002) *Coronary Heart Disease: Estimating the Impact of Changes in Risk Factors*, The Stationery Office, London.

Nied, R.J. and Franklin, B. (2002) Promoting and prescribing exercise for the elderly. *American Family Physician*, **65** (3), 419–426.

Nicholl, J.P., Coleman, P. and Williams, B.T. (1995) The epidemiology of sports and exercise related injury in the United Kingdom. *British Journal of Sports Medicine*, **29**, 232–238.

Resnick, B. (2001) A prediction model of aerobic exercise in older adults living in a continuing care retirement community. *Journal of Ageing and Health*, **13** (2), 287–310.

Riddoch, C. (2005) Physical activity. In (ed. L. Ewels), *Key Topics in Public Health*, Churchill Livingstone, Edinburgh, pp. 103–117, Chapter 6.

Sarafino, E.P. (2006) *Health Psychology: Biopsychosocial Interactions*, 5th edn, John Wiley & Sons Inc., Hoboken, NJ.

Schneider, S., Seither, B., Tünges, S. and Schmitt, H. (2006) Sports injuries: population base representative data on incidence, diagnosis, sequelae, and high risk groups. *British Journal of Sports Medicine*, **40** (4), 334–339.

Shephard, R.J. (1994) *Aerobic Fitness and Health*, Human Kinetics, Champaign, IL.

Shephard, R.J. (2001) Relative vs. absolute intensity of exercise in a dose-response context. *Medical Science Sports Exercise*, **33** (6), S400–S418.

Shephard, R.J. (2002) A health Canada/CDC conference on 'Communicating Physical Activity and Health Messages: Science into Practice'. *American Journal of Preventative Medicine*, **23** (3), 221–225.

Shephard, R.J. (2004) Exercise and men's health. In (eds R.S. Kirby, C.C. Carson, M.G. Kirby and R.N. Farah), *Men's Health*, 2nd edn, Taylor & Francis, London, pp. 39–54, Chapter 4.

Sherry, E. (1998) Epidemiology of sporting injuries. In (eds E. Sherry and S.F. Wilson) *Oxford Handbook of Sports Medicine*, Oxford University Press, Oxford, pp. 16–33, Chapter 2.

Simon, C., Everitt, H. and Kendrick, T. (2005) *General Practice*, 2nd edn, Oxford University Press, Oxford.

Taylor, C. and Cooper, M. (2003) Insights into adolescents health and eating disorders, (eds S. Grandis, G. Long, A. Glasper and P. Jackson), *Foundation Studies for Nursing: Using Enquiry Based Learning*, Palgrave, Basingstoke, pp. 115–137, Chapter 4.

Taylor, C., Lillis, C. and LeMone, P. (2005) *Fundamentals of Nursing: The Art and Science of Nursing*, 5th edn, Lippincott, Philadelphia.

Will, P.M., Demko, T.M. and George, D.L. (1996) Prescribing exercise for health: a simple framework for primary care. *American Family Physician*, **53** (2), 579–585.

World Health Organization (2002) *World Health Report*, WHO, Geneva.

Word List

Word/phrase	Meaning
Addiction	The physical and psychological dependence on using a substance, i.e. tobacco or alcohol
Adverse drug event	Harm resulting from medical intervention related to a drug
Adverse healthcare event	An event or omission arising during clinical care and causing physical or psychological injury to a patient
Allergic response	An exaggerated immune response to an antigen resulting in release of histamine, inflammation and tissue damage
Allergy	An immune response due to hypersensitivity to an antigen
Anaphylaxis	A hypersensitivity reaction
Anthropometry	Measures of the human body
Anti-discriminatory practice	Acknowledging the sources of oppression in a person's life and actively seeking to reduce them.
Anxiety	A vague, uneasy feeling of discomfort or dread, accompanied by an autonomic response
Assumption	Something that is taken for granted without any proof
Attitudes	Mental stance that is composed of several beliefs. Often involves a negative or positive judgement towards a person, object or idea
Autonomy	An individual's freedom to make choices about themselves and about issues that concern them. The term self-rule is central to the concept of autonomy
Bacillus	Rod-shaped bacterium
Bariatric surgery	Surgery on the stomach and/or intestines to help the person with extreme obesity lose weight
Behaviour	Observable response of an individual to external stimuli
Beliefs	Interpretations or conclusions that are accepted as accurate

Beneficence	Ethical principle regarding the duty to promote good and prevent harm
Blame culture	An organizational culture which inhibits openness regarding reporting incidents as staff are fearful of being personally penalized for making errors
cGMP	Cyclic guanosine monophosphate, a molecule that facilitates vasodilation leading to erection
Coccus	A spherical bacterium
Cognition	The mental process or faculty by which knowledge is acquired
Cognitive skills	Intellectual skills that can include problem solving, critical thinking and decision making
Communication	Communication is the complex, active process of relating to individuals and groups, which may include health team members, by written, verbal and non-verbal means. The goal is to understand and be understood and involves the transmission of ideas, messages, emotions and information by various means, between individuals and groups. Therapeutic communication promotes caring relationships between nurses and patients
Competency	Ability, qualities and capacity to function in a particular way.
Compliance	The degree to which the patient follows the recommendations made by nurses and other healthcare professionals (this is also sometimes called adherence)
Concept(s)	Vehicle of thought. Abstract ideas or mental images of reality
Conceptual framework (model)	Structure that links global concepts together to form a unified whole
Conceptualization	Process of developing and refining abstract ideas
Concordance	An agreement between the patient and the nurse or another healthcare professional about how medicines should be taken and used. This term replaces compliance
Construct	Abstraction or mental representation inferred from situations, events or behaviours
Coping	A complex of behavioural, cognitive and physiological responses that aims to prevent or minimize unpleasant or harmful experiences that challenge one's personal resources

Counselling	The process of helping an individual to recognize and cope with problems that may cause stress. An attempt to develop interpersonal growth with the aim of promoting personal growth
Criteria	Standards that are used to evaluate whether the behaviour demonstrated indicates accomplishment of the goal
Critical thinking	A purposeful, deliberate method of thinking used in a search for meaning
Cryptorchidism	Undescended testes – a congenital male abnormality
Cultural competence	Process through which the nurse provides care that is appropriate to the patient's cultural context
Cultural diversity	Individual differences among people that result from racial, ethnic and cultural variables
Culture	Dynamic and integrated structures of knowledge, beliefs, behaviours, ideas, attitudes, values, habits, customs, language, symbols, rituals, ceremonies and practices that are unique to a particular group of people
Decision making	The consideration and selection of interventions that facilitate the achievement of a desired outcome
Delegation	Process of transferring a selected nursing task in a situation to an individual who is competent to perform that task
Democratic leadership style	Style of leadership (also called participative leadership) that is based on the belief that every group member should have input into the development of goals and problem solving
Demography	The study of populations. Statistics related to distribution by age and place of residence, mortality and morbidity
Deontology	Ethical theory that considers the intrinsic moral significance of an act itself as the criterion for determination of good
Detumescence	Loss of turgidity and erection
Diploid	A diploid cell contains two copies of each chromosome.
Disability	A lack of ability to perform an activity a normal person can perform

Disease	An alteration in body function resulting in a reduction of capabilities in the ability to perform the activities of living, or contributing to the shortening of the normal life span
Distress	Experienced when stressors evoke an ineffective response
Duty	Obligation created either by law or contract, or by any voluntary action
Efficacy	The extent to which nursing and/or medical interventions achieve health improvements under ideal conditions
Epidemic	The situation in which the occurrence of a health problem had increased quickly
Empowerment	Process of enabling others to do for themselves
Ethical dilemma	Situation that occurs when there is a conflict between two or more ethical principles
Ethical principles	Tenets that direct or govern actions
Ethical reasoning	Process of thinking through what one ought to do in an orderly, systematic manner in order to provide justification of actions based on principles
Ethics	Branch of philosophy concerned with determining right from wrong on the basis of a body of knowledge
Ethnicity	Culture group's perception of themselves (group identify) and others' perception of them
Ethnocentrism	Assumption of cultural superiority and an inability to accept other cultures' ways; a tendency to look at the world through the perspective of your own culture
Ethnography	A type of qualitative research whose approach involves anthropology, in which a person's culture is examined by studying the meanings of the actions and events of the culture's members
Ethnomethodology	A type of qualitative methodology in which interpretations of ethnography are made in a particular social world
Equity	Fair distribution of resources or benefits
Eustress	Type of stress that result in positive outcomes
Euthanasia	Intended action or lack of action causing the merciful death of someone suffering from a terminal illness or incurable condition; derived from the Greek work *euthanatos*, which literally means 'good or gentle death'

Evidence-based practice	Integration of best available research with clinical expertise in order to make decisions about patient care
Fear	Anxiety caused by consciously recognized and realistic danger. It can be a perceived threat, real or imagined
Fidelity	Ethical concept that means faithfulness and keeping promises
Gender (biology sex)	Biological structure of person's genitals that designates them as male, female or intersexed
Gender identify	View of oneself as male or female in relationship to others
Gender role	Masculine or feminine role adopted by a person; often culturally and socially determined
General medical services	In the United Kingdom this is the contract under which GP practices provide medical care or services to those patients who are registered with them
Group dynamics	Study of the events that take place during small-group interaction and the development of sub-groups
Haploid	A haploid cell contains only one copy of each chromosome
Hazard	Anything that can cause harm
Healing	Process of recovery from illness, accident or disability
Healing touch	Energy-based therapeutic modality that alters the energy fields through the use of touch, thereby affecting physical, mental, emotional and spiritual health
Health	Process through which a person seeks to maintain an equilibrium that promotes stability and comfort, includes physiological, psychological, sociocultural, intellectual and spiritual well-being
Health Care Commission	Promotes improvement in quality of the NHS and independent healthcare. Assesses performance of healthcare organizations, awarding annual ratings
Health and Safety Executive	A statutory body which reports to the Health and Safety Commission, with day-to-day responsibility for making arrangements for the enforcement of safety legislation to ensure that risks to health and safety due to work activities are properly controlled

Health promotion	Process undertaken to increase levels of wellness in individuals, families and communities
Health Protection Agency	An independent body that protects the health and well-being of the population of the United Kingdom, particularly with regard to infectious diseases, chemical hazards, poisons and radiation
Health-seeking behaviours	Activities that are directed towards attaining and maintaining a state of well-being
Heterosexism	Perspective of assumption that people are heterosexual
Heterosexual	Describes sexual activity between a man and a woman
Holism	The belief that individuals function as complete units that cannot be reduced to the sum of their parts
Holistic nursing	Nursing practice that has as its aim the healing of the whole person
Homosexuality	Sexual activity between two members of the same sex
Hopelessness	A subjective state in which an individual sees limited or no alternatives or personal choices available and is unable to mobilize energy on own behalf
Hypothesis	Statement of an asserted relationship between dependent variables
Iatrogenic disease	A condition or disease that is caused by medical or surgical intervention, for example, the side effects of some drugs
Identity	What sets one person apart as a unique individual; it may include a person's name, gender, ethnic identify, family status, occupation and various roles
Illness	Inability of an individual's adaptive responses to maintain physical and emotional balance that subsequently results in impairment in functional abilities
Illness stage	Time interval when a patient is presenting or manifesting specific signs and symptoms of an infectious agent
Implied contract	Contract that recognizes a relationship between parties for services
Incidence	Refers to the prevalence of a disease in a population or community. The predictive value

	of the same test can be different when applied to people of differing ages
Individualism	A predominant cultural type that focuses on an independent lifestyle that flourishes in urban settings
Infection	Entry of a harmful microbe into the body and subsequent multiplication in the tissues
Informed consent	Patient understands the reason for the proposed intervention, its benefits and risks, and agrees to the treatment often by signing a consent form
Interpersonal communication	Process that occurs between two people in face-to-face encounters, over the telephone or through other communication media
Intuition	Knowing something without evidence, the learning of things without the conscious use of reasoning
Intersexed	A general term used for a variety of conditions in which a person is born with a reproductive or sexual anatomy that does not seem to fit the typical definitions of female or male.
Interview	Therapeutic interaction that has a specific purpose
Intrapersonal communication	Messages one sends to oneself, including 'self-talk' or communication with oneself
Justice	Ethical principle based on the concept of fairness that is extended to each individual
Knowledge and skills framework	Describes the knowledge and skills required by NHS staff to deliver quality services in their work. It also supports personal development and career progression
Leadership	Interpersonal process that involves motivating and guiding others to achieve goals
Leadership theory	Conceptual support framework for leadership
Leading question	A question that influences the patient to give a specific answer
Learning	Process of assimilating information with a resultant change in behaviour
Learning plateau	Way in which an individual incorporates new information
Lesbian	Female who has affectional and sexual tendencies toward females
Liability	Obligation one has incurred or might incur through any act or failure to act
Life events	Major occurrences in a person's life that require some element of psychological adjustment
Lifestyle	The values and behaviours that have been taken on by a person in daily life

Living will	Document prepared by a competent adult that provides direction regarding medical care should the person become incapacitated or otherwise unable to make decisions personally
Locus of control	A person's perception of the sources of control over events and situations affecting the person's life
Malaise	A feeling of being generally unwell
Medication error	Any preventable harm that may cause or lead to inappropriate medication use or patient harm while the medication is in the control of the healthcare professional, patient or customer
Mentor	A knowledgeable person; someone with insight; someone to trust and confide in, who helps a person to clarify thinking
Micro-organism	Bacteria, fungi, protozoa and viruses that are too small to be seen by the human eye
Minority group	Group of people who constitute less than numerical majority of the population and who, because of their cultural or physical characteristics, are labelled and treated differently from others in the society
Mitosis	Eukaryotic cell division into two diploid daughter cells
Morality	Behaviour in accordance with custom or tradition that usually reflects personal or religious beliefs
Morbidity	The condition, illness, injury or disability
Mortality	Refers to death often associated with large population
Motivation	The internal drive or externally arising stimulus to action or thought
Mourning	Period of time during which grief is expressed and resolution and integration of the loss occur
National Institute for Health and Clinical Excellence	An independent organization responsible for providing national guidance on the promotion of good health and the prevention and treatment of ill health
National Service Frameworks	One of a range of measures to raise quality and decrease variations in service; they contain long-term strategies
Need	Anything that is absolutely essential for existence

Negligence	Failure of an individual to provide the care in a situation that a reasonable person would ordinarily provide in a similar circumstance
Negotiation	A method of conflict management whereby the parties decide what they must retain and what they are willing to give up in order to reach a compromise position
Non-maleficence	Ethical principle that means the duty to cause no harm to others
Nursing	An art and a science that assists individuals to learn to care for themselves whenever possible; it also involves caring for others when they are unable to meet their own needs
Nursing leadership	Interpersonal process in nursing that involves motivating and guiding others to achieve goals
Nursing research	Systematic application of formalized methods for generating valid and dependable information about the phenomenon of concern to the discipline of nursing
Objective data	Observable and measurable data that is obtained through both standard assessment techniques performed during the physical examination and laboratory and diagnostic tests
Open-ended questions	Interview technique that encourages the patient to elaborate about a particular concern or problem
Open family system	A family system that interacts with the environment and in doing so maintains growth and balance
Pain	State in which an individual experiences and reports the presence of physical discomfort; may range in intensity from uncomfortable sensation to severe discomfort. Pain is what the patient says it is, existing whenever s/he says it does
Pandemic	A worldwide outbreak of an infectious disease
Paradigm	A pattern of collective understandings and assumptions about reality and the world
Paraverbal communication	The way in which a person speaks, including voice tone, pitch and inflection

Paraverbal cue	Verbal message accompanied by cues, such as tone and pitch, speed, inflection, volume of voice and other non-language vocalizations
Participative leadership style	Leadership style where every person's viewpoints are considered as valuable and everybody has an equal voice in making decisions
Passive euthanasia	Process of cooperating with the patient's dying process
Paternalism	Practice by which healthcare providers decide what is 'best' for patients and then attempt to coerce patients to act against their own choices
Perception	Person's sense and understanding of the world.
Personality	The cognitive, affective or behavioural predispositions of people in different situations, over a period of time
PDE 5	Phosphodiesterase type 5, a substance responsible for the breakdown of cGMP leading to detumescence
PGE_1	Prostaglandin E_1, a neurotransmitter resulting in erection
Phenomenon	Observable fact or event that can be perceived through the senses and is susceptible to description and explanation
Philosophy	Statement of beliefs that is the foundation for one's thoughts and actions
Portfolio	A collection of evidence which is selected from a personal portfolio for a particular purpose
Power	Ability to do or act, resulting in the achievement of desired results
Prejudice	A negative belief that is generalized about a group and this leads to prejudgement
Prevalence	The total number of cases existing at a given period of time
Polypharmacy	The prescribing of four or more drugs.
Profession	Group (vocational or occupational) that requires specialized education and intellectual knowledge
Professional organizations	Members engaged in the same professional pursuit, often with similar goals and concerns
Professional regulation	Process by which nursing ensures that its members act in the public interest by providing a unique service that society has entrusted to them

Professional standards	Authoritative statements developed by the profession by which quality of practice, service and/or education can be judged
Qualitative research	Systematic collection and analysis of subjective narrative materials, using procedures for which there tends to be a minimum of research-imposed control
Quality assurance framework	Traditional approach to quality management in which monitoring and evaluation focus on individual performance, deviation from standards and problem solving
Quality improvement	A process for change using a multidisciplinary approach to problem identification and resolution
Quantitative research	Systematic collection of numerical information, often under conditions of considerable control
Rapport	Mutual trust and understanding in a relationship
Racism	Discrimination directed towards individuals who are misperceived to be inferior because of biological factors
Radiation	Loss of heat in the form of infrared rays
Rationale	Explanation based on the theories and scientific principles of natural and behavioural sciences and the humanities
Reflection	The process of thinking over what has happened and why, what you may have learnt and you might do differently, what needs to be preserved and strengthened. There are reflective models that can help you to reflect effectively and in a meaningful manner
Reflective diary	A personal aid to reflection, a document used to structure and record reflective accounts
Relationship	An interaction of individuals over a period of time
Religion	A system of beliefs and practices that usually involves a community of like-minded people
Research	Systematic method of exploring, describing, explaining, relating or establishing the existence of a phenomenon, the factors that cause changes in the phenomenon, and how the phenomenon influences other phenomena
Risk	The chance of something happening that will have an impact on individuals and/or organizations. Risk is measured in terms of likelihood and consequence

Risk management	A method of reducing risks of adverse events occurring in organizations by systematically assessing, reviewing and seeking ways to prevent the occurrence of risks
Role	Set of expected behaviours associated with a person's status or position
Role ambiguity	Role expectations that are unclear. People do not know what or how to do what is expected of them
Role conflict	When the expectations of one role compete with the expectations of other roles
Screening	The act of discovering unknown or undisclosed disease risk or actual disease in order to intervene in an attempt to prevent the occurrence or progression of the disease
Scope of practice	Legal boundaries of practice for healthcare providers as defined in statute
Self-concept	The collection of ideas, feelings and beliefs one has about oneself
Self-esteem	A sense of pride in oneself; self-love
Sexual dysfunction	Physical inability to perform sexually, but can also be a psychological inability to perform sexually
Sexual health	Ability to form mutually consensual, developmental-appropriate sexual relationships that are safe and respectful of self and others; includes emotional, physical and psychological components
Sexuality	Human characteristic that refers not just to gender but to all the aspects of being male or female, including feelings, attitudes, beliefs and behaviour
Sexual orientation	Individual's preference for ways of expressing sexual feelings
Sick role	A set of social expectations met by an ill person, such as being exempt from the usual social role responsibilities and being obligated to get well and to seek competent help
Skill	The ability to carry out or perform a task well
Socialization	The ways in which people learn about the ways of a group or society in an attempt to become a functioning partner
Sociocultural	Involving social and cultural features or processes

Spirituality	Relationship with one's self, a sense of connection with others and a relationship with a higher power or divine source
Standard of care	Delineates the extent and character of the nurse's duty to the patient; defined by organizational policy or professional standards of practice
Stress	Body's reaction to any stimulus
Stressors	Circumstances or events that a person perceives as threatening or harmful to them
Subjective data	Data from the patient's point of view, including feelings, perceptions and concerns
Surveillance	Systematic observation of the occurrence of disease in a population
Teaching	Active process in which one individual shares information with another as a means to facilitate behavioural changes
Teaching-learning process	Planned interaction promoting a behavioural change that is not a result of maturation or coincidence
Teaching strategies	Techniques employed by the teacher to promote learning
Team	Group of individuals who work together to achieve a common goal
Theory	Set of concepts and propositions that provide an orderly way to view phenomena
Therapeutic communication	Use of communication for the purpose of creating a beneficial outcome for the patient
Therapeutic range	Achievement of constant therapeutic blood level of a medication within a safe range
Therapeutic touch	Holistic technique that consists of assessing alterations in a person's energy fields and using the hands to direct energy to achieve a balanced state
Therapeutic use of self	Process in which nurses deliberately plan their actions and approach the relationship with a specific goal in mind before interacting with the patient
Transcultural nursing	Formal area of study and practice focused on comparative analysis of different cultures and subcultures with respect to cultural care, health and illness beliefs, and values and practices with the goal of providing healthcare within the context of the patient's culture

Transgender	Person who dresses and engages in roles of the person of the opposite gender
Tumescence	Vasodilation of the corpora cavernosa brings about an erection
Utility	Ethical principle that states that an act must result in the greatest amount of good for the greatest number of people involved in a situation
Values	Principles that influence the development of beliefs and attitudes
Variable	A characteristic that is measurable on people, objects or events that may change in quantity or quality
Veracity	Ethical principle that means that one should be truthful, neither lying nor deceiving others
Whistle-blowing	Calling attention to the unethical, illegal or incompetent actions of others

Index

Note: Page references in *italics* refer to Figures; those in **bold** refer to Tables